S0-AWS-329

WITHDRAWN

Cultural Encyclopedia of Vegetarianism

Cultural Encyclopedia of Vegetarianism

Margaret Puskar-Pasewicz, Editor

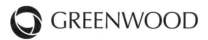

GREENWOOD

AN IMPRINT OF ABC-CLIO, LLC
Santa Barbara, California • Denver, Colorado • Oxford, England

RADO COLLEGE LIBRARY
COLORADO SPRINGS, COLORADO

Copyright 2010 by Margaret Puskar-Pasewicz

All rights reserved. No part of this publication may be reproduced, stored in a retrieval system, or transmitted, in any form or by any means, electronic, mechanical, photocopying, recording, or otherwise, except for the inclusion of brief quotations in a review, without prior permission in writing from the publisher.

Library of Congress Cataloging-in-Publication Data

Cultural encyclopedia of vegetarianism / Margaret Puskar-Pasewicz, editor.
    p. cm.
  Includes bibliographical references and index.
  ISBN 978-0-313-37556-9 (hard copy : alk. paper) — ISBN 978-0-313-37557-6 (ebook)
1. Vegetarianism—Encyclopedias.   I. Puskar-Pasewicz, Margaret.
  TX392.C85   2010
  641.5'636—dc22   2010022838

ISBN: 978-0-313-37556-9
EISBN: 978-0-313-37557-6

14 13 12 11 10   1 2 3   4 5

This book is also available on the World Wide Web as an eBook.
Visit www.abc-clio.com for details.

Greenwood
An Imprint of ABC-CLIO, LLC

ABC-CLIO, LLC
130 Cremona Drive, P.O. Box 1911
Santa Barbara, California 93116-1911

This book is printed on acid-free paper ∞

Manufactured in the United States of America

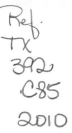
Ref.
TX
392
C85
2010

Contents

Preface

Throughout time and across cultures, food has always represented more than merely the fulfillment of a physiological necessity. The ways that human beings produce, market, prepare, and consume food provide valuable insight into our conceptions of sickness and health, morality, personal identity, recreation, and family life. As individuals and as members of a global society, our attitudes toward food also have profound meanings and consequences.

Because food plays such a central role in all of our daily lives, the prohibition of a specific food or drink can be particularly revealing. Calls to avoid meat consumption represent one of the oldest and most culturally significant food taboos in world history. In spite of the recent explosion of scholarship on food consumption and practices as well as the establishment of new academic programs on food studies across the country, very little work has appeared on vegetarianism. Furthermore, both popular and scholarly accounts of vegetarianism, particularly its development in the United States, are riddled with myths and misconceptions. Ignoring the longer history of vegetarianism in the United States buries its importance as both a social movement and a cultural force.

Perhaps the greatest and most harmful misunderstanding that many Americans have about vegetarianism is that it is a new or even distinctly modern invention. While it is certainly true that rationales for adopting vegetarianism and the ways these ideals are put into practice in daily life can vary significantly, it is both inaccurate and naive to assume that vegetarianism's recent popularity in the United States is disconnected from the past. This encyclopedia is largely intended as a step toward filling this notable historical gap. Indeed, vegetarianism has a long history in the United States, going back to the early 19th century.

Although vegetarianism in the United States is commonly associated with the 1960s and 1970s, a burgeoning vegetarian movement existed by the time of the Civil War. Nineteenth-century advocates focused primarily on the moral and physiological rationales for vegetarianism as opposed to ethical concerns for the treatment of nonhuman animals. In spite of the existence of numerous societies, periodicals, and institutions dedicated to promoting vegetarianism throughout the 19th century, this early history has been largely obscured or, more often, ignored. This encyclopedia seeks to compile and explain the most important ideas, people, groups, trends, practices, and themes associated with vegetarianism, primarily in the United States, throughout its history. It is the first encyclopedia to focus on the cultural aspects of vegetarianism.

This volume also examines modern vegetarianism's origins in the religious and ethical prohibitions of flesh in ancient times. The origins of vegetarianism can be most clearly traced back to the development of the ancient Eastern religions, namely, Hinduism, Buddhism, and Jainism, and to the philosophers of the Greco-Roman world, most notably Pythagoras and his followers. A meatless regimen was typically referred to in the West as the "Pythagorean diet" until the coining of the phrase "vegetarianism" in 1847. Restrictions on animal food emerged earlier within Judaism, but total abstention from meat and fish was never established as a universal doctrine. Both Jews and Christians today still uphold some restrictions on meat, either year-round or during specific times of the year.

A valuable and unique contribution of this book is its dual focus on the cultural and historical aspects of vegetarianism. This book is intended for students and general readers interested in the growth of vegetarianism and how it has influenced popular culture in the United States. As a result, entries span a diverse range of topics from Mohandas Gandhi to punk rock to global warming. Equally important, since American vegetarianism did not emerge in isolation from the rest of the world—in fact, it was largely influenced by other cultures and places—the encyclopedia also covers a broad geographic area including Asia and Europe, where vegetarianism has had a longer history, as well as containing more detailed country entries. Each of the more than 90 alphabetically ordered entries supplies a brief historical background and includes cross-references to related entries and suggestions for further reading.

The chronology identifies major events related to vegetarianism. The alphabetical and topical lists of entries enable readers to quickly locate specific terms as well as to browse entries of potential interest by scholars from a variety of fields such as history, law, English, sociology, philosophy, physics, nutrition, and religious studies. In addition, illustrations and sidebars, with excerpts from works and people discussed in the entries plus other information complementary to the entries, are included throughout the text to enhance readers' understanding of the subject. The selected bibliography identifies important books, articles, and Web sites that can be used for further research on vegetarianism.

The purpose of this volume is not to advocate for or against vegetarianism but instead to shed light on its historical and cultural significance. Nonetheless, an important theme alluded to throughout the book is the global implications of a vegetarian diet. Or, put another way, it is crucial that we begin to understand the cost to ourselves, our environment, and our fellow animals if we continue down the same path of mass meat production that we have been on for over 100 years. As the works of numerous scholars over the last four decades have demonstrated, world hunger is not the result of our inability to produce sufficient food.

As Frances Moore Lappé, a best-selling author and longtime activist, has argued since the publication of her 1971 work, *Diet for a Small Planet,* increased food production will not end the problem of hunger and malnutrition in the United States and around the world. Instead, she and others argue that there is actually an abundance of food but that our means of food production, distribution, and consumption result in unfathomable amounts of waste. For example, as much as 50 percent of the grain currently cultivated around the world goes to feeding livestock as opposed to feeding people directly. Although a lot of farm animals are eventually used for human consumption, this is an incredibly inefficient system of producing adequate nourishment for our large global population. Even by the optimistic estimates given by the U.S. Department of Agriculture, for every seven pounds of grain and soy fed to farm animals, people receive one pound of food.

If alleviating world hunger is not sufficient to motivate us to rethink our consumption of meat and fish, our current diet's astounding toll on our bodies should at least give us pause. Obesity and diabetes, especially among children, are now rampant throughout the United States and increasingly so in nations that are adopting our high-fat, high-sugar diet. While total abstention from meat would not provide a perfect solution to these problems, reducing our intake of meat and other animal products such as cheese would certainly have some salubrious effects on our collective health. I hope that the entries in this encyclopedia prompt readers to consider how their daily decisions about what to eat and what not to eat have staggering consequences for our world.

Acknowledgments

Throughout this project, I have benefited from the assistance of numerous colleagues—old and new—for which I am very grateful. I am indebted to all of the contributors for their willingness to share their expertise as well as their encouragement. I owe a special debt of gratitude to Jerry Friedman, who from an early stage often went above and beyond in terms of helping to identify contributors, making sure his entries were as accurate and up-to-date as possible, and reminding me of the importance of language in discussions about animals. Sam Calvert provided valuable insight at several important stages of the project, and I enjoyed sharing stories about our mutual experiences of being snowed in this past winter. In studying the history of vegetarianism, as in any subject from the past, it is sometimes difficult to separate the truth from the myth; I am grateful to Tom Hertweck, and Adam Shprintzen who responded promptly to my e-mails to confirm details related to the history of the Philadelphia Bible Christian Church. Special thanks also go to my colleague and friend Susan M. Ferentinos, who read and sent countless e-mails that enabled me to finish this project, and Wendi Schnaufer at Greenwood Press/ABC-CLIO for providing me with this valuable opportunity. Last, but certainly not least, I'm grateful to all of my family, especially my husband, John, and our two beagles, Alle and Schenley, for their unfailing patience and affection.

Introduction

Food has become a wildly popular theme in 21st-century American culture. From the establishment of the Food Network to the proliferation of new cookbooks and the creation of video games where virtual chefs can hone their culinary skills, it is clear that citizens of the 21st century are preoccupied with the subject of food. This obsession with food consumption and practices, however, is hardly a new development in the United States.

Throughout their history, Americans have expressed deep concerns and anxieties about the food that they eat and how it is eaten. European colonists not only struggled at times to cultivate sufficient food for survival but also wrestled with food's religious, cultural, and social meanings. Food functioned—then and now—as a way to help immigrants maintain connections to their pasts. Nonetheless, the diverse plant and animal life of the Americas also offered important contrasts to African, European, and Caribbean foodways and food practices. By the end of the 18th century, some colonists even viewed food as a means of forging a distinct American identity, as demonstrated by the famous boycotts against English goods, most notably tea.

The rapid political, social, and economic changes of the early 19th century further complicated Americans' already-complex relationship with food. Individuals' physical health was equated with the state of their moral well-being, so that everyday decisions about food took on much greater significance. At the time, medical professionals (both orthodox and unorthodox) and social reformers such as Bronson and William A. Alcott, Sylvester Graham, and the Rev. William Metcalfe of the Philadelphia Bible Christian Church warned against the dangers of gluttony in general and, in particular, the evils of certain foods and drinks such as alcohol, tobacco, and meat. In particular, many reformers believed that meat consumption tended to be overstimulating and made people, typically men, more violent and sexually aggressive, which led to other social problems.

Reinforced by the evangelical fervor of the period as well as widespread criticism of the poor state of medical therapeutics, vegetarianism emerged amid a number of interrelated movements all aimed at moral reform. Like the popular temperance movement against alcohol consumption and the far more controversial antislavery movement, early vegetarians initially argued merely for a reduction in Americans' daily meat consumption but later changed to a more radical stance of total abstention. In 1850, the American Vegetarian Society was organized to promote the moral and physiological benefits of vegetarianism and lasted for over a decade. (The society took its name from its English counterpart, the Vegetarian Society, which coined the term "vegetarian" in 1847.) Thus began an enduring trend in the history of U.S. social reform to advocate prohibition as a means to improve the country's seemingly declining moral and physical health.

By the turn of the 20th century, proponents of vegetarianism increasingly relied on evidence from new developments in the fields of the medical and social sciences and slightly less on moral arguments to bolster their calls for total abstention from meat. Also strongly influenced by public concerns about food purity and the mass production of meat (made famous in Upton Sinclair's 1906 novel *The Jungle*), a new national organization known as the Vegetarian Society of America formed in 1886. In addition, dozens of state and local vegetarian societies as well as meatless restaurants and sanitariums sprung up across the country. With the onset of World Wars I and II, day-to-day decisions about food consumption once again became a symbol of patriotism. Consumers, mainly wives and mothers, who abstained from "luxury" items such as meat or at least restricted their family's consumption of these items were seen as vital contributors to the nation's war efforts abroad. At the same time that early 20th-century Americans celebrated their growing sense of technological and cultural superiority over the rest of the world, which included the high availability and consumption of beef in the United States, concerns about the nation's declining moral and physical health emerged with greater resonance.

In the 1950s and early 1960s, civil rights activism on behalf of African Americans (and later women, homosexuals, Chicanos, and other minority groups) brought social reform back to the forefront of American political life. Inspired by these earlier efforts, as well as the countercultural movement of the late 1960s that called for challenges to traditional forms of authority and the formation of new communal societies, a small minority of Americans adopted vegetarianism. Although often mistaken as the time of its genesis, the late 1960s and 1970s more accurately represented a resurgence of vegetarianism. Public interest in vegetarianism also sparked renewed concerns about the safety of America's system of mass food production and provided a catalyst for the food revolution of the last four decades.

The 1970s and 1980s also witnessed the formulation of new theories about the rights of animals. The work of scholars such as Peter Singer, Tom Regan, and Gary L. Francione prompted many people inside and outside of the United States to reconsider human beings' relationships to animals. As a result of these and other trends previously discussed, numerous organizations emerged in these decades to promote the rights of animals.

Much of vegetarianism's current appeal in American society reflects the cultural influence of animal rights groups as well as older animal welfare organizations such as the Humane Society of the United States. Even groups popularly depicted as dangerous or radical, such as Ingrid Newkirk's People for the Ethical Treatment of Animals (PETA), have launched very successful campaigns in recent years to raise awareness of the ethical and medical issues related to meat consumption.

Perhaps the most notable indication of the movement's increasing significance in recent decades has been the vociferous attacks on vegetarianism, both in interpersonal relationships and in the public arena. Due to its associations with the social experimentation and radical politics of the 1960s, many critics have viewed vegetarianism as a rejection of one of the quintessential rituals of American suburban life: the family dinner of red meat and potatoes. Even in the early 21st century, it is not uncommon for vegetarians to be ridiculed as "health food nuts" or effeminate, and their diet as nothing more than "rabbit food." These stereotypes are reinforced by the million-dollar efforts of large-scale, industrial meat companies and associations to portray vegetarianism as extreme and even unhealthy.

In spite of this backlash, a vegetarian lifestyle has become more socially acceptable than ever before in U.S. history. The thriving production of vegetarian cookbooks and the ever-growing array of meat substitutes that line the shelves of mainstream grocery stores also attest to the fact that it is easier than ever to adopt a meatless diet. In very recent years, national fast food chains—which typically served as the targets of food reformers—have acknowledged the widespread popularity of vegetarianism and started to promote meatless options, such as the Burger King's veggie burger. Finally, the rapid growth of vegetarian restaurants, the organic food industry, and community-supported agriculture (CSA) also attest to vegetarianism's cultural significance in the United States and beyond.

Margaret Puskar-Pasewicz

Chronology

ca. 599–483 BC	Vegetarian ideas develop within Hinduism, Buddhism, and Jainism in India
ca. 580–540 BC	Ethical vegetarianism emerges in Greece, most notably through the work of Pythagoras (ca. 570–490 BC) and his followers
1691	Thomas Tryon's *A Bill of Fare of Seventy Five Noble Dishes,* the first English-language meatless cookbook, is published
1809	Bible Christian Church is founded in Salford, England, by Rev. William Cowherd
1811	John Frank Newton's *The Return to Nature; or a Defence of the Vegetable Regimen* is published
1812	Martha Brotherton's *Vegetable Cookery, A New System of Vegetable Cookery* is published. Brotherton and her husband are active members of the (English) Bible Christian Church
1813	English Romantic poet Percy Bysshe Shelley publishes *A Vindication of Natural Diet*
June 1817	Rev. William Metcalfe and 40 members of the Bible Christian Church emigrate from England to establish a church in Philadelphia
1822	One of the earliest pieces of animal rights legislation, The Cruel Treatment of Cattle Act (aka Martin's Act), is passed in the United Kingdom
1824	Society for the Prevention of Cruelty to Animals (SPCA) is founded in England

1837	Organization of the American Physiological Society is founded in Boston, Massachusetts
1838	Gerrit Mulder, a Dutch physician and self-taught chemist, discovers protein as part of a larger effort by mid-19th-century medical scientists to separate foods into distinct categories
1839	Sylvester Graham's *Lectures on the Science of Human Life* is published
1843–1844	Vegetarian communal society known as Fruitlands is established in Massachusetts by Bronson Alcott
1844	William A. Alcott's *A Vegetable Diet Defended* is published
July 1845– September 1847	Henry David Thoreau lives at Walden Pond; the experience is the basis for his book *Walden* (1854)
September 30, 1847	Term "vegetarian" is coined, and the Vegetarian Society of the United Kingdom, which still exists in the 21st century, is formed
May 15, 1850	The American Vegetarian Society (AVS) is formed, with William A. Alcott elected as the group's first president
1859	Alcott dies, and Metcalfe replaces him as the AVS president
1855–1857	A vegetarian colony in Kansas, organized by Henry S. Clubb, is established and fails
1861–1865	U.S. Civil War
1862	Metcalfe dies
1863	Seventh-day Adventism is established by Ellen G. White and her husband, James White, in Battle Creek, Michigan.
April 10, 1866	American Society for the Prevention of Cruelty to Animals (ASPCA) is founded by Henry Bergh in New York City
September 5, 1866	The Whites open the Western Health Reform Institute based on Seventh-day Adventist dietary principles in Battle Creek, Michigan. It eventually becomes known as the Battle Creek Sanitarium under the leadership of John H. Kellogg in the mid-1870s
1867	Important anticruelty laws are passed in New York City
1868	George T. Angell starts the Massachusetts Society for the Prevention of Cruelty to Animals (MSPCA)

1869	Anticruelty laws are passed in Massachusetts
1871	Anticruelty laws exist in cities from the East Coast to California
1876	Clubb becomes pastor of the Philadelphia Bible Christian Church
1885	First vegetarian restaurant in the United States opens on West 23rd Street in New York City
1886	Vegetarian Society of America (VSA), led by Clubb, is the second national organization in the United States founded to promote vegetarianism
1892	Henry S. Salt's influential work *Animals' Rights: Considered in Relation to Social Progress* follows his other best-known work, *A Plea for Vegetarianism* (1886)
1893	Ella Eaton Kellogg's *Science in the Kitchen*, in which she uses domestic science principles to promote a vegetarian diet, is published
1893	Third International Vegetarian Congress, in conjunction with the World's Fair, is held in Chicago
1899	First issue of Bernarr Macfadden's *Physical Culture* is published
ca. 1900s	Several vegetarian athletes win national and international athletic competitions
1903	The House of David establishes a vegetarian community in Benton Harbor, Michigan, which continues to exist today
1907	Yale University study concludes that vegetarian athletes have more stamina than do nonvegetarian athletes
1908	The International Vegetarian Union, comprised of vegetarian organizations around the world, is founded
1910	*250 Meatless Menus and Recipes* by Eugene Christian and Molly Griswold Christian is published
1911	The first vitamin, vitamin B, is discovered
1914–1918	As part of the U.S. government's domestic efforts during World War I, the Food Administration encourages restrictions on meat as well as promoting meat substitutes to citizens on the home front
1921	Clubb dies, and the Philadelphia Bible Christian Church ceases operation
1935	Members of the House of David establish a new vegetarian community in Waco, Texas, which will become

	infamous for its violent confrontation with the U.S. government in 1993
1941–1945	The United States' formal entry into World War II prompts renewed government campaigns for citizens to limit or abstain from meat
1944	Donald Watson creates the term "vegan" as a distinct designation from "vegetarian" and organizes the Vegan Society in England
1949	Well-known vegetarian advocate and physician Herbert Shelton establishes the American Natural Hygiene Society
1954	Humane Society of the United States (HSUS) is founded
ca. 1960s	Countercultural movement is born in the United States that prompts a renewed interest in vegetarianism
1960	H. Jay Dinshah founds the American Vegan Society
1971	Frances Moore Lappé's book *Diet for a Small Planet* is published. It will become a best seller.
1971	Vegetarian communal society known as "the Farm" is organized in Summertown, Tennessee
1974	North American Vegetarian Society is organized
1975	Philosopher Peter Singer's canonical work on animal rights, *Animal Liberation,* is published
1976	The American Liberation Front forms in the United Kingdom
1977	*The Moosewood Cookbook* by Mollie Katzen is published and becomes one of the biggest-selling cookbooks ever
1980	People for the Ethical Treatment of Animals (PETA) is founded by Ingrid Newkirk and Alex Pacheco
1983	Tom Regan's *The Case for Animal Rights* is published
1985	Neal D. Barnard establishes the Physicians Committee for Responsible Medicine (PCRM)
1986	Lorri Houston and Gene Baur start the Farm Sanctuary after rescuing a living sheep from a pile of dead animals at a stockyard
1990	Carol J. Adams's seminal work *The Sexual Politics of Meat: A Feminist-Vegetarian Critical Theory* is published
1992	"Flexitarian," a term for someone who practices a more permissive type of vegetarian diet, is coined

1994	The character of Darlene Connor on the hit television show *Roseanne* adopts vegetarianism in the episode "Lanford Daze"
1995	On the popular and long-running cartoon *The Simpsons,* daughter Lisa becomes a vegetarian
1995	After lobbying from students, campus organizations, and the community, the University of California at Berkeley becomes the first college to offer vegan options at every meal
1996	Gary L. Francione, the first professor to teach animal rights theory in an American law school, publishes *Rain without Thunder: The Ideology of the Animal Rights Movement*
1996	Talk show host Oprah Winfrey and Howard F. Lyman (aka the Mad Cowboy) are unsuccessfully sued by a group of cattle ranchers after Winfrey states on her program that she will no longer eat hamburgers
1998	Renowned pediatrician Benjamin Spock endorses a vegetarian diet for children as well as pregnant women
2001	As a result of a successful class-action lawsuit, McDonald's admits to using cow fat in their so-called vegetarian french fries
2003	First case of bovine spongiform encephalopathy, aka mad cow disease, is reported in the United States, in Mabton, Washington
2007	U.S. Centers for Disease Control and Prevention study reveals that approximately 367,000 young Americans, or roughly 1 in every 200 people younger than 18, practice vegetarianism
2007	Consumption of meat around the world reaches 284 million tons, compared to 71 million tons in 1961

List of Entries

Topical List of Entries

Agriculture

Advertising
Africa
Agribusiness
Agriculture, Community-Supported
Asia
Baur, Gene
Colonies, Communal Societies, and Utopias
Consumer Products
Europe
France
Germany
Global Warming
Health Food Stores and Food Cooperatives
Houston, Lorri
India
Katzen, Mollie
Lappé, Frances Moore
Lyman, Howard F.
Meat and Violence
Netherlands, The
Newkirk, Ingrid
Organic Foods and Technology
Pacelle, Wayne
Pacheco, Alex
People for the Ethical Treatment of Animals
Physiological Benefits
Policy
Reform

Religion and Spirituality

Societies, Organizations, and Institutions

ACTIVISM AND PROTESTS

Activists are those who take action to make sweeping policy changes in society, business, and politics or who act on a case-by-case basis in furtherance of such policies. Public demonstrations, such as protests, are the most widely recognized form of activism, but activism encompasses a broad range of advocacy including public discussion, applications of one's profession, engaging in boycotts, and direct action. An activist campaign can specifically advance a policy, such as by handing out literature, or it can indirectly advance a policy, such as by lobbying the government to remove opponents' benefits. Vegetarian activists believe that abstaining from animal flesh provides religious, nutritional, or moral advantages, and vegan activists believe that nonhuman animals deserve to live free from all forms of human domination. Mutually, they believe that the greatest social problems, such as war and violence, disease, hunger, and pollution, will be drastically reduced the more society progresses to a plant-based diet. Accordingly, they take action to stimulate discussion and to cause change in public policy.

Democratic societies with rich histories of free speech draw the most activism, which helps to explain why most vegetarian and vegan activism is in Europe and the United States. Vegans and vegetarians have learned from the history of labor and women's rights and from civil rights activism.

History In the ancient world, theistic beliefs brought about vegetarian and vegan advocacy. Mahavira (ca. 599–527 BC), a prominent Jain sage, and Siddhartha Gautama (ca. 563–483 BC), the historical Buddha, propounded nonviolence (*ahimsa*) to all animals as essential for leading an enlightened life. Ahimsa remains as a core tenet in both religions. Apollonius of Tyana (ca. 3 BC–AD 97) was a then-famous neo-Pythagorean sage who advocated consuming only plants. Theism continued to be the principal reason for vegetarian and vegan advocacy in early U.S. history. William Metcalfe (1788–1862), a leader of the Bible Christian Church, preached vegetarianism in Pennsylvania. Folk hero Johnny Appleseed

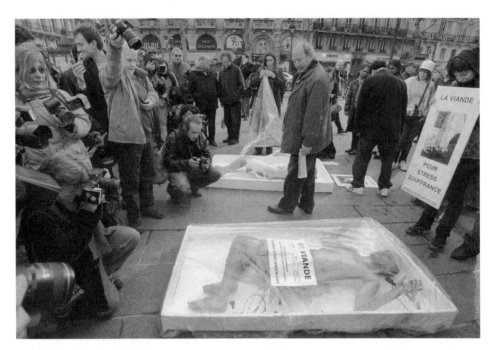

Activists lay on the pavement and pose as packaged meat on Thursday February 22, 2007, to promote vegetarianism in Paris. The poster at right reads Meat. Fear. Stress. Suffering. (AP Photo/Christophe Ena)

(John Chapman, 1774–1845) was also a preacher who spread his religious beliefs that it was wrong to harm animals for food or any other reason.

In the mid- and late 1800s, health became the principal rationale for vegetarianism advocacy. Sylvester Graham used his powerful oration to promote health through vegetarianism. His tireless advocacy attracted a following of Grahamites and influenced contemporary and later health reformers, such as the physicians William A. Alcott (1798–1859) and Herbert Shelton (1895–1985). Unlike Graham, Alcott advocated a vegan diet. Shelton became the premier natural hygienist, advocating superior nutrition through vegan and ideally raw food. He lectured around the United States, wrote several books on veganism and nutrition, and ran for U.S. president in 1956 with the American Vegetarian Party. An important part of Graham, Alcott, and Shelton's activism was helping to legitimize nutrition as a science before the mainstream medical community began to relate diet to disease.

Vegetarian and vegan societies started appearing in the wake of Graham's and Shelton's calls for change. Vegetarians in Philadelphia founded the Vegetarian Society of America (VSA) in 1886, organized lectures on health and social meals, and published a journal called *Food, Home and Garden*. At that time, Philadelphia was believed to have the highest population of vegetarians. The VSA participated in the World's Fair in Chicago (1893) to expose the public to vegetarianism. An International Vegetarian Congress was held at the fair, attracting delegates from international vegetarian groups. In 1944, Donald Watson (1910–2005) founded the Vegan Society in England. Watson, who coined the term "vegan," started the vegan movement because he believed that abstinence from exploiting non-humans was morally compelling and that vegetarianism was merely a stepping-stone to veganism. The compelling nature of vegan ideology has kept its activism prominent ever since. Inspired by Watson's group, H. Jay Dinshah (1933–2000) founded the American Vegan Society in 1960 to promote veganism through conventions, educational programs, and publications.

Following the publication of Ruth Harrison's book *Animal Machines: The New Factory Farming Industry* (1964), an article by Brigid Brophy in the (U.K.) *Sunday Times* (1965), Roslind and Stanley Godlovitch's book *Animals, Men and Morals* (1971), and Peter Singer's book *Animal Liberation* (1975), the modern animal rights movement began. Animal rights, originating as a secular rather than theistic ideology, concludes that nonhuman animals have a right to life and liberty and that, consequently, veganism is the only moral diet for humans. Although not all vegans espouse animal rights, animal rights advocates necessarily advocate veganism, making a natural alliance between animal rights and vegan activists. In 1975, the International Vegetarian Union's World Vegetarian Congress was held in the U.S. for the first time. Attending animal rights activists collaborated with health activists, and in 1981 they organized the Action for Life Conference. There, the activists officially launched the animal rights movement in the United States.

Environmentalism is currently creating a fourth epicenter for vegan activism. The Food and Agriculture Organization (FAO) of the United Nations published *Livestock's Long Shadow: Environmental Issues and Options* (2006), which explains why using animals for food is the largest source of damage to land, water, and air. Other publications had detailed the adverse effect of raising animals as food long before *Livestock,* but *Livestock* received the greatest exposure, probably because of its connection to the United Nations. With climate change being the subject of world debate and the FAO publication detailing the relationship between environment and diet, environmental activists are bringing veganism to the world agenda.

Diverse Strategies Vegetarian and vegan advocacy had a paradigm shift in the early 1970s and again in the 1980s. First, Connie Salamone and Nellie Shriver separated from vegan societies that they believed were too passive. Then Salamone and Shriver engaged in vegan advocacy by using protests, street theater, and other economical tactics. Their model became popular for vegan activism because it received a lot of exposure with relatively little time, money, and other resources. The second shift came a decade later when members of the Animal Liberation Front (ALF) broke into several slaughterhouses and vivisection laboratories. After ALF communiqué's and videotapes were released, protests erupted across the United States. ALF videos continue to draw people into activism.

Grassroots activism, populated by experienced and beginning activists, has blossomed since the early 1990s. Calling itself "L.A.'s largest Earth Day Festival," WorldFest is run entirely by volunteers. Taking place annually since 1999, it draws up to 20,000 people to a festival of food, music, and speakers. Grassroots activists formed Vegan Toastmasters International, a chapter of Toastmasters, to develop public speaking skills among vegans. Filmmaker Eric Prescott has made the documentary *I'm Vegan* (2009) to show the world what mainstream vegans are like and to neutralize unfair criticism against them. As with other social justice movements, the combined work of grassroots activists is greater than that of high-profile organizations, but this is difficult to gauge because the grassroots rarely attract the media, so their accomplishments are seldom recorded.

Animal rights groups and vegetarian and vegan societies have become the hubs of activism where most of the high-profile campaigns are developed and most of the media attention is directed. Groups like Compassion Over Killing (COK) have achieved remarkable success with scant resources. Based in Washington, D.C., COK was founded in 1995 as a high school club. Relying on volunteers, COK investigated the powerful United Egg Producers (UEP) after it started marketing its eggs as "animal care certified." COK secretly filmed the deplorable conditions where UEP members' hens were kept and then beat UEP in court, forcing them to stop deceiving consumers. Some activist groups have chosen the Internet as their principal medium. Vegan Outreach, founded in 1993, is active through its expansive Web site and its "Why Vegan" booklet. Vegan Outreach claims that volunteers have distributed over 10 million booklets. Activists run veganfreaks.net as a place for vegans to socialize and debate issues. Some commercial Web sites, like craigslist.org, have established their own vegan fora, where the general public can converse with activists.

Individuals and groups sometimes take direct action. Direct action is a tactic where one intervenes for the authorities when the authorities are unavailable or unwilling to act. Since 1977, the Sea Shepherd Conservation Society has taken activism to the high seas, taking a direct-action approach to protect whales and other marine animals under the United Nation's "World Charter for Nature" because national authorities have refused to so. In its tenure, the society has sunk unoccupied whaling ships, sabotaged whale hunts, saving thousands of lives, and accumulated evidence as an attempt to force national authorities to prosecute and stop whalers. In 2010, its captain, Peter Bethune, boarded a Japanese whaling security ship to place its captain under arrest for his earlier sinking of a society ship, *Ady Gil,* and the attempted murder of the *Ady Gil's* crew. The Japanese responded by arresting him. Volunteer members of the society are typically drawn from the vegan activist community.

Professionals as Activists Professionals of all types have applied their skills to vegan activism, destroying the stereotype of vegan activists as rebels on the lunatic fringe. Philosophers such as Steve Best, Paola Cavalieri, and Tom Regan and authors including Carol Adams, Joan Dunayer, and John Robbins have published hard-hitting and dynamic treatises on animal rights and veganism. Professor of psychology Melanie Joy published a book on "carnism," a term she coined as the inverse to "veganism," to describe the ideology of eating animals.

Present-day medical professionals are more outspoken than in past decades. Benjamin Spock (1903–1998), a revolutionary pediatrician, advocated veganism for children. Founded in 1985, the Physicians Committee for Responsible

Medicine is an activist medical organization that researches and publishes studies on the advantages of a vegan diet and occasionally goes to court to expose fraud within the meat and dairy industries. It has proved through peer-reviewed studies that a vegan diet is superior to the American Diabetes Association's recommended nonvegan diet for people suffering from diabetes.

Filmmakers have been activists since films debuted. Advocacy films like *Charlotte's Web* (1973) and *Babe* (1995) have used fairy-tale appeal to question the use of animals as food. *Year of the Dog* (2007) was a story about how one person became aware of and reacted to the institutional cruelty to nonhumans. In nonfiction, *Earthlings* (2003) is an encyclopedic film that shows the abuse that inspired veganism, and *Meet Your Meat* (2003) shows undercover footage of slaughterhouses. Raw-food vegan activists made *Raw for 30 Days* (2007), which follows diabetics reversing their disease by changing their diet.

Some people have managed to make activism their profession. Since 1990, Howard Lyman, a former cattle rancher, has devoted his life to promoting veganism. "Go Vegan with Bob Linden" is the first dedicated vegan radio program, established in 2001, with an international audience through its Web site. Several entrepreneurs, like Native Foods restaurant founder Tanya Petranova and the producer of VegTV, Marie Oser, incorporate animal rights or advocacy of a plant-based diet into their businesses. Professional activism is steadily growing in society, evidenced by the growth of advocacy publications, films, businesses, and individuals sustaining their livelihood solely on activism.

Universities and High Schools Academia, as a center of intellectual energy, is fertile with organized and spontaneous activism. In 2003, University of California, Los Angeles (UCLA) students formed Bruins for Animals, maintaining a pro-vegan and antivivisection presence in one of the largest vivisecting universities. Six years later, the group received an award for their diligent work promoting veganism in the UCLA community. Across the United States, professors also contribute to activism through numerous ethics and law courses that specifically address the moral and legal relationship between human and nonhuman animals.

English teacher Karen Coyne founded the Compassion in Action Club in California for high school students to learn about a vegan diet and to introduce students to activism. Eleven-year-old Emilie Reiley organized students at her Lanikai, Hawaii, elementary school and successfully petitioned for the school to provide vegan meals. Schools are not always supportive. In 1999, Utah high school student John Ouimette was forced by his administrators to remove his shirt because of its message, "Vegans Have First Amendment Rights." People for the Ethical Treatment of Animals (PETA) provides outreach material to teens through its PETA2 offshoot.

The effect of vegetarian and vegan activism in the educational system is unknown, although a survey conducted in 2004 by Aramark discovered that 25 percent of 100,000 U.S. college students wanted vegan meals available on campus. For comparison, an estimated 7 percent of U.S. residents are vegetarian, and fewer than 1 percent are vegan.

Protests and Boycotts When activists don't make progress with sympathetic techniques, they sometimes turn to confrontation. Protests and boycotts can take a tremendous amount of organizing and perseverance, but they tend to get the most publicity. Publicity, in turn, can persuade the public to support the activists' campaign.

A large part of activism in the late 20th century targeted the supply side of flesh industries. McDonald's was frequently targeted in a series of protests from the late 1980s through the 1990s. Torching effigies of mascot Ronald McDonald became a popular tactic, sometimes stopping business for hours. In some cases, activists occupied its restaurants, including one protest when hundreds of activists attending a national convention blocked one restaurant's doors. In Los Angeles, activists took dead calves, discarded by nearby milk factories, and brought them to McDonald's restaurants. Activists held a funeral for one in a McDonald's parking lot, and at another protest, activists displayed a dead calf in the back of a pickup truck while circling through the drive-through lane.

Some campaigns have involved the general public in boycotts with good results. There has been a constant boycott against Canadian industries, like tourism and maple syrup, because of Canada's annual killing of baby harp seals. The boycott had made modest progress since its 1990 inception, but that changed in 2003 after Canada announced that it would kill one million babies in the following three years. Activists responded, and in 2009 their efforts caused the European Union to boycott Canada's seal products and the U.S. legislature to condemn the killings. Also in 2009, COK and Mercy for Animals jointly called for a boycott of Boca Burgers because eggs were used in their veggie burgers. Less than one month after the boycott's beginning, Boca Burgers pledged to remove eggs from all of their products.

Individuals and small groups can be effective. In 2000, lifelong activist lauren Ornelas [sic] organized a campaign against duck slaughter. Following investigations of major duck-killing businesses, Ornelas and other activists used constant pressure, including protests, to persuade markets and their customers not to buy duck meat. As a result, Trader Joe's stopped selling duck meat, Whole Foods Market no longer buys duck meat from the investigated companies, and Pier 1 Imports stopped selling duck feathers.

Many vegans believe that their success in protests and boycotts has unfairly brought government oppression. For several years, Viva!USA protested Honeybaked Ham before Thanksgiving. In 2003, Viva!USA activists Caitlin Childs and Christopher Freeman were arrested while protesting because they recorded the license plate number of a plainclothes Department of Homeland Security agent who was filming them. In the subsequent winning lawsuit against the Department of Homeland Security, the Georgia American Civil Liberties Union discovered that the Georgia Bureau of Investigation and other government agencies and departments had spied on and infiltrated peaceful animal rights groups.

Litigation's Mixed Results Activists participated in a major victory against McDonald's in 2001. McDonald's admitted to putting cow fat in its french fries that it marketed as vegetarian. The class-action lawsuit resulted in a $12.5 million settlement against McDonald's, with half awarded to vegetarian groups. Yet in another case, Jerold Friedman lost his computer technician job because his employer demanded that he be vaccinated and he refused because vaccines contain animal derivatives. Seeking to protect vegans from employment discrimination, he sued, alleging that his employer unlawfully discriminated against his secular religion of ethical veganism. In 2004, the California Court of Appeal contradicted federal and California precedents with its ruling that in order for a religion to be recognized under the law, it must have more similarity with traditional monotheistic religions, such as a component of otherworldliness.

With the growing field of animal law, activists have an increasing selection of animal-advocate attorneys to protect the rights of vegans and to remove subsidies enjoyed by the killing industries. Animal law, which attempts to apply property law benevolently to nonhumans, is now taught in 110 U.S. law schools according to the Animal Legal Defense Fund, and 140 law schools have student chapters of the fund.

Worldwide View Belgian activists are unique in getting state funding for vegan outreach. After they submitted a sociocultural adult education plan to their government, they received a five-year subsidy to promote vegan food and reduce animal consumption. Further, the Belgian City of Ghent adopted the activists' campaign for "Donderdag Veggiedag" (Thursday Veggie Day), when one day each week the city encourages its residents not to eat animals.

Many nations have small and growing vegan-advocacy organizations, like Animal Friends Croatia and Brazilian VEDDAS, which run campaigns and demonstrations for veganism and against all forms of animal cruelty. Austrians were so effective that in May 2008, 10 activists were jailed for three months without charges for their vegan advocacy. In 2007, Israeli activists successfully persuaded their supreme court to ban foie gras. Grassroots Bulgarian activists have protested against Meat Mania festivals. The Czech Republic, France, and Italy share an annual Veggie Pride March, Brazil has an annual Vegan Festival, and New Zealand has an annual Vegetarian Film Festival.

Despite being a largely vegetarian region, diet-related activism in India and East Asia is in its nascent stage, but signs are that it's growing. The Indian Vegan Society promotes Western-style activism, and it sponsored the 11th annual International Vegan Festival in 2007. As in India, there is some activism in East Asia. Through the years of its empire, the Chinese were obligate vegetarians. Now, mimicking the West, flesh eating is becoming more popular, but in 2003, PETA started its vegan campaigns in the Asia-Pacific region.

See also Advertising; Ahimsa; Alternative and Holistic Medicine; American Vegetarian Society; Animal Liberation Front; Animal Rights and Animal Welfare; Asia; Consumer Products; Dinshah, H. Jay; Ethical Vegetarianism; Europe; Global Warming; India; International Vegetarian Union; Meat and Violence; Meatless Diets before Vegetarianism; Metcalfe, Rev. William; People for the Ethical Treatment of Animals; Physiological Benefits; Policy; Reform; Religious Beliefs and Practices; Television and Films; Veganism; Vegetarians and Vegans, Celebrity; Vegetarians and Vegans, Noted; Vegetarian Society of America; Watson, Donald.

Further Reading

Adams, Carol. *The Sexual Politics of Meat: A Feminist-Vegetarian Critical Theory.* New York: Continuum, 1999.

Association against Animal Factories. www.vgt.at.

Ball, Matt, and Friedrich, Bruce. *The Animal Activist's Handbook.* New York: Lantern Books, 2009.

Bidwell, Victoria. Timeline for the Life & Hard Times of Dr. Shelton. www.soilandhealth. org/02/0201hyglibcat/shelton.bio.bidwell.htm.

Cavalieri, Paola. *The Animal Question: Why Nonhuman Animals Deserve Human Rights.* New York: Oxford University Press, 2004.

Compassion in Action Club. www.theciaclub.com.

Compassion Over Killing. www.cok.net.

DeRose, Chris. *In Your Face.* Dennard, AR: Duncan, 1997.

Dunayer, Joan. *Animal Equality: Language and Liberation.* Derwood, MD: Ryce, 2001.

Ethical Vegetarian Alternative. www.vegetarisme.be.

Ethical Vegetarianism, Animal Rights Defense and Society. veddas.blogspot.com.

Farm Animal Reform Movement. farmusa.org.

Go Vegan with Bob Linden. www.goveganradio.com.

Graham, Sylvester. *Lectures on the Science of Human Life.* Boston: Marsh, Capen, Lyon, & Webb, 1839.

Iacobbo, Karen, and Michael Iacobbo. *Vegetarian America, A History.* Westport, CT: Praeger, 2004.

International Vegetarian Union. ivu.org.

Jones, Christopher, ed. *Philostratus: The Life of Apollonius of Tyana.* Cambridge, MA: Harvard University Press, 2005.

Mann, Keith. *From Dusk 'til Dawn.* London: Puppy Pincher Press, 2007.

Regan, Tom. *The Case for Animal Rights.* Berkeley: University of California Press, 2004.

Robbins, John. *Diet for a New America.* Tiburon, CA: H.J. Kramer, 1998.

Rodger, George. "Interview with Donald Watson—Vegan Founder." www.foodsforlife. org.uk/people/donald-watson-vegan/donald-watson.html.

Sea Shepherd. www.seashepherd.org.

Shelton, Herbert. *Superior Nutrition.* San Antonio, TX: Dr. Shelton's Health School, 1976.

Singer, Peter. *Animal Liberation.* New York: Harper Perennial, 2001.

Torres, Bob, and Jenna Torres. *Vegan Freak: Being Vegan in a Non-Vegan World.* Colton, NY: Tofu Hound Press, 2005.

Vegan Outreach. www.veganoutreach.org.

Jerold D. Friedman

ADVERTISING

Vegetarian-related advertising generally focuses most intently on specific food products rather than on vegetarianism as a lifestyle or particular belief system. Such advertising relies predominantly on health concerns and product quality, though environmentalism and animal rights are often evoked. Health-based advertising cites the benefits of vegetarian products and the costs of meat-based diets, especially in relation to heart disease and cholesterol levels and in response to public health scares, such as so-called mad cow disease.

Closely tied to health-based advertising are claims of better flavors and textures, especially of "faux meat" meat substitutes, which are greatly improved over similar products of early vintage, as well as the increased convenience of vegetarian foods, including entire lines of frozen or preprepared foods. These advertising tactics have led to huge sales increases for soy protein, nondairy, and similar "heart-healthy" products.

Environmental advertising broaches the conservation of resources through locally grown food as opposed to food that is grown and transported across the nation or globe. It also focuses on the intense damage done to groundwater, air quality, and soil by factory farms and plays on the growing market trend toward local, organic food products.

Consumer research firms like Mintel Intelligence and Target Marketing place the vegetarian market in the range of 18 million people in the United States alone with annual sales at $1.6 billion to $2.8 billion, increasing steadily over the past decade. Substantial growth of the market is attributable in part to the development and promotion of vegetarian products by global companies like Kraft and Kellogg's, which have the resources to develop, test, and then sell vegetarian products to vast markets while also offering coupons, discounts, and free samples to attract curious consumers. Smaller companies have also capitalized on market growth by updating package appearances and increasing visibility in mainstream supermarkets.

While market research describes the full-time vegetarian as female and college-educated with an average age of 47, advertising by mainstream companies is often aimed at so-called trade-off consumers—those across the age and economic spectrum who decrease their meat intake for health or economic reasons without necessarily identifying themselves or their diets as vegetarian. Such broad-based marketing is evident as more supermarkets integrate vegetarian food items into the general product selection rather than segregating them into health food sections.

This mainstreaming of vegetarianism and vegetarian foods has emphasized vegetarianism as a diet rather than as an ethical system. Nevertheless, many of the principles that have characterized vegetarianism throughout history, for example, recognition of the connection between human, animal, and plant kingdoms, have continued to be a vital part of modern advertising, including the use of soy-based inks, corporate donations to environmental causes, and a Web-based product presence that emphasizes personal and community involvement and holistic or "green" living. Product tie-ins with broadcast television and publishing have worked well to create integrated marketing approaches and cross-selling opportunities. For committed vegetarians, this mainstreaming has posed some risks because there is no regulated definition of "vegetarian" and thus far no standard vegetarian symbol to notify consumers whether a product is completely or partially free of animal flesh, products, and/or by-products.

See also Agribusiness; Agriculture, Community-Supported; Consumer Products; Global Warming; Organic Foods and Technology; Policy.

Further Reading

Formichelli, Linda. "Market Focus—Vegetarians: The Meatless Market." Target Marketing. http://www.targetmarketingmag.com/article/the-meatless-market-403185_1.html.

Mogelonsky, Marcia. "New Product Trends Category Analysis: Advancing Vegetarianism." Prepared Foods. http://www.preparedfoods.com/Articles/Feature_Article/c4b127 9255788010VgnVCM100000f932a8c0.

Milton W. Wendland

AFRICA

Throughout history, African cuisine has centered on the consumption of vegetables and grains. Vegetable- and grain-based dishes have traditionally been the focal point of most African meals. The vegetarian lifestyle in Africa, as it pertains to the ethical treatment of animals and humans' obligation to them, isn't a commonly held belief except among small segments of the population living throughout the continent. Africa's diverse population is composed of a multitude of races and religions, including Muslims and Hindus, who adhere to vegetarian practices because of their religious beliefs or abstain from eating meat on holy days.

African vegetarian cooking can be traced back hundreds of years. Many early Africans were nomadic people. The first nomadic pastoral society developed in the period from 8500 to 6500 BC in the area of the southern Levant. The food they ate and the way they prepared it reflected a more vegetarian lifestyle. Historically, nonwhites have had a long history of eating vegan and vegetarian dishes and using alternative sources of protein, while Europeans embraced a more meat-based diet and also viewed the daily consumption of meat as a sign of wealth.

Since earliest times, fruits, grains, and vegetables have been an important part of African cookery. Many early African peoples did not plant crops but survived by eating the roots, berries, and leaves that they gathered. Trees and plants that bore fruit such as the locust bean, plantain, mango, and papaya provided a large part of the nomads' diet. In certain parts of Africa, food is sometimes scarce, so African cooks also developed the ability to create dishes out of whatever ingredients they had available during the season. As time went by, more and more Africans cultivated the land and planted crops. Millet was one of the first grains used as food for people and livestock. Over the years, millet has been cultivated from a wild weed to the staple crop familiar today. Millet is popular because it is drought- and disease-resistant and can grow in different types of soil. It is a staple food in North Africa where it is often mixed with water and cooked to make a mushy porridge.

Many people who live in Ghana and other West African countries are from families who have been farmers for hundreds of years. Today's farmers cultivate much of the land using methods that their ancestors developed. Some fields are still tilled with wood-handled hoes. During the harvest time, in many areas of Africa the grain is threshed by beating it with paddles. Women grind corn and millet into flour and meal by pounding the kernels with a wooden pestle in a hollow tree trunk. An especially high grade of millet is finely ground into a flour called teff. Teff flour makes wonderful pancake-like bread called injera.

The use of wild yams for food may go back as far as when millet was first planted. In Africa, yams have become such an important part of the diet that they are seen as having almost mystical qualities. The yam is included in many ceremonies, as part of the meal and as decorations—from the celebration of a new birth to a memorial for the death of an elder. Elaborate festivals honoring the yam were created in Ghana and other West African countries. Harvest celebrations that recognize the yam are still held in Africa.

African yams are thick, oblong tubers usually a little over a foot long. Tubers are plants that have short, thick, fleshy stems that grow underground. Yams and white potatoes are two of the many types of tubers. African yams come in many shapes, colors, and sizes. African Igname yams can weigh as much as 100 pounds. Some varieties of yams have a slightly buttery taste when boiled and a texture similar to the Yukon Gold variety of potato. Cocoyams are a smaller type of yam, usually about the size of an American sweet potato. Some food historians believe that the misconception that a sweet potato is a yam may stem from the substitution in name and use of the sweet potato for the African yam by slave cooks in America.

Sesame seeds are another early food from Africa; they were traded throughout the continent and the Eastern world starting around 2000 BC. The seeds have a nutlike flavor and are used as a thickening agent and as a cooking oil. Fruits of many varieties also grow on the African continent. Wild oranges and lemons were found in Senegambia as early as the mid-15th century by Portuguese travelers. Dates and figs have been available since before biblical times. The fruit of the tamarind, besides being made into a refreshing beverage called *dakhar* in modern Senegal, is also used medicinally as a mild laxative. And tamarind is a common ingredient in many commercially prepared meat sauces. Watermelons are native to many of Africa's tropical regions. Pumpkins and calabashes are edible gourds that were found in the famous cities of Timbuktu and Gao on the Niger River in Africa. The dried gourds were made into dishes, spoons, and food-storage vessels.

Palm trees grow in most parts of Africa. The palm tree produces coconuts, dates, palm nuts, and palm oil, which are used as the basis for soups and stews as well as for making household products. Africa is also the home of the legendary baobab tree, which produces an edible fruit. This tree's trunk can grow as thick as 30 feet in diameter. The bark of the tree is used to make rope, cloth, paper, and medicine. The nuts from the tree are ground into a flour used to thicken sauces. Large truffles, which are mushroom-like plants, grow on or near the roots of trees, and they're tasty when peeled and cooked over coals or used in broths.

Simple, delicious vegetarian dishes that use natural ingredients are a trait of African cooking. African dishes can also be spicy. In ancient times, salt was hard to come by and was highly prized as a way of preserving food. Peppers, such as the *melegueta* and guinea pepper, were more abundant and were used to make spicy, flavorful dishes. Seasoning foods with peppers eventually became a trademark of African recipes.

Africans usually eat large meals only twice a day—at noon and in the evening. Small snacks are eaten throughout the day, such as a piece of bread, fresh fruit, or fried plantains. In African cities, street vendors sell snacks in open-air markets. Sweet snacks like those commonly eaten in America are seldom eaten in Africa.

Outside the cities, the people in the countryside grow all of their own fruits and vegetables in small gardens. Poultry, fish, and meat are less available and more expensive in the markets than fruits and vegetables, which is one reason why soups and stews are a regular part of the diet. It is not uncommon for African recipes to be meatless. Traditionally, meat was not served in large quantities and was usually reserved for special celebrations. In many African recipes, meat is not the focal point of the dish as is often the case with American meals. Vegetable-based stews are sometimes served with a starchy doughlike dish called *fu fu*. Pinches of fu fu dough are used to scoop up the soup or stew. Some of the staples of the African diet include bananas, yams, sweet potatoes, cassava (another tuber, or root, plant), and plantains. Plantains look like large, green bananas but have starchy properties similar to a potato. Plantains are delicious, especially when cooked over hot coals or sliced thinly and fried. The availability in Africa of a variety of fresh fruits, grains, and vegetables is due to some of the richest soil on earth combined with a steady stream of tropical rainfall. This fertile continent has produced some of the most deliciously unique vegetarian recipes in the world.

See also International Vegetarian Union; Meatless Diets before Vegetarianism; Religious Beliefs and Practices.

Further Reading

Gregerson, Jon. *Vegetarianism—A History.* Fremont, CA: Jain Publishing, 1994.

International Vegetarian Union. "IVU in Africa." http://www.ivu.org/africa/index.html.

Medearis, Angela Shelf. *The Ethnic Vegetarian—Traditional and Modern Recipes from Africa, America, and the Caribbean.* New York: Rodale, 2004.

Angela Shelf Medearis

AFRICAN HEBREW ISRAELITES

The African Hebrew Israelites of Jerusalem, also known as the Kingdom of Yah, are a transnational community of several thousand individuals with roots in Chicago, Illinois, and a village located in the Israeli city of Dimona. Their lifestyle is fundamentally based on practices of holistic and regenerative health, and they follow a strict vegan diet according to their interpretation of the Bible. They point to veganism as a necessary foundation for optimal health, peaceful interaction, and spiritual enlightenment. In addition, members wear clothing made only of natural fibers, exercise regularly, receive massages, and do not smoke or drink alcohol, except for naturally fermented wines they produce themselves. In 1998, physicians visited the community of more than 2,000 men, women, and children in Israel. They found that only 6 percent of members suffered from high blood pressure, compared with 30 percent of African Americans, and only 5 percent of members were obese, compared with 32 percent of African American men and nearly half of African American women. Since the community was formed, no members have died from any newly developed long-term chronic disease.

The Kingdom of Yah traces its ancestry to the tribe of Judah—Jews who were brought from West Africa to America during the trans-Atlantic slave trade. Ben Ammi Ben-Israel, the founder and spiritual leader of the community, attests that in 1966—when he was named Ben Carter and worked as a Chicago metallurgist—the angel Gabriel appeared to him in a vision and told him to establish the prophetic Kingdom of God in the Holy Land of Israel. In 1967, Ben-Israel led nearly 400 others from Chicago to Liberia, where they aimed to cleanse themselves of the negative attributes that they had acquired since the outset of their captivity.

After two years in extremely difficult living conditions, an initial group of 39 members arrived in Israel, where they were transported by Israeli government officials to the Negev Desert town of Dimona. The Israeli Chief Rabbinite altered the Law of Return in order to deny them automatic citizenship, and Ben-Israel and his community refused to undergo an official conversion to Judaism. Over the following decades, a bitter and hostile struggle between Israeli officials and the Kingdom of Yah ensued. Meanwhile, the community in Dimona and several other Israeli towns increased in size, primarily through illegal immigration and the growth of large, polygamous families. In the 1990s, the Israeli government granted them temporary-resident status until 2003, when the Israeli Interior Ministry finally offered the community permanent residency.

With the conflict between the Kingdom of Yah and the Israeli government now largely diffused, the community has become a valued part of the nation's culture. More than 100 of the youth have served in the Israeli Defense Forces, and community members have created their own music genre called Songs of Deliverance and have performed across Israel and throughout the world. They have also represented Israel in national and international sports, as well as academic and musical competitions. They operate a factory in Dimona that produces soy products, as well as several vegetarian soul-food restaurants and catering facilities in Israel and in a growing number of U.S. cities. They are respected for their dedication to veganism and holistic health, and members across the world take part in events like the Sugarless and Live Food weeks seasonally. Representatives from the community have also organized programs related to environmentally sustainable international development, regenerative health, and peace. Projects include a partnership with the Ghanaian Ministry of Health and the establishment of an organic agricultural demonstration village in that nation, a social enterprise organization in Kenya that provides communities with the tools to construct water wells, and the Ben Ammi Institute for a New Humanity, a venture with the Southern Christian

Leadership Conference that teaches holistic and nonviolent conflict resolution skills to families and communities.

See also Africa; Alternative and Holistic Medicine; Bible and Biblical Arguments; Colonies, Communal Societies, and Utopias; Ethnic and Racial Groups, U.S.; Physiological Benefits; Religious Beliefs and Practices; Restaurants.

Further Reading

The African Hebrew Israelites. http://africanhebrewisraelitesofjerusalem.com/.

Cohen, Benyamin. "The Prince and I." *American Jewish Life Magazine,* March 1, 2007.

Israel Ministry of Foreign Affairs. "The Hebrew Israelite Community." http://www.mfa.gov. il/mfa/facts%20about%20israel/people/the%20black%20hebrews.

Jackson, John L., Jr. "African Hebrew Israelites: American Black Community Finds Spiritual Home in the Negev." http://www.myjewishlearning.com/israel/Contemporary_Life/ Society_and_Religious_Issues/African_Hebrew_Israelites.shtml.

Michaeli, Ethan. "Another Exodus: The Hebrew Israelites from Chicago to Dimona." In *Black Zion: African American Religious Encounters with Judaism,* edited by Yvonne Patricia Chireau and Nathaniel Deutsch, 73–90. New York: Oxford University Press, 2000.

Garrett Broad

AGRIBUSINESS

Agribusiness refers to the way in which food production is integrated into a larger industrial economic system. The term was first introduced in 1955 by John Davis to signal the shift away from small-scale family farming and agricultural activity toward a large-scale, industrial agrofood system. Unlike agriculture, agribusiness describes the myriad industries and businesses, from equipment and supply manufacturers to growers, processors, and distributors, necessary for modern food provisioning. Agribusiness is considered to be adverse to vegetarian culture. Vegetarians claim that the commodification of food and the prioritization of economic earnings over all else have led to significant consequences for people, animals, and the planet.

The classic model of agribusiness centers on the vertical integration of all stages in the food-production process, in which the growing, processing, selling, and marketing of foodstuffs are managed by a single corporate entity. Agribusiness operates by controlling commodities globally. Today, agricultural activities are under the control of highly concentrated, transnational, corporate ownership and management. This requires that food production comprise a wide network of entanglements spanning both the private and public sectors, including landowners, corporate shareholders, financiers, laborers, farmers, contract farmers, fertilizer and chemical manufacturers, wholesalers, marketers, retail sellers, government agencies, laws and regulators, lobbyists, seed suppliers, scientific and technological researchers, and so on. For this reason, agribusiness has been used as shorthand for corporate farming to highlight the domination of capitalist business interests in feeding the world.

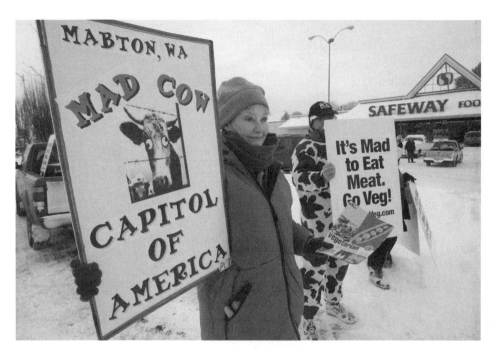

Protesters with People for the Ethical Treatment of Animals protest in 2004 near Mabton, Washington, the location of the farm where the first case of mad cow disease in the United States was discovered that year. The protesters handed out "Vegetarian Starter Kit" booklets in front of a grocery store. (AP Photo/Ted S. Warren)

The mechanization of agriculture has turned farming into an industrial operation that is characterized as inefficient and unsustainable. Mass-producing crops drives down prices, although government subsidies help offset these losses. This makes it difficult for small farmers to continue their work. At the same time, commodity-crop production contributes to soil erosion and depletion and requires high inputs of fertilizer and fossil fuels. Corporations, with stakes in other industries, promote genetically modified seeds to help minimize these difficulties and keep yields stable, even though the long-term consequences are unknown.

Above all, vegetarians oppose intensive livestock production. Some of the largest agrofood corporations include meat and dairy producers, including Cargill, Oscar Mayer, Smithfield, Tyson, and Dean Foods. Each year billions of animals are raised for food, frequently under the most gruesome conditions. Many of these animals live in very restrictive indoor settings, with little room to move around or opportunity to socialize with other animals. Because they are confined, animals are subject to invasive physical procedures to prevent injurious behavior toward themselves or others. They are also given nontherapeutic doses of antibiotics and/or hormones to limit medical issues caused by such unsanitary conditions. Concentrated animal feeding operations are further said to pollute the surrounding air and groundwater, while slaughterhouses are among the most dangerous workplaces in America.

See also Agriculture, Community-Supported; Consumer Products; Global Warming; Organic Foods and Technology.

Further Reading

Belasco, Warren, and Roger Horowitz, eds. *Food Chains: From Farmyard to Shopping.* Philadelphia: University of Pennsylvania Press, 2008.

Magdoff, Fred, John Bellamy Foster, and Frederick Buttell, eds. *Hungry for Profit: The Agribusiness Threat to Farmers, Food, and the Environment.* New York: Monthly Review Press, 2000.

Stull, Donald, and Michael Broadway. *Slaughterhouse Blues: The Meat and Poultry Industry in North America.* Belmont, CA: Thompson, 2004.

Jen Wrye

AGRICULTURE, COMMUNITY-SUPPORTED

Community-supported agriculture (CSA) is a partnership between a farmer and a group of consumers in which consumers pay in advance for a share of the harvest. Shareholders absorb some of agriculture's inherent risks, providing farms with stable markets and income early in the season. In return, consumers receive shares of diverse, high-quality, affordable produce throughout the growing season, and an opportunity to build new relationships with farmers, farms, food, and each other. Though some CSA shares now include foods derived from animals, CSA's foundations lie in plant-based food production, distribution, and consumption. Shares are typically designed for a household of four on a vegetarian diet, making them particularly well suited for vegetarians, vegans, and others who eat vegetable-rich diets.

The CSA concept centers around ideals of small-farm viability, short food supply chains, environmentally sound agriculture, diets rich in plant-based foods, and vibrant local economies. Traditionally, CSAs have sought to be inclusive and accessible. Thus, many offer payment plans or sliding-scale share prices, and nonprofit organizations lead approximately 10 percent of America's CSAs.

Approximately 90 percent of CSA farms offer organically or biodynamically produced foods. All offer produce harvested at peak ripeness. Shares may also include rare regional vegetable varieties not often found in supermarkets, which have health, culinary, aesthetic, or flavor qualities that members value. Some farms offer extras, above the cost of the vegetable share, including fruit, meat, eggs, and dairy products, and some CSAs contract with multiple farms to achieve this product range.

The CSA concept migrated to the United States from Germany and Switzerland, and in 1986 the country's first two CSAs were founded simultaneously in Massachusetts and New Hampshire. Similar European models had emerged in the 1970s, inspired by Chilean cooperative farms and by Rudolf Steiner's writings on biodynamic agriculture. A Japanese model, *teikei* ("partnership"), partnered farmers and consumers in the 1960s, but its influence on the development of European and American CSA models remains uncertain.

Farmers lead roughly 75 percent of America's CSAs, and the rest are coordinated by member core groups. Some farms host the weekly distribution and have members harvest their own shares. Farmers for most urban CSAs deliver to a central distribution site and organize seasonal farm visits for members. Labor, either in farm or administrative duties, is often a membership requirement.

Share prices range from roughly $300 to $700 for 20–25 weeks. CSAs comprise 10 to 1,000 or more shareholders, whom researchers characterize as highly educated people of varying income levels. As shares include a diversity and quantity of vegetables new to many consumers, newsletters have become key modes of information exchange on preparing and preserving the week's share.

An estimated 1,300–2,000 American CSA farms, concentrated around the coasts and the Great Lakes, provide food for approximately 270,000 member households. Under many different names and models, the broader CSA concept is growing worldwide. Its strongest roots are in Japan (16 million consumers), western Europe (more than 250,000 consumers in the United Kingdom, France, and the Netherlands alone), and Canada (30,000 consumer members). Though fewer in number, CSA ventures have also been identified in Malaysia, Morocco, Mali, Benin, Togo, Latvia, and Romania.

See also Africa; Agribusiness; Asia; Consumer Products; Europe; Health Food Stores and Food Cooperatives; Organic Foods and Technology; Reform.

Further Reading

Adam, Katherine L. *Community Supported Agriculture.* Fayetteville, AR: ATTRA—National Sustainable Agriculture Information Service, 2006.

Groh, Trauger, and Steven McFadden. *Farms of Tomorrow Revisited: Community Supported Farms—Farm Supported Communities.* Kimberton, PA: Biodynamic Farming and Gardening Association, 1998.

Henderson, Elizabeth, and Robyn Van En. *Sharing the Harvest: A Citizen's Guide to Community Supported Agriculture.* White River Junction, VT: Chelsea Green, 2007.

Shayna Cohen

AHIMSA

Ahimsa is a doctrine of Jainism, Buddhism, and Hinduism that affirms that all forms of life are sacred, and thus it prohibits violence in thoughts, words, and actions under any circumstances. Jainism is an ancient dharmic religion from India. Ahimsa supports the belief that all life forms, including plants and animals, are equal, possess souls, and are capable of attaining salvation. The term "ahimsa" itself is Sanskrit for nonviolence, literally the avoidance of violence (himsa).

Ahimsa is also one of the *yamas* (a rule or code of conduct for living) of ashtanga yoga (a system of yoga recorded by the sage Vamana Rishi) and was popularized in the West by Mahatma Gandhi. Gandhi's peaceful protests were based on the nonviolent principles of ahimsa. Examples of ahimsa include Hindu monks who sweep in front of them as they walk, to avoid injuring insects; a young Jain's refusal to participate in gossip or use paper (as it hurts trees); or the decision to commit oneself to a vegetarian or vegan lifestyle. Frequently, people mistake ahimsa as a synonym for vegetarianism. Though practicing vegetarianism is a way of practicing ahimsa, it is not the only requirement for doing so. Ahimsa encompasses much more than a vegetarian diet. The principles of vegetarianism, however, dovetail nicely with those of ahimsa, and these two concepts are conceptually linked.

When eating meat, especially before prepackaged foods became the norm, the consumer had to consider where to find the animal to be eaten, as well as how to kill, cook, eat, and/or preserve it. Therefore, the entire process of eating animals was considered himsa because one had to think and speak about killing the animal, as well as perform the act of killing itself. According to the doctrine of ahimsa, when people consume the flesh of a dead animal, they not only commit an act of himsa, but they also become infected by the pain of the dead animal. When they eat meat, they also ingest the feelings of violence and pain contained in that animal's final experience.

The *Mahabharata,* one of the defining historical and cultural texts for Indians, particularly Hindus, also applies the notion of ahimsa to abstention from meat. According to the *Mahabharata,* which first appeared as a unified text in AD 350, "The purchaser of flesh performs himsa by his wealth; he who eats flesh does so by enjoying its taste; the killer does himsa by actually tying and killing the animal. Thus, there are three forms of killing. He who brings flesh or sends for it, he who cuts of the limbs of an animal, and he who purchases, sells, or cooks flesh and eats it—all of these are to be considered meat-eaters" (115:40). Since the work clearly equates the killing and consumption of animals for food as an act of violence, vegetarianism has long been practiced by Hindus, and Hindus, along with Buddhists, will continue to practice vegetarianism as long as ahimsa serves as one of their guiding tenets.

See also Animal Rights and Animal Welfare; Antivivisection; Dinshah, H. Jay; Eastern Religions, Influences of; Ethical Vegetarianism; Francione, Gary L.; Gandhi, Mohandas; India; Jainism; Religious Beliefs and Practices; Veganism.

Further Reading

Balsys, Bodo. *Ahimsa: Buddhism and the Vegetarian Ideal.* New Delhi, India: Munshiram Manoharlal, 2004.
Sethia, Tara. *Ahimsa, Anekanta and Jainism.* New Delhi, India: Motilal Banarsidass, 2004.
Shepherd, Mark. *Gandhi Today: A Report on India's Gandhi Movement and Its Experiments in Nonviolence and Small Scale Alternatives.* Friday Harbor, WA: Simple Productions, 1987.
Tobias, Michael. *Life Force: The World of Jainism.* Fremont, CA: Jain Publishing, 2000.

Jen Westmoreland Bouchard

ALCOTT, WILLIAM A. (1798–1859)

William A. Alcott was a physician and early vegetarian reformer. He was elected the first president of the American Vegetarian Society in 1850 and wrote several books on health, vegetarianism, and education. Alcott was born in Wolcott, Connecticut, and began his medical training in 1822. In 1825, Alcott completed his training by attending a course of lectures at Yale Medical College. He espoused practical measures to ensure his patients' good health: fresh air, mild food, and as little medication as possible. Advocates of plain food such as Alcott warned against the consumption of spices, sugar, and raw vegetables to avoid overstimulation, or overheating, of the body.

In the mid-1830s, he rose to prominence after publishing several advice manuals for young men and women on how to create a healthy and happy home. In them, Alcott combined advice about how young married people should interact with one another with advice on domestic economy, chastity, and health. He saw his work as treating not just the body but also the spirit. The body and spirit were seen as interconnected by many 19th-century reformers, who believed that the health of the body indicated a good soul and an ability to withstand psychological trauma.

In 1839, after a lifelong aversion to meat and fish, Alcott became a confirmed vegetarian and abstained from all animal-derived foods, including milk. Alcott not only believed that a vegetarian diet would benefit anyone's physical health but also argued that vegetarianism was beneficial to society as a whole. This argument was based on the notion of love holiness, which asserted that individual actions created a chain of benevolence. By abstaining from animal food, vegetarians would not have to engage in acts of violence against animals and thus would avoid any temptation to give in to the baser passions. Thus, a vegetarian could move beyond the simple human need of obtaining food and instead focus on the higher things, including cultivating morality and a spiritual life.

Alcott remained close to his cousin, the transcendentalist Bronson Alcott, during their adult lives. Bronson was also an advocate of the concept of love holiness, and the two of them were involved in several similar ventures. In 1843, Bronson, the father of author Louisa May, founded an experimental community in Massachusetts called Fruitlands. There, he implemented many of the ideas shared by his cousin, including vegetarianism, love holiness, and simple clothing. While William Alcott did not join his cousin's venture, he followed its progress and demise closely. He corresponded regularly with his cousin, and each read the other's published works.

Alcott continued his advocacy of a vegetarian diet and was a prominent spokesman for the movement. At the inaugural meeting in 1850 of the American Vegetarian Society, Alcott was elected president. Prior to his election, he focused his publishing efforts on describing the superiority of the vegetarian diet. The society was the idea of Rev. William Metcalfe (the leader of the vegetarian Philadelphia Bible Christian Church) and Sylvester Graham. Graham was among the best-known diet reformers of the mid-19th century and pioneered the use of less refined flour for heartier and more nutritious bread. The first meeting was dedicated to the promotion of vegetarianism as a superior diet and lifestyle, and the focus of the commentary was on the health to be gained by avoiding meat. Alcott argued that vegetarianism was suitable for all people. Regardless of an individual's initial health, a vegetarian diet would improve it. Avoiding animal protein would allow people to be more vigorous and physically active. In addition, it would benefit people's souls, as they would be able to suppress the animal passions that are inherent in eating another creature. The meeting was regarded as a success, and its proceedings were published and disseminated among vegetarian and reform circles.

For the next nine years, Alcott lived in Auburndale, Massachusetts, and espoused a strict form of vegetarianism that involved eating a limited selection of vegetables without any condiments, jams and jellies, or butter. He also tended to avoid wearing a hat or shoes, which he argued was more natural and thus healthier. He died in 1859, at age 60, from tuberculosis, which he had lived with since his childhood.

See also Alternative and Holistic Medicine; American Vegetarian Society; Bible Christians, Philadelphia; Graham, Sylvester; Meatless Diets before Vegetarianism; Metcalfe, Rev. William; Physiological Benefits; Religious Beliefs and Practices.

Further Reading

Alcott, William A. *Vegetable Diet Defended.* London: J. Chapman, 1844.

Alcott, William A. *The Young Housekeeper, or Thoughts on Food and Cookery.* Boston: Waite, Pierce and Company, 1846. http://digital.lib.msu.edu/projects/cookbooks/html/books/book_15.cfm.

Iacobbo, Karen, and Michael Iacobbo. *Vegetarian America: A History.* Westport, CT: Praeger, 2004.

International Vegetarian Union. "History of Vegetarian Societies in North America—1837–1908." http://www.ivu.org/history/societies/usa.html.

Preece, Rod. *Sins of the Flesh: A History of Ethical Vegetarian Thought.* Vancouver, British Columbia: University of British Columbia Press, 2008.

Salomon, Louis B. "The Least-Remembered Alcott." *New England Quarterly* 34, no. 1 (March 1961): 87–93.

Spencer, Colin. *Vegetarianism: A History.* New York: Four Walls, Eight Windows, 2002.

Gwynne K. Langley Rivers

ALTERNATIVE AND HOLISTIC MEDICINE

Since the late 1700s and early 1800s, alternative and holistic medicine advocates have been among the most active and ardent promoters of vegetarianism. As critics of mainstream orthodox medical practice in the 19th century, reformers such as Sylvester Graham and John Harvey Kellogg made vegetarianism a cardinal principle, based on a combination of philosophical and scientific evidence. Likewise, a wide range of alternative medical systems including hydropathy and naturopathy promoted vegetarianism as a central component of a holistic approach to health and wellness throughout the 20th century. In each of these cases, vegetarianism and health have intersected with philosophies of bodily or spiritual purity and broader movements for social reform.

Like many 19th-century Jacksonian movements, vegetarianism was a reaction to industrialization's encroachment into everyday life. Sylvester Graham (1794–1851), minister, lecturer, and hygiene crusader, was the best-known figure of the 1830s and 1840s popular health reform movement, which melded spirituality and personal health and held individuals responsible for their own well-being. Graham's influence in promoting vegetarianism was so vast that he is considered by many to be the father of movement in the United States. Graham and the physician William A. Alcott (1798–1859)—the two most prominent spokesmen for vegetarianism at the time—were recruited to the cause by the Bible Christian Church, a sect founded in Manchester, England, in the early 1800s. In 1817, William Metcalfe (1788–1862), a Bible Christian Church minister, preached vegetarianism in Philadelphia. Graham and Alcott were among the early vegetarian converts. Alcott was also influenced by his cousin, the transcendentalist Bronson Alcott who was the father of author Louisa May Alcott and founder of the vegetarian commune Fruitlands.

By the 1830s, Graham and Alcott were joined by well-known surgeon and Dartmouth professor Reuben Mussey (1780–1866) as crusaders for the transformation of vegetarianism from a predominantly Christian moral orientation to a scientific and physical preoccupation. In 1837, Graham and Alcott founded the American Physiological Society (APS) in Boston. The organization promoted the teaching of physiology, anatomy, and especially diet. The society's members liberally drew from a wealth of popular literature on hygiene from the 18th and early 19th century, along with the physiological research of London physicians George Cheyne and William Lambe and French scientists Marie-Francois Xavier Bichat and Francois-Joseph Victor Broussias.

Graham and his fellow health reformers blended religion, science, philosophy, and politics in establishing a scientific rationale for vegetarianism. Grahamites—also known as Pythagoreans and eventually as vegetarians after 1847—employed a physiological rationale for modifying behavior, but they believed Americans suffered from an increased incidence of disease because they engaged in immoral behavior that was inherently unphysiological and unhealthful. Their complex theory of physiology depicted the body as a fragile organism vulnerable to overstimulation. The program of reform, known as Grahamism, prescribed a vegetarian diet, which also restricted dairy products and stimulants such as coffee and tea. Emphasis was also placed on sexual restraint, a proper balance between rest and exercise, and cleanliness.

According to early vegetarian advocates, medicine was not needed as long as one followed the strict rules governing diet and behavior. Graham's gospel constituted a radical departure from the traditional emphasis on moderation in medical thought, but, above all, Grahamism promoted vegetarianism as the original,

God-appointed diet of humankind, prescribed by Genesis 1:29. Alcott promoted the idea that vegetarianism provided the basis for all reform, whether civil, social, moral, or religious. The vegetarian diet (also called the natural or meatless diet) was not surprisingly, then, an integral part of other reform movements of the period—including temperance, women's suffrage, women's dress reform, and abolition.

In 1850, feminists and abolitionist leaders were among the health reformers gathered at the first American Vegetarian Convention, which established the American Vegetarian Society (AVS). The AVS was modeled on the still-existing Vegetarian Society of the United Kingdom, which had been created in 1847. Alcott was made president, Graham and nine other men were appointed as vice presidents, and Metcalfe became the correspondence secretary and editor of the society's *American Vegetarian and Health Journal.* The AVS nourished affiliate organizations, including the New York Vegetarian Society, and helped to spread the Grahamite gospel, but by 1854 the organization was on unstable ground with Graham's early death and a lack of funds to support the society's fledgling journal.

In the antebellum period, information about vegetarianism continued to flow to the public through alternative medicine channels. After Graham's death, proponents of hydropathy, or the water cure, played a particularly important role in sustaining interest by endorsing vegetarianism's preventive orientation as a complement to water, the hydropathic healing agent for disease. Russell T. Trall (1812–1877), another vice president of the AVS and dean of the hydropathy profession, became one of the most prolific promoters of vegetarianism, as a crusading editor and touring lecturer; the head of hydropathy's leading educational institution, the Hygeio-Therapeutic College; and the writer of popular pro-vegetarian books including *The Scientific Basis of Vegetarianism.* Vegetarianism was also regularly promoted in the profession's chief periodical, the *Water-Cure Journal,* which began publication in 1845 and by the 1860s reached tens of thousands of readers. Joel Shew, who had opened the country's first water-cure establishment in 1843 in Lebanon Springs, New York, featured a vegetarian diet as an essential part of the health regimen, as did other popular health establishments, including the renowned Jackson Sanitarium in Dansville, New York, which treated over 20,000 people from 1858 until its closing in the early twentieth century. James Caleb Jackson (1811–1895), who had served as a vice president for the AVS, expanded on the work of Graham and Trall and by 1858 opened an institution that was a forerunner of holistic health at a time when the word "holistic" had not been thought of yet. Jackson called for vegetarianism as a Christian duty essential for purity and physical perfection and spread the vegetarian message beyond the sanitarium in his books and magazines.

Guests at the Glen Haven Water-Cure, where Jackson worked prior to starting his own establishment in Dansville, included a young woman named Ellen G. White (1827–1915) and her husband, James White (1821–1881), founders of the Seventh-day Adventist Church. In 1866, the Whites opened a water-cure institution of their own, the Western Health Reform Institute in Battle Creek, Michigan. In 1872, the Whites hired physician John Harvey Kellogg (1852–1943), the man who would build the little water cure into a legendary institution. By the late 1870s, Kellogg had rechristened the institute and established the Battle Creek Sanitarium Health Food Company to produce Jackson's granola, the whole-grain cereals that bore his name, and the graham crackers named after the vegetarian health reform trailblazer. Kellogg lectured about the scientific basis for vegetarianism and its various health benefits for decades, despite facing harsh criticism from the medical establishment, which continued to marginalize vegetarian advocates. At its height, Kellogg's Battle Creek Sanitarium served vegetarian meals to over 7,000 guests a year.

Vegetarianism had become a tenet of many alternative medicine advocates by the dawn of the 20th century, but as the popularity of hydropathy waned, a new generation of athletes and critics of conventional medicine continued to champion the vegetarian diet. One of the most popular showmen of the day, Bernarr Macfadden (1868–1955), built a vast publishing empire based on an approach to health known as physical culture, which included an emphasis on exercise, fasting, pure food, and vegetarianism. In 1899, Macfadden published the first issue of *Physical Culture* magazine, which heavily criticized the use of drugs in mainstream medicine and provided a forum for vegetarian views. *Physical Culture* eventually reached a circulation of 500,000 and regularly featured a photo of Macfadden's muscled physique on its cover.

Another prominent advocate of vegetarianism, Benedict Lust (1872–1945), opened the American School of Naturopathy in midtown Manhattan in 1901 and established two health-cure resorts shortly thereafter in New Jersey and Florida. The resorts offered guests an exhaustive menu of alternative therapies including sun and light baths, massage, hydropathy, exercise programs, and vegetarian diets. Under the banner of naturopathy, Lust's followers offered virtually any conventional or unconventional health practice that promoted natural healing.

Lust, like Macfadden, loathed the medical establishment. Macfadden had suggested that the American Medical Association (AMA) represented a threat to the life and health of citizens with its monopolistic power over individual doctors, but Lust went further in critiquing what he considered the scientific fallacies of conventional medicine, including the germ theory of Louis Pasteur, vaccinations, and vivisection (the use of live animals in experimental medicine). Morris Fishbein, editor of the *Journal of the American Medical Association,* responded by moving against the growing interest in natural health, including vegetarianism. Fishbein wrote in his 1927 book, *The New Medical Follies,* that Lust's system, including the promotion of vegetarian diets, was nothing more than an attempt to capitalize on people's ills for the purpose of financial gain. As alternative medicine faced an assault led by the AMA, vegetarianism suffered a series of similar blows between the 1930s and 1960s. The AMA's consumer magazine, *Hygeia,* called vegetarians "food faddists," associated vegetarianism with religious fanaticism, and referred to the vegetarian diet as a "freak diet." Meanwhile, press coverage of vegetarianism declined dramatically.

Advocates of alternative medicine, including Herbert Shelton (1895–1985), still continued to advocate the same type of Grahamite regimen that had inspired earlier health reformers. Shelton, like drugless doctors before him, did not practice medicine but instructed his clients on nutritional healing and preventive dietary measures. Along with establishing the American Natural Hygiene Society in 1949, Shelton founded *Dr. Shelton's Hygienic Review,* which championed vegan and vegetarian diets for several decades.

On the heels of the 1960s countercultural embrace of vegetarianism as a viable ecological and healthful choice, the holistic health movement of the 1970s helped to reestablish the ties between vegetarianism and alternative medicine. When the word "holistic" was introduced into medicine in the 1970s, practitioners of alternative medicine immediately embraced it as an ideal that distinguished them from conventional medicine. With an emphasis on using natural therapies, preventive measures, patient education, and an ecological whole-person approach to healing, vegetarianism proved a perfect fit. The integration of the physical, mental, and spiritual levels of being in holism recalled the tenets of Grahamism, and vegetarianism comfortably found a place as a central tenet in each.

In the final three decades of the 20th century, mounting evidence of the health benefits of a vegetarian diet helped transform vegetarianism from a predominantly political and philosophical movement into a commercially viable industry and cultural phenomenon measured by a growing number of books, magazines, and Internet resources. *Vegetarian Times,* founded by Paul Obis, grew from an independent four-page newsletter read by a small community of vegetarians in 1974 into a mainstream commercial periodical with a circulation of over 220,000 by 2006. Several other magazines published by vegetarian interest groups also prioritized reporting on health news, including developments in the field of alternative and holistic medicine. Health and lifestyle blogs and Web sites including VegSource.com and Vegetarian Resource Group's vrg.org also began featuring videos, podcasts, and pages of information on the health benefits of vegetarianism.

Vegetarianism, like alternative and holistic medicine, has undergone a revolution of sorts in recent decades, with different variations achieving mainstream status, while activists and extremists remain on the cultural fringe. Since the 1970s, the gradual validation of vegetarian diets by conventional health and government organizations including the American Dietetic Association and U.S. Department of Agriculture has contributed to greater social acceptance. Nevertheless, scientific studies showing that a vegetarian diet can be helpful in preventing or reversing arthritis, diabetes, heart disease, and cancer have rarely been disseminated by the mass media or acknowledged by the medical establishment. In the early 21st century, the relationship between vegetarianism, alternative medicine, and health remains controversial.

See also Alcott, William A.; American Vegetarian Society; Battle Creek Sanitarium; Bible and Biblical Arguments; Bible Christians, English; Bible Christians, Philadelphia; Colonies, Communal Societies, and Utopias; Consumer Products; Graham, Sylvester; Health Food Stores and Food Cooperatives; Internet, The; Kellogg, John Harvey; Macfadden, Bernarr; Metcalfe, Rev. William; Physical Fitness and Athleticism; Physiological Benefits; Policy; Reform; Transcendentalism.

Further Reading

Iacobbo, Karen, and Michael Iacobbo. *Vegetarian America: A History.* Westport, CT: Praeger, 2004.

Maurer, Donna. *Vegetarianism: Movement or Moment?* Philadelphia: Temple University Press, 2002.

Nissenbaum, Stephen. *Sex, Diet and Debility in Jacksonian America: Sylvester Graham and Health Reform.* Westport, CT: Greenwood, 1980.

Whorton, James C. *Crusaders for Fitness: The History of American Health Reformers.* Princeton, NJ: Princeton University Press, 1984.

Whorton, James C. *Nature Cures: The History of Alternative Medicine in America.* New York: Oxford University Press, 2002.

Eric Boyle

AMERICAN VEGETARIAN SOCIETY (1850–1862)

The American Vegetarian Society (AVS) was the first national vegetarian organization founded in the United States. Formed under the leadership of several health reformers—physician William A. Alcott, Sylvester Graham, and the founder of the Philadelphia Bible Christian Church, Rev. William Metcalfe—the society was established at the first American Vegetarian Convention in New York City's Clinton Hall on May 15, 1850. The first national vegetarian convention included prominent women and men involved in a variety of antebellum reform movements, all of whom had a common desire to advocate for a meat-free diet. Inspired by the successful foundation of the Vegetarian Society in England (now known as the Vegetarian Society of the United Kingdom) in 1847, American dietary reformers decided to codify the principles of vegetarianism in the United States. Members of the AVS emphasized the lifestyle's health benefits while connecting a vegetable diet with varying reform movements. The diet was positioned as a vehicle to achieve success in diverse social movements including abolition, women's suffrage, economic equity, and health reform. With these principles in mind, the American Vegetarian Convention voted in favor of the founding of a national society aimed at promoting the diffusion of vegetarian ideals through lectures, printed publications, and local organizations. The convention's attendees produced a "Declaration of Sentiments and Resolutions" aimed at spreading awareness of the health and social benefits of a vegetarian diet and resolved to build a nationwide vegetarian organization to manage the growth of that ideal. Alcott, a longtime advocate of meatless dietetics, was elected the society's first president, a role that he filled from 1850 until his death in 1859.

This new organization, named the American Vegetarian Society, held its first meeting in Philadelphia in September 1850. At this time the AVS published the first edition of its periodical, the *American Vegetarian and Health Journal,* which became a monthly publication by 1851. The journal served as the public voice of the AVS, advocating for vegetarianism while also connecting the diet to larger reform movements such as women's rights, abolitionism, and the nascent animal rights movement. Information about the organization also was diffused by the popular press, receiving coverage from most major, urban, daily newspapers. T.L. Nichols's *Water-Cure Journal*—a popular health and welfare publication that emphasized a variety of home health treatments—also consistently reported on the activities of the AVS.

In addition to utilizing the printed word, the AVS held yearly meetings and festival meals to celebrate and spread awareness of the diet. These celebrations drew prominent reformers ranging from abolitionist and *New York Tribune* publisher Horace Greeley to famed women's suffragist Susan B. Anthony. Elaborate, multicourse vegetarian meals were served, often followed by pro-vegetarian speeches and musical entertainment. The growth of the national organization gave birth to numerous localized, affiliate associations including the largest, the New York Vegetarian Society, founded in 1852.

Despite its best efforts, by 1854 the AVS's popularity and influence began to wane. The organization continued holding annual meetings and festivals, but its publishing arm discontinued. In October 1854, the AVS printed the final issue of the *American Vegetarian and Health Journal.* In its place the *Water-Cure Journal* continued reporting regularly on AVS activities. At its annual meeting in 1854 the society debated the merits of its existence, ultimately deciding to continue activities. However, the AVS had reached the height of its size, popularity, and influence. By 1857, the AVS began the process of cooperation and integration with the Vegetarian Society based in Great Britain, as each organization's bylaws included honorary membership for vegetarians in foreign countries. While this organizational shift was at first more symbolic, it set the stage for the eventual conjoining of the two organizations. Comembership ensured that the *Vegetarian Messenger,* the monthly publication of the Vegetarian Society, became the de facto publication of the AVS, as its members received free subscriptions, and the journal included coverage of vegetarian activities in the United States.

In March 1859, Alcott died, leaving the AVS without one of its founders and most notable proponents. In response, members of the organization turned to American vegetarianism's past for a leader to take over the organization. William Metcalfe, one of the earliest proponents of meat abstention in the United States, took over the presidency of the AVS in its waning years. Annual meetings were no longer held in elaborate, public buildings but rather in Philadelphia's Bible Christian Church. With the AVS facing financial hardships, free memberships were no longer available to Americans, and many American vegetarians decided to join the British society instead in order to continue receiving copies of the *Vegetarian Messenger.* Membership numbers in the AVS continued to drop significantly, leading to its dissolution following the organization's 12th annual meeting in 1862. American vegetarians would be without a national organization for more than 20 years. The organization that would follow, however, was connected to the life span of the AVS. The Vegetarian Society of America—founded in 1886—was established under the leadership of Henry S. Clubb, a former active member of the AVS and leader of the Philadelphia Bible Christian Church.

See also Alcott, William A.; Alternative and Holistic Medicine; Bible Christians, English; Bible Christians, Philadelphia; Clubb, Henry S.; Graham, Sylvester; Metcalfe, Rev. William; Periodicals; Physiological Benefits; Reform; Vegetarian Society of America; Vegetarian Society of the United Kingdom.

Further Reading

Iacobbo, Karen, and Michael Iacobbo. *Vegetarian America: A History.* Westport, CT: Praeger, 2004.

The Philadelphia Bible Christian Church. *History of the Philadelphia Bible-Christian Church for the First Century of Its Existence from 1817 to 1917.* Philadelphia: J.B. Lippincott, 1922. www.ivu.org/history/usa19/history_of_bible_christian_church.pdf.

Preece, Rod. *Sins of the Flesh: A History of Ethical Vegetarian Thought.* Seattle: University of Washington Press, 2008.

Puskar-Pasewicz, Margaret. "'For the Good of the Whole': Vegetarianism in Nineteenth-Century America." PhD diss., Indiana University, 2003.

Silver-Isenstadt, Jean L. *Shameless: The Visionary Life of Mary Gove Nichols.* Baltimore: Johns Hopkins University Press, 2002.

Whorton, James C. "'Tempest in a Flesh-Pot!': The Formulation of a Physiological Rationale for Vegetarianism." In *Sickness and Health in America: Readings in the History of Medicine and Public Health*, edited by Judith Walzer Leavitt and Ronald L. Numbers. Madison: University of Wisconsin Press, 1977, 315–330.

Williams, Susan. *Food in the United States, 1820s–1890.* Westport, CT: Greenwood, 2006.

Adam D. Shprintzen

ANIMAL LIBERATION FRONT

The Animal Liberation Front (ALF) is a decentralized, nonhierarchical animal liberation movement that consists of a series of small autonomous and anonymous cells operating in at least 20 countries around the world. The ALF is an abolitionist movement that aims to end all forms of animal exploitation through the use of direct action. The principal forms of direct action employed by the ALF are economic sabotage—primarily property damage, vandalism, and arson—of laboratories, factory farms (intensive industrial farming units), and fur farms, and the rescue and rehabilitation of animals confined in such sites of exploitation. The ALF also aims to educate the public about systemic violence against animals. Toward this end, the ALF frequently releases footage of experiments and other forms of animal abuse, obtained during raids. Because of the tremendous risk of indictment and imprisonment posed by their actions, ALF activists are compelled to carry out actions covertly.

The ALF was formed in the United Kingdom in 1976 by antihunt activist Ronnie Lee and is an outgrowth of a hunt saboteur group, Band of Mercy, established by Lee and fellow activist Cliff Goodman four years earlier. Lee and Goodman developed Band of Mercy as an extension of the Hunt Saboteurs Association (founded in 1963) but took its name from another hunt saboteur group (established by Catherine Smithies in 1824 as the youth branch of the Royal Society for the Prevention of Cruelty to Animals). A year after its modern refounding, Band of Mercy expanded its mission to include the abolition of vivisection as well as hunting. In an even more significant break with its forerunners, Band of Mercy abandoned legal direct action and opted instead for its illegal counterpart, which its members considered to be a more effective means of resistance. Whereas earlier antihunting groups had typically employed tactics such as sounding horns,

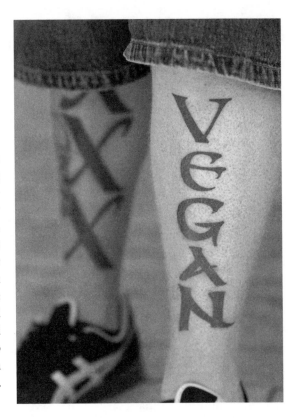

Tattoos of the word "vegan" and "XXX" cover the leg of a young man who did not want to be identified at the Total Liberation Tour in Salt Lake City, Utah, 2004. The letter X or variations such as "XXX" are popular symbols for straightedge, a subculture of punk rock that became associated in the 1990s with militant veganism and animal rights activism. The FBI had said that the tour would feature top leaders of the Animal Liberation Front and Earth Liberation Front. (AP Photo/Fred Hayes)

obstructing roads, igniting smoke bombs, and distracting dogs with false scents, Band of Mercy opted instead for the destruction of vessels, vehicles, and equipment used to maim and kill animals. Band of Mercy committed its first act of arson on November 10, 1973, when its members burned down a laboratory under construction at Milton Keynes. In 1974, police arrested Lee and Goodman after a raid on Oxford Laboratory Animal Colonies in Bicester, and they were sentenced to three years in prison. Goodman subsequently became a police informer; Lee expanded his organization, which he now dubbed the Animal Liberation Front, after his release.

Since its formation in 1976, the ALF has been responsible for tens of millions of dollars in damage to various exploitative industries. Spokespersons for the ALF suggest that while legal protest has its place, animal exploiters are more likely to actually close down their operations as a result of costly property damage, escalating insurance costs, or the loss of insurance altogether.

The ALF is perhaps best known for its activities in the United States. Its exact origins in the United States are disputed. Some point to the release of two dolphins from a research facility in Hawaii in 1977 as the first American ALF action, while Ingrid Newkirk, cofounder of People for the Ethical Treatment of Animals (PETA), traces the origins of ALF in the United States to a raid on a Howard University laboratory on Christmas Eve in 1982, when activists rescued 24 cats whose legs had been crippled for the purposes of an experiment. Newkirk specifically attributes the cat rescue and the development of the ALF in the United States to a former female police officer from the Montgomery County Police Force in Maryland; to protect this person's identity, Newkirk has pseudonymously named her "Valerie." Valerie is credited with setting up and offering financial support to other cells throughout the country and for leading other famous rescues and raids. Among the most well known of these actions is the 1985 rescue from a University of California Riverside laboratory of "Britches," a baby macaque monkey who was kept in solitary confinement in a wire cage and whose eyes had been sewn shut for blindness experiments; in addition, a device called a "Tri-Sensory Aid" had been attached to Britches's head that was so heavy that it prevented him from holding up his head. A more recent victory claimed by the ALF in the United States is the liberation of 300 captive mink from McMullin Mink Farm in South Jordan, Utah, in August 2008.

Because of its militant stance and its use of direct action, the ALF has also stirred tremendous controversy within and outside the animal welfare, rights, and liberation movements. The main source of contention is whether the direct-action tactics employed by the ALF constitute violence or terrorism. In "The ALF Primer," the ALF asserts that it is unequivocally opposed to violence against all human and nonhuman animals: "The ALF does not, in any way, condone violence against any animal, human or non-human. Any action involving violence is by its definition not an ALF action, and any person involved is not an ALF member." Despite the ALF's explicit denunciation of violence against all sentient beings, in January 2005 the U.S. Department of Homeland Security officially labeled the ALF a terrorist threat. The following year, then–U.S. president George W. Bush signed the Animal Enterprise Terrorism Act (AETA), which designates property damage as well as any "operations interfering with any animal enterprise" as acts of terrorism. Although the ALF is not named in the AETA, it is undoubtedly its principal target. Critics of AETA insist that its real aim is not to protect the public from injury and harm but rather to protect the interests of multibillion-dollar corporations that turn a hefty profit from engaging in exploitative practices toward animals. ALF proponents also highlight the irony of deeming the ALF a terrorist threat when it is committed to avoiding and preventing harm to all sentient beings, while Western governments are responsible for the deaths not only of billions of nonhuman animals each year but also of activists such as Barry Horne. Horne died in a U.K. prison hospital on November 5, 2001, after a 68-day hunger strike, which he had embarked on to protest the British government's support for vivisection. As a result of its characterization as a terrorist threat, and the correspondingly harsh penalties imposed on convicted ALF activists, advocates of the ALF see it as a target of government repression. Despite the tremendous risk attached to its activities, however, the ALF continues to defend, on ethical and political grounds, its right to break laws when necessary to counter the effects of a "lawful" state apparatus that sanctions and administrates the commission of mass atrocities against helpless animals.

Excerpt from a Manifesto for Animal Liberation

We need a far richer and more radical concept of abolitionism that draws from and revitalizes the strength and power of the nineteenth century anti-human slavery movement that erupted in the US (and of course earlier in the UK). Unlike the pale imitation and caricature espoused by Franciombes, the version of abolitionism we champion is far more in tune with the radicalism, pluralism, and alliance politics (imperfect and impermanent as it was) of nineteenth-century abolitionism. But eschewing nostalgia and outmoded political models, this approach also draws from numerous other contemporary theories and political movements. We recognize the need for radical social change and we understand that the fight against speciesism, capitalism, the state, and hierarchy in all forms will be waged on many different fronts simultaneously.

... We endorse a form of abolition that (1) defends the use of high-pressure direct action tactics, along with illegal raids, rescues, and sabotage attacks; (2) views capitalism as an inherently irrational, exploitative, and destructive system, and sees the state as a corrupt tool whose function is to advance the economic and military interests of the corporate domination system and to repress opposition to its agenda; (3) has a broad, critical understanding of how different forms of oppression are interrelated, seeing human animal, nonhuman animal, and earth liberation as inseparable projects; and, thus, (4) promotes an anti-capitalist alliance politics with other rights, justice, and liberation movements who share the common goal of dismantling all systems of hierarchical domination and rebuilding societies through decentralization and democratization processes.

We form this new group out of the need for a radical social approach to veganism and animal rights that transcends bourgeois liberalism; the need for a global Left that renounces speciesism and all other ancient and lingering prejudices and forms of oppression; the need for post-hierarchical worldviews and democratic and ecological societies; and the need for total liberation and revolutionary transformation.

Source: Stephen Best. "Manifesto for Radical Abolitionism: Total Liberation by Any Means Necessary." November 13, 2009. http://www.animalliberationfront.com/ALFront/Manifesto-TotalLib.htm.

Some welfare and rights organizations, such as the Humane Society of the United States, have also denounced the ALF, in part out of concern that its illegal tactics bring only negative public attention to, and thereby undermine the legitimacy of, the animal liberation movement. Other critics of the ALF question whether it can properly call itself a nonviolent movement when it engages in vandalism and property destruction. While a number of activists and scholars suggest that such tactics should be considered violent, ALF activists and supporters deny that the destruction of inanimate objects constitutes violence. Instead, they contend that by destroying buildings, vehicles, computers, and other property in raids and liberations, they in fact curb the enactment of violence against sentient beings.

Another criticism of the ALF that is voiced within some sectors of the animal liberation movement is that it provides a venue for the expression of stereotypically masculine aggression. Supporters of the ALF counter this claim by suggesting that that the anonymity required by ALF members provides women with an opportunity to engage in actions without suffering gender discrimination. Others align the ALF with radical feminist, ecofeminist, and especially anarcha-feminist ethics and politics for, among other things, operating in a nonhierarchical framework (which, for example, prevents the male usurpation of decision-making powers) and being dedicated to the prevention of violence against the most vulnerable victims of patriarchal and capitalist brutality—namely, women, children, and nonhuman animals.

With its members both condemned as terrorists and celebrated as freedom fighters, the ALF remains one of the most controversial direct-action movements in the world. Whether it is considered a leader in the animal liberation movement or a renegade group with no place in it at all, it appears that as long as the United States and other governments continue to legalize and institutionalize violence against animals, while increasingly diminishing the public's capacity to speak and act out against such brutality, the ALF and its allies will consider it necessary to continue to carry out illegal direct action to end animal exploitation.

See also Activism and Protests; Animal Rights and Animal Welfare; Antivivisection; Ecofeminism; Newkirk, Ingrid; Policy.

Further Reading

"The ALF Primer." http://www.animalliberationfront.com/ALFront/ALFPrime.htm.

Animal Enterprise Terrorism Act. November 2006. http://frwebgate.access.gpo.gov/cgi-bin/getdoc.cgi?dbname=109_cong_bills&docid=f:s3880enr.txt.pdf.

Best, Steven, and Anthony J. Nocella II. *Terrorists or Freedom Fighters? Reflections on the Liberation of Animals.* New York: Lantern Books, 2004.

Keith, Shannon. *Behind the Mask: The Story of the People Who Risk Everything for Animals.* Documentary. Uncaged Films, DVD, 2006.

Newkirk, Ingrid. *Free the Animals: The Amazing True Story of the Animal Liberation Front.* New York: Lantern Books, 2000.

Zipporah Weisberg

ANIMAL RIGHTS AND ANIMAL WELFARE

The terms "animal rights" and "animal welfare" represent two significant ways of understanding and describing the relationship between humans and animals. Although features of the two overlap and their precise definitions are the subject of dispute, in general "animal welfare" accepts the basic principle that humans may use animals for their own purposes, as long as those animals are treated humanely and protected from unnecessary suffering or cruelty. The phrase "animal rights," in contrast, embraces a spectrum of beliefs that challenges the unquestioned use of nonhuman animals for human purposes. An animal welfare advocate might work to improve the conditions under which animals used in laboratory experiments are kept, for instance, demanding larger cages or the use of anesthesia during certain procedures. A supporter of animal rights would likely reject the idea of animal experimentation as a legitimate practice and instead seek its abolition.

Individuals concerned with animal welfare typically cite animals' ability to feel pain as a basis for their beliefs but consider it unnecessary, unrealistic, or impractical to alter fundamentally the ways in which humans have traditionally interacted with animals. Medical and scientific breakthroughs achieved through animal experimentation, the need for food and materials like leather and wool, and the importance of animals to rural and agricultural economies all represent important aspects of the human-animal relationship, according to the basic philosophy of animal welfare. Some theories of animal rights, however, contend that animals possess many of the same inherent, natural rights as humans, such as the right to live one's own life or the right not to be considered property. Other theories, especially those derived from the philosophy of utilitarianism, do not ascribe individual rights to animals but suggest that humans should nonetheless avoid using them for their own purposes, since the aggregate suffering of animals exploited for human ends does not outweigh any potential benefit to humanity. Because they do not assert that animals possess any natural rights, many proponents of this utilitarian position prefer the term "animal liberation" to "animal rights."

The tradition of animal welfare is a long one, with roots in ancient Hebrew religious texts. Several passages in the Old Testament can be interpreted as outlining basic human obligations to domestic animals, and the book of Genesis established the concept of dominion, the idea that humans have authority over all animal life but are expected by God to use this authority responsibly. These ideas were absorbed and continued by the subsequent teachings of Christianity and Islam, and the fundamental belief that humans may use animals for their own ends as long as they minimize unnecessary suffering has since become a nearly universal aspect of Western culture. Still, the basic tenets of animal welfare were not legally codified until the 19th century, beginning in Britain with an 1822 act prohibiting the cruel treatment of some domestic animals. Growing interest in animal welfare led British advocates to form the Society for the Prevention of Cruelty to Animals (SPCA) in 1824 (it later became the RSPCA when Queen Victoria's imprimatur allowed the group to add the word "Royal"), and a similar organization, the ASPCA, was founded in the United States in 1866. Animal welfare societies flourished during the Victorian era, with independent and autonomous SPCAs opening in many European cities and American states alongside other groups dedicated to improving the treatment of horses, dogs, and cats or opposing vivisection, the use of animals in laboratory experiments. Although interest and membership in many of these organizations waned somewhat during the first half of the 20th century, there was a resurgent interest in animal welfare after World War II. This has been especially evident through the enactment of national animal-protection and anticruelty laws in numerous countries.

The animal rights position is much more recent, since even the concept of individual, natural rights for humans was generally developed only in the 17th and 18th centuries. Essays and books on the topic of rights for animals began appearing in the 1790s, with one of the first cogent arguments in favor of equal consideration for animals made by Briton Lewis Gompertz in his 1824 treatise *Moral Inquiries on the Situation of Man and of Brutes*. Few took Gompertz seriously at the time, and only during the 1890s did some individuals begin seriously advocating individual rights for animals and linking the idea to specific issues like vivisection, hunting, and vegetarianism. Books like Henry Salt's 1892 *Animals' Rights, Considered in Relation to Social Progress* and J. Howard Moore's 1906 *The Universal Kinship* strongly endorsed the basic principle that animals possessed at least some fundamental rights. Interest in animals' rights also declined through much of the 20th century, but during the 1970s the modern animal rights movement emerged from the liberation movements of the previous decade, spurred by important books by activists and philosophers like Richard Ryder, Peter Singer, and Tom Regan. This resurgent movement explicitly likened the treatment of animals to that of historically oppressed human populations and suggested that vegetarianism was not merely a dietary choice but indeed a moral obligation.

Despite the contributions of individual activists and thinkers, for many people the animal rights and animal welfare positions are associated with organizations, particularly the larger, well-financed, and politically connected national and international nonprofit groups. Among the most visible animal welfare institutions are the traditional anticruelty societies like the RSPCA in Britain and the ASPCA in the United States. These groups engage in a broad array of activities related to protecting animals from cruelty or abuse, especially pets and domestic animals like dogs, cats, and horses. They also work to enforce existing animal-protection laws, while securing additional protection through promoting new legislation. Campaigns undertaken by animal welfare organizations include efforts to rescue animals during natural disasters, end dogfighting, expose so-called puppy mills and other large-scale dog-breeding operations, improve conditions for carriage horses, and promote the adoption of stray animals. Most animal welfare societies stop short of specifically advocating vegetarianism and typically do not fundamentally oppose the use of animals for human consumption. Many do work, however, to improve the conditions under which food animals are raised and slaughtered.

The largest and most visible organization dedicated solely to the animal rights position is People for the Ethical Treatment of Animals (PETA). Like the welfare societies, it works on multiple fronts, though its scope extends well beyond domestic animals to include zoo animals, animals used in the production of clothing, and wildlife. PETA's mission statement and promotional materials explicitly state that animals are "not ours to use," and increasing public awareness of the

"A Bird in the Cage"

Tom Regan's writings, including *The Case for Animal Rights* (1983), profoundly shaped the animal liberation movement and contributed significantly to the passage of animal-protection laws. In this excerpt from an autobiographical essay, "A Bird in the Cage," Regan explains how the loss of his dog, Gleco, represented a critical moment in his understanding of animal rights and prompted him to become a vegetarian.

Earlier on the day we returned home, Gleco was killed—hit by a car while darting across a road.

Faced with this incalculable loss, Nancy [his wife] and I lapsed into a period of intense, shared grief. For days we cried at the mere mention or memory of Gleco. Earlier that summer, while thinking about Gandhi and pacifism, I had encountered the rude question of the ethics of meat eating. Once severed from any essential connection with pacifism, the rational arguments seemed to be there. My head had begun to grasp a moral truth that required a change in behavior. Reason demanded that I become a vegetarian. But it was the sense of irrevocable loss that added the power of feeling to the requirements of logic.

What Gleco's death forced upon me was the realization that my emotional attachment to a particular dog was a contingent feature of the world. Of my world. Except for a set of circumstances over which I had no control, I would have loved some other dog (Jock, perhaps, or the poor creature at the mercy of the med student). And given some other conditions, over which again I had no control, I would never have even known Gleco at all. I understood, in a flash it seemed, that my powerful feelings for this particular dog, for Gleco, had to include other dogs. Indeed, every other dog. Any stopping point short of every dog was, and had to be, rationally and emotionally arbitrary.

And not just dogs. Wherever in the world there is life that feels, a being whose welfare can be affected by what we do (or fail to do), there love and compassion, justice and protection must find a home.

Source: http://www.tomregan-animalrights.com/regan_bird.html.

animal rights position is among its basic goals. It has undertaken public and often-controversial campaigns against the use of animals in medical experiments and has been highly critical of the cosmetics, fast food, and fur industries, among others. Straddling the line between the traditional animal welfare and animal rights positions are associations like the Humane Society of the United States, the largest American animal advocacy organization. The Humane Society engages in many traditional welfare activities like animal rescue and improving the humane treatment of domestic animals, but it also specifically advocates a vegetarian diet as a significant means for reducing the suffering of farm animals and addresses issues related to wild animals as well.

While the phrase "animal rights" is frequently used by both the public and the media as a generic term for any form of animal advocacy, it is clear that the animal welfare position still dominates Western culture. Cable television networks like Animal Planet, best-selling memoirs about living with animals, and an increased general interest in pets are all indications that the lives of humans and animals are as entwined as ever but also serve to reinforce traditional assumptions about the proper relationship between the two. Animal rights advocates, meanwhile, are sometimes portrayed as misanthropes or even dangerous extremists, with the high-profile actions of groups like PETA offered as proof of just how outside the mainstream they are. These perceptions are exacerbated by the occasional guerrilla tactics of radical groups like the Animal Liberation Front, whose activities receive substantial attention from the media but generate ambivalence within the animal rights community.

Although vegetarians appear to have some shared interests with the animal rights and animal welfare movements, historically the overlap has been relatively limited, with most individuals adopting vegetarianism typically doing so for reasons of health, religion, or other issues unrelated to animals. Both animal welfare and animal rights present powerful arguments in favor of a meatless or vegan diet, however, and since the 1970s these connections have been increasingly explored and strengthened. Interest in the treatment of farm animals has grown as agriculture continues to industrialize, and some vegetarians cite factory farming practices like hog confinements and battery cages for hens as influencing their decision to give up meat. Animal rights advocates in particular have worked to associate their position with dietary decisions and have often made vegetarianism and veganism a crucial element of both their philosophy and their activism.

See also Activism and Protests; Agribusiness; Animal Liberation Front; Antivivisection; Bible and Biblical Arguments; Dinshah, H. Jay; Ecofeminism; Ethical Vegetarianism; Francione, Gary L.; Gandhi, Mohandas; Newkirk, Ingrid; People for the Ethical Treatment of Animals; Policy; Reform; Salt, Henry S.; Singer, Peter; United Kingdom; Veganism; World Wars in England.

Further Reading

Beers, Diane L. *For the Prevention of Cruelty: The History and Legacy of Animal Rights Activism in the United States.* Athens, OH: Swallow Press, 2006.

Francione, Gary L. *Introduction to Animal Rights: Your Child or the Dog?* Philadelphia: Temple University Press, 2000.

Midgely, Mary. *Animals and Why They Matter.* Athens: University of Georgia Press, 1983.

Phelps, Norm. *The Longest Struggle: Animal Advocacy from Pythagoras to PETA.* New York: Lantern Books, 2007.

Regan, Tom. *The Case for Animal Rights.* Berkeley: University of California Press, 1983.

Ryder, Richard D. *Animal Revolution: Changing Attitudes towards Speciesism.* Rev. ed. New York: Berg, 2000.

Scully, Matthew. *Dominion: The Power of Man, the Suffering of Animals, and the Call to Mercy.* New York: St. Martin's, 2003.

Singer, Peter. *Animal Liberation: A New Ethics for Our Treatment of Animals.* New York: Avon Books, 1975.

Gary K. Jarvis

ANTIVIVISECTION

Antivivisection is a 19th-century term denoting opposition to the use of live animals in medical or scientific experiments. Although anatomists, physiologists, and other scientists have used living animals in their research for centuries, criticism prior to the 18th century was limited by both the relative infrequency of experiments and the lack of any organized opposition. During the second half of the 19th century, the number of experiments began expanding exponentially, however, as the realms of science and medicine became increasingly professionalized. In response, some existing animal-protection societies became increasingly vocal in their opposition, while other animal welfare advocates formed organizations such as Britain's Victoria Street Society and the American Anti-Vivisection Society specifically to expose the practice and lobby against it. Some antivivisectionists—particularly British leader Frances Power Cobbe—were openly hostile to vegetarianism, but a significant overlap existed between the two movements. Especially during the late 19th century, it was not uncommon for organizations devoted to diet reform and those seeking an end to animal experimentation to share members, ideas, and resources. The initial antivivisection movement peaked around the turn of the 20th century, and public opposition waned somewhat as animal experimentation appeared to promise significant advances in disease prevention and surgical techniques.

A renewed antivivisection impulse emerged beginning in the 1970s, closely aligned with the modern animal rights movement and spurred by well-publicized exposés of experiments at the American Museum of Natural History in New York, the Institute for Behavioral Research in Silver Spring, Maryland, and the University of Pennsylvania's Head Injury Clinic in Philadelphia. These examples, and the subsequent organization of animal rights organizations like People for the Ethical Treatment of Animals—itself a direct outgrowth of the Silver Spring monkeys case—led to increasingly numerous and visible campaigns against the use of animals in experiments, as new activists worked alongside the long-standing antivivisection organizations. Experiments by scientists and other researchers drew increased scrutiny from activists, the public, and government regulators.

Beginning in the 1980s, antivivisection activism spread beyond scientific laboratories to also expose and question the ways in which animals were used in the development of consumer products. Corporations that tested products like cosmetics on animals were especially affected, as activists publicized routine but little-known practices like the Draize test, in which potentially harmful substances are applied to the skin or eyes of rabbits to check for irritation. Although many companies continue to use animal testing, others began to seek alternatives, specifically marketing themselves and their products as cruelty-free or animal-free.

Mainstream animal welfare organizations do not necessarily oppose the use of animals in product tests and scientific experimentation, but virtually all support legislation and ethical codes of conduct that require laboratory animals to receive humane treatment. Animal rights organizations typically oppose these uses of animals altogether, though many also work to improve existing treatment and conditions. Most antivivisection protest is peaceful and has been quite effective in raising awareness about animal experimentation and testing. Frequently, however, the most visible actions are taken by more radical individuals at the fringes of the animal rights and animal liberation movements who conduct guerrilla-style raids in the name of groups like the Animal Liberation Front. Midnight break-ins to free laboratory animals or the vandalism of facilities and equipment often generate considerable publicity and attention for the cause, although some believe they risk alienating the public rather than encouraging broad acceptance of antivivisection goals.

See also Activism and Protests; Animal Liberation Front; Animal Rights and Animal Welfare; Consumer Products; Kingsford, Anna; People for the Ethical Treatment of Animals; Reform.

Further Reading

Monamy, Vaughn. *Animal Experimentation: A Guide to the Issues*. 2nd ed. Cambridge: Cambridge University Press, 2009.

Rudacille, Deborah. *The Scalpel and the Butterfly: The War between Animal Research and Animal Protection*. New York: Farrar, Straus and Giroux, 2000.

Turner, James. *Reckoning with the Beast: Animals, Pain, and Humanity in the Victorian Mind*. Baltimore: Johns Hopkins University Press, 1980.

Gary K. Jarvis

ASIA

The vast and diverse continent of Asia is considered the cradle of Eastern vegetarianism. The customs of Asian vegetarians vary with religious, ethical, geographic, and economic ideologies. Ancient Indian religious faiths—Hinduism, Jainism, and Buddhism—are based on nonviolence; Taoism and Confucianism in China, as well as the Manichaeism of Central Asia, all favored or insisted on a vegetarian diet.

The Silk Road network and the ancient Indian Ocean trade routes were important paths for commercial, cultural, and religious exchange between people from China, Southeast Asia, India, Persia, and Mediterranean countries. For centuries, vegetables, fruits, grains, and cooking techniques traveled along with traders from one civilization to another. All of these profoundly influenced the cuisines of Asia. The countries along the trade routes also shared an incredible legacy of religious interchange.

With its chosen middle path and flexibility, Buddhist teachings spread across Asia, and in each new culture it reached, these teachings were adopted by blending them with the existing belief systems to fit the local mentality. Unlike the ancient Indian faiths, Taoist vegetarianism was not based on respect for animal life but rather on the view that certain animal foods might interfere with bodily harmony. All of these religious teachings had a tremendous impact on the vegetarian way of life in Asia and eventually the rest of the world.

East Asia   China has a long history of vegetarianism going back to the ancient Sage Kings around 2300 BC. Their spiritual way of life was Tao, a faith based on inner spiritualism, compassion, and vegetarianism. Taoism and Confucianism were the dominant faiths when Buddhism was introduced to China. Buddhism transformed itself and the concepts and values of Taoism and Confucianism. Vegetarianism was assimilated into Chinese Buddhism, and it spread under royal patronage. The Su diet of the Buddhists avoids meat, fish, dairy products, dried lily stem, onions, chives, garlic, and leeks and is based on Buddhist reluctance to take life and Taoist concerns with gaining immortality. Mahayana Buddhism is found mainly in China, Japan, and Vietnam.

During the Imperial era, vegetarian cuisine was enriched by vegetables that arrived along the Silk Road as well as crops cultivated in China. The Chinese emperor Liang of Wu (464–569) was a major advocate of the vegetarianism in Chinese Buddhism. During the Tang period (635–705), various laws, including a ban on all slaughter and fishing, were instituted, and vegetarian feasts were held by Tang emperors for Taoist and Buddhist monks.

Because of their adherence to traditional values, many contemporary Chinese people at one time or another during their lives take vows not to eat meat and observe two meatless days every lunar month. Vows are sometimes made as a part of religious initiations into Buddhist and Taoist vegetarian associations. Vows to avoid meat have usually been of limited duration. Lifetime abstinence from flesh has been far less common, done mostly by clergy and devout women and widows. Today, vegetarianism is still found especially in monasteries.

Both Buddhism and Shintoism had an effect on Japanese food preferences. Shinto is a blend of many local and regional traditions that became a formal institution in the sixth century. The ancient Japanese diet consisted of fresh vegetables, rice, and other cereals along with fish and shellfish but little meat. With the arrival of Buddhism, there was a royal ban on hunting and fishing. In the 13th century, Zen monks from China popularized a cuisine called *Shojin Ryori* in Japan that uses no animal products. This culinary tradition is still alive in Zen temples of Kyoto, Nikko, and Kamakura. Many dishes incorporating *Shojin* ingredients are also prepared by the Japanese in modern times. In the late 19th century, Gensai Ishizuka's book on *seisyoku* (macrobiotics), based on ancient Chinese philosophy and Taoism, promoted vegetarian food and a little fish. In the 20th century, lacto-ovo vegetarian cuisine inspired by the Seventh-day Adventist tradition from the United States became popular in Japan. The Japanese Vegetarian Society was founded in 1993 to pursue animal rights, environmental issues, and human health.

Taiwanese follow a combination of Buddhism, Confucianism, and Taoism, and most of the Buddhist population avoids eating all meat, seafood, onions, leeks, and garlic. Because of the island nation's subtropical location, Taiwan has an abundant supply of fresh fruits and vegetables. Mongolians primarily eat dairy products, meat, and animal fats. Buddhism had a strong influence on Korean cuisine, especially Korean temple cuisine. As in Japan, however, seafood is quite prevalent in Korean cuisine.

South Asia Vegetarianism has a substantial presence in South Asia. Throughout its history, South Asia has gone through significant changes with the developments of religions, namely, Hinduism Jainism, and Buddhism, as well as waves of foreign invasions that greatly influenced and shaped the gastronomy of this region. A 2003 study reported by the *Journal of Nutrition* showed that South Asians, with the exception of Pakistanis, consume the least amount of meat in the world. India, the largest nation in the region, has the largest concentration of vegetarians in the world. According to a 2006 survey by *The Hindu* and CNN-IBN, more Indian women and young children and those above the age of 55 are likely to be vegetarians. The study concludes that 31 percent of Indians are vegetarians, and another 9 percent also consume eggs. These results have remained more or less stable over the years. A 1998 survey showed that around 30 percent of the Indian population was vegetarian. Vegetarianism in India is a function of inherited cultural practices, religion, community, and regional location rather than individual beliefs. Indian vegetarianism is based on the principle of *ahimsa,* meaning respect for life.

Since early times, the three indigenous religions of India have upheld respect for life and actively encouraged adherents to give up animal killing and eating. Although meat eating was not popular during Vedic times, the practice was not restricted. Cows were respected, but they were ritually sacrificed and their meat was consumed under the supervision of a Brahmin priest. Jainism and Buddhism developed between 600 BC and 500 BC partially as a reaction against animal sacrifices. With generous royal support, Jainism and Buddhism spread all over ancient India, and the concept of vegetarianism gained popularity. Jainism and Buddhism condemned the excessive use of animal sacrifice and influenced Hinduism, which gradually moved to a ban animal slaughter and meat eating. Vegetarianism was on the rise with the spread of the Hindu *bhakthi* movement and eventually prevailed as a symbol of prestige and piety in Indian society. Among Hindus in South India, several groups are vegetarian, including Brahmins, several Vaishnava sects, and several non-Brahmin sects. All followers of Jainism are strict vegetarians. The abundance and variety of plant food available in India also contributed to its popularity.

Today vegetarianism in India is a traditional way of living, based mainly on religious considerations. Most Indian vegetarians are lacto-vegetarians, followed by lacto-ovo vegetarians, and a small number are vegans. Indian vegetarian food includes certain animal products, such as milk, butter, and yogurt, because no killing of the animal is involved in the extraction of these products, and they provide both protein and calcium. On most days, even traditional nonvegetarians eat a vegetarian diet. Even when meat is served in a meal, it is served as side dishes.

Just as in India, vegetarianism in Sri Lanka developed with the introduction of Buddhism and Jainism. In the third century BC, Sri Lanka became a predominantly Buddhist nation with the conversion of King Devanampiya-Tissa. Consumption of animal food was minimal under Buddhist kings, and fishing and hunting were the occupation of the people with low social status. King Amandagamani (AD 79–89) was the first to issue an order prohibiting killing of animals.

The principle of nonviolence was highly respected, but Buddhists were more pragmatic; they conformed to the local conditions and accommodated indigenous beliefs and practices as well as local food habits. By the 16th century, with the arrival of colonialism, consumption of animal foods was on the rise in Sri Lanka. Modern vegetarianism in Sri Lanka had its beginning around 100 years ago with the formation of vegetarian societies. The trend in favor of a vegetarian way of life is gaining momentum.

Vegetables are the most important food group in Nepali cuisine. Nepal is one of the poorest countries in the world and not everyone can afford meat. Upperclass Hindus avoid meat for religious reasons. Meat, poultry, and fish are served only occasionally, mostly during celebrations. Bangladesh is home to a large population of Hindus, and the Vashinavites observe a vegetarian diet that includes fish. Because of its high price, meat is not common everyday, even among nonvegetarians.

Pakistan is a largely Muslim country and predominantly nonvegetarian. The Pakistan Vegetarian Society was established in 2001 by Murad Khan as a nonprofit voluntary organization. Its primary objectives are to promote humanitarian and nutritional aspects of vegetarianism through research and education and to link individuals and organizations that believe in the principles of vegetarianism.

Southeast Asia   Southeast Asians are extremely diverse, follow several religions, and are not generally vegetarian. Rice, fish, and vegetables are the staples; though meat is highly valued, meat flavors do not dominate except for grilled meats. The poor consume meat only on special occasions. People of Malaysia, Philippines, and Brunei mostly consume nonvegetarian food. Theravada Buddhism practiced in varying intensities is the dominant religion of mainland countries in this region. Monks are banned from killing animals, but they consume meat offered by devotees. In Myanmar, food offerings during the holy period of Lenten are meatless. Women and the elderly generally observe vegetarian fasts.

Thailand's 10-day vegetarian festival is an annual event, and the festival's sacred rituals are supposed to bring good luck. Thai with Chinese ancestry strictly observe the 10-day vegetarian or vegan diet. New Buddhist movements such as Santi Asoke with its emphasis on environmental concerns require followers to be vegetarian. More Theravada Buddhists are taking on the Mahayana practice of fasting a few days a month.

Central and West Asia   Central Asian and Russian cuisines have similar ingredients, dishes, and customs. Vegetarianism appeared in Russia in the 14th century but was forbidden for many years. The Eurasian Vegetarian Society publishes a vegetarian magazine and arranges talks by well-known Russian vegetarians. The nomads of the Central Asian steppe live by their livestock, and the cuisines of arid West Asian countries are a fusion of Turkish, Arabian, North African, and Persian, mostly nonvegetarian.

The International Vegetarian Union is a growing global network of independent organizations that promotes vegetarianism worldwide. The Asian Vegetarian Union, a member of the International Vegetarian Union, was launched in 2000 to promote vegetarianism in Asian countries. Russia, South Asia, Southeast Asia, and East Asia have a substantial presence in this organization. With the formation vegetarian societies, a vegetarian way of life is gaining momentum.

See also Eastern Religions, Influences of; Ethical Vegetarianism; Ethnic and Racial Groups, U.S.; India; International Vegetarian Union; Jainism; Meatless Diets before Vegetarianism; Reform; Religious Beliefs and Practices; Social Acceptance.

Further Reading

Chapple, Christopher. *Nonviolence to Animals, Earth, and Self in Asian Traditions.* Albany: State University of New York Press, 1993.

Simoons, Frederick J. *Eat Not This Flesh: Food Avoidances from Prehistory to the Present.* Madison: University of Wisconsin Press, 1994.

Simoons, Frederick J. *Food in China: A Cultural and Historical Inquiry.* Boca Raton, FL: CRC Press, 1991.

Thompson, David. *Thai Food.* Berkeley, CA: Ten Speed Press, 2002.

Walters, Kerry S., and Lisa Portmess, eds. *Religious Vegetarianism: From Hesiod to the Dalai Lama.* Albany: State University of New York Press, 2001.

Yadaav, Yogendra, and Sanjay Kumar. "The Food Habits of a Nation." *The Hindu,* August 14, 2006.

Ammini Ramachandran

ATTWOOD, CHARLES RAYMOND (1932–1998)

Charles R. Attwood was an American pediatrician and an advocate of vegetarianism who is best known for his devotion to improving the health and welfare of children. As a best-selling author and popular lecturer, Attwood worked tirelessly to raise awareness of the importance of vegetarianism and exercise.

Born near New Edinburg, Arkansas, Attwood graduated from Hendrix College in 1953, earned his MD from the University of Arkansas School of Medicine in 1958, and interned at Brook General Hospital in San Antonio, Texas. After serving in the U.S. Army as a pediatrician and completing his pediatric residency at Letterman General Hospital in San Francisco, Attwood opened a private practice in Millbury, California. In 1972, he moved to Crowley, Louisiana, where he established a highly successful pediatric practice.

Attwood was a fellow of the American Academy of Pediatrics, member of the American Academy of Nutrition, and a consultant to the Center for Science in the Public Interest. In addition to his popular books, journal articles, and lectures, Attwood produced a popular audio series. In 1997, Attwood won the Telly Award for the video *Mooove Over Milk* and was recognized by the Cleveland Clinic as an expert in the prevention of coronary artery disease. In 1998, he was scheduled to be the keynote speaker at the Twelfth Annual Asian Cardiology Congress, but he died of a malignant brain tumor before the conference took place.

Supporters of vegan diets credit Attwood's activism and reputation as key factors in convincing many physicians that a vegetarian diet could be safe and healthy at all stages of human life. It was not until 1996 that the U.S. Dietary Guidelines for Americans included the acknowledgment that a vegetarian diet could be healthy. In 1996, Attwood was instrumental in organizing opposition to Gerber Baby Food because the fruits and vegetables in their products were diluted with water, sugar, and starches. The publicity generated by Attwood and his colleagues led to significant change in the formulation of baby foods. In the 1990s, Attwood became involved in cases where social workers from the California Department of Children's Services removed the children of parents who were following strict vegetarian diets. Attwood was instrumental in defending some vegetarian parents but was concerned that others were unsuccessful in custody cases based on claims that vegetarian parents were negligent.

Attwood's influential book *Low-Fat Prescription for Kids* (1995) provided a low-fat diet based on vegetables, fruits, legumes, and whole grains. According to Attwood, a low-fat, vegetarian diet reduced the risk of premature heart disease, stroke, certain cancers, and diabetes. Benjamin Spock endorsed Attwood's book and incorporated his dietary program in the final edition of *Dr. Spock's Baby and Child Care* (1998). Attwood's last book, *A Vegetarian Doctor Speaks Out* (1998), was based on essays written for VegSource.com, a popular vegetarian Web site that he helped establish. Attwood was a critic of what he considered dangerous fad diets. In particular, he condemned diets that blamed obesity on carbohydrates.

See also Alternative and Holistic Medicine; Childbearing and Infant Feeding; Childrearing; Ethical Vegetarianism; Physiological Benefits; Policy; Reform; Social Acceptance; Veganism.

Further Reading

Attwood, Charles R. *Dr. Attwood's Low-Fat Prescription for Kids.* New York: Viking, 1995.
Attwood, Charles R. *A Vegetarian Doctor Speaks Out.* Prescott, AZ: Hohm, 1998.
VegSource. http://www.vegsource.com.

Lois N. Magner

AUSTRALIA

The earliest vegetarian society in Australia was founded in Melbourne in 1886, with a constitution largely based on that of the Vegetarian Society of the UK, of which some of the founders had previously been members. The membership of the society, which was aimed at promoting abstention from flesh foods, mainly comprised religious and teetotaling men; although there were female members, they did not play a significant role in leadership and organization. Records of organized vegetarianism in Australia in the first half of the 20th century are sparse before the reconstitution of the Australian Vegetarian Society in 1948; however, organizations such as the Seventh-day Adventists, Women's Christian Temperance Union, and Theosophists continued to promote a vegetarian diet and lifestyle. The new society was founded partly on a religious basis and partly on the basis of animal welfare concerns. The society immediately began publication of a newsletter called the *Australian Vegetarian*.

Between the late 1950s and the mid 1970s, vegetarian societies operated largely independently in the different states of Australia. The first congress, held in 1985, was affiliated with the International Vegetarian Union. The International Vegetarian Union and in 1987 the Western Australian society was founded as an offshoot of the Theosophical Society. This organization subsequently developed and became fully independent from the theosophical movement. In 1991, vegetarian societies in New South Wales and Victoria combined their local newsletters to publish the *New Vegetarian* magazine. Both the Western Australian society's newsletter and the Natural Health Society of Australia merged with the *New Vegetarian* magazine to form the *New Vegetarian and Natural Health* magazine. In Australia, there is now a national magazine that helps to connect the numerous vibrant societies, some of which are affiliated with the International Vegetarian Union.

Vegetarianism in Australia today is more closely tied to animal welfare concerns and health consciousness than it is to religion. Although Australia's beef industry was not greatly affected directly by international health scares over mad cow disease and foot and mouth disease, there was significant fear, particularly regarding mad cow disease, following an outbreak in Japan, and there has been activism for reform of animal husbandry and meat-production practices. Young Australians, like young people throughout the developed world, have, it seems, been influenced by an increasing awareness of both the dangers and the cruelties inherent in the modern meat industries. Vegetarianism, as a lifestyle choice with political and philosophical implications, has to a certain extent become chic, and the social acceptance of the vegetarian lifestyle has led to proliferation of information on vegetarianism, as well as of restaurants and foodstuffs catering to a vegetarian and vegan clientele. This chicness, however, exists only among urban Australians. Australia has a sizable rural, agricultural population, and pastoral farming and meat industries employ a significant segment of the population. To a certain extent, uninformed and in some cases offensive prejudices that vegetarianism is linked with being left-wing politically, being unpatriotic or un-Australian, or being effete, urban, and pretentious still run strong in some sectors of Australian society.

Further Reading

Crook, Edgar. "Vegetarianism in Australia: A History." http://www.ivu.org/history/australia/index.html.

Matthew Winston

B

BACKLASH

Backlash against vegetarian and vegan diets and lifestyles is widespread, often pernicious, and present in both interpersonal and cultural contexts. Backlash often takes the guise of nutritional and health concerns but also extends to extremist portrayals and verbal attacks. Backlash in the interpersonal context is often masked as puzzlement over exactly what a vegetarian or vegan eats, concern that a plant-based diet is not nutritionally sufficient, dismay when encountering unexpected nonanimal foods, or outright anger at the vegetarians or vegans for supposedly ruining the family meal or imposing their views on others. Backlash often takes the form of interrogating the vegetarian or vegan to locate perceived inconsistencies or gaps in logic, such as pointing at leather shoes as inconsistent or reasoning that vegetarians do not eat beings that feel pain and plants feel pain, and therefore vegetarians should not eat plants.

Backlash of this sort also occurs on the cultural level, often emerging in the form of pseudo-scientific and -historical arguments. Such assertions focus on mistaken notions that humans have always eaten animals, that only animal flesh can provide certain nutrients like protein and iron, and that vegetarian and vegan diets are dangerous for children, pregnant women, athletes, or the elderly. Most historical and scientific research, however, has demonstrated that such concerns are largely unfounded and—in the case of nutritional and health concerns—false, because proper vegetarian and vegan diets have been followed successfully in populations around the world for centuries.

Backlash, however, often goes much further than simple misinformation or misdirected concern. Far-fetched and extremist backlash takes many forms. One popular Web site (vegetariansareevil.com) lists "famous vegetarians" like Adolf Hitler, Charles Manson, and the Antichrist to suggest that vegetarians are pernicious by nature and that vegetarianism is a form of child abuse that is "forced upon helpless child victims." It defines vegetarianism textually and visually as a militant religion akin to Muslim terrorists and states that vegetarians are more violently aggressive because they are "always hungry." This sort of backlash is akin to that used against several social movements of the 20th century, which attempted to link a plant-based diet to disruptive, radical, or violent politics.

Though perhaps comical to a degree, such misinformed notions filter into the larger culture and appear in more legitimate fora. A 2009 *Time* magazine article asked, "Is Vegetarian a Teen Eating Disorder?" and cited research from the *Journal of the American Dietetic Association,* which found that teenage vegetarians choose their diets for weight-loss purposes rather than for ethical, environmental, or health reasons and exhibit higher rates of binge eating and of laxative and diuretic abuse. The article perpetuated the air of suspicion around vegetarianism generally by suggesting that overindulging or binge eating could result from feeling hungry and specifically by warning parents and physicians to be "extra vigilant" whenever a teenager adopts a vegetarian diet.

Similar studies or concerns arise every few years, as with a similar 2003 *Time* magazine article that queried, "Where's the Beef (in the Teenage Diet)?" noting the trend among teenagers to consider vegetarianism "cool." In response, the National Cattleman's Beef Association launched "Cool 2B Real," a Web site that promoted the eating of cows in a vibrant, hip Web format complete with surveys featuring questions like "What kind of beef do you most like to eat with your friends?" Although the Web site is no longer active, likely due to disinterest, the message behind it remains popular. The "real" part of the campaign presages a later pop culture incident in which singer Jessica Simpson brandished a T-shirt emblazoned "Real Girls Eat Meat," drawing criticism from women's rights groups and from animal rights groups like People for the Ethical Treatment of Animals. In both cases, critics pointed out the underlying misogynistic message in suggesting that females are not real unless they eat animals. Similar ploys have been used in a variety of marketing scenarios, from Wendy's infamous commercial featuring the petite elderly woman demanding to know "Where's the beef?" to the more recent Burger King ad featuring various men reprising Helen Reddy's feminist classic, "I Am Woman" as they refused "chick food" and demanded to "eat like men."

Backlash is also evident in popular culinary shows and publishing tie-ins, like the Travel Channel's *Anthony Bourdain: No Reservations* and the related book, *Kitchen Confidential.* Bourdain has been an outspoken critic not only of vegetarianism and veganism but also of animal rights generally and has referred to vegetarians as "the enemy of everything good and decent in the human spirit" and to vegans as a "Hezbollah-like splinter faction" of vegetarianism (70). Similarly, in popular cooking contest shows like Food Network's *Next Food Network Star* and Bravo's *Top Chef,* in which chefs are challenged to prepare dishes under a variety of conditions and using a variety of common and novel ingredients, vegetarian cooking challenges are presented as quirky and usually elicit groans of dismay from contestants.

Pseudoscientific and moral concerns about vegetarianism tend to be grounded in incomplete understandings of sacred texts, Darwinian evolution, and ontology (the study of existence). For example, animal eaters cite biblical passages purported to give humans dominion over the animal kingdom (Gen. 1:26) or the specious logic that humans have evolved to the top of the food chain and that since lower animals eat other animals, then the top of the food chain should be able to do the same. Philosophical arguments against vegetarianism might also assert that because animals are nonrational or amoral beings, in contrast to humans, humans are therefore justified in using these lesser beings to their advantage.

Such backlash is not limited to avowed animal eaters. Even among vegetarians and vegans themselves, there is disagreement whether vegetarian and vegan refer simply to dietary choices or to larger moral-ethical commitments to the environment, nature, and/or animal rights and to what extent those commitments must be upheld. The growth of humane or free-range farming has reopened age-old debates over animal cruelty, particularly with respect to eggs, honey, and dairy products, while the availability of meat substitutes that appear and taste like animal products has raised concerns over faux vegetarians or those who follow the strict letter of the vegetarian or vegan diet by not consuming animals but fail in principle because they continue to use animal-resembling and animal-tasting products.

See also Activism and Protests; Agribusiness; Bible and Biblical Arguments; Childbearing and Infant Feeding; Childrearing; Consumer Products; Meat and Violence; Organic Foods and Technology; People for the Ethical Treatment of Animals; Physical Fitness and Athleticism; Physiological Benefits; Social Acceptance; Youth.

Further Reading

American Dietetic Association. "Position of the American Dietetic Association: Vegetarian Diets." *Journal of the American Dietetic Association* 109, no. 7 (July 2009): 1266–82.

Bourdain, Anthony. *Kitchen Confidential. Updated Edition: Adventures in the Culinary Underbelly*. New York: Ecco Press, 2007.

Iacobbo, Karen, and Michael Iacobbo. *Vegetarians and Vegans in America Today*. Westport, CT: Praeger, 2006.

Torres, Bob, and Jenna Torres. *Vegan Freak: Being Vegan in a Non-Vegan World*. Colton, NY: Tofu Hound Press, 2005.

Milton W. Wendland

BARNARD, NEAL (1953~)

Neal D. Barnard is an American physician, psychiatrist, clinical researcher, author, and leading advocate for veganism, ethical biomedical research, and animal rights. Barnard's interests range from demonstrating the impact of diet on human health to finding alternatives to the use of live animals in medical education, testing, and research.

Although Barnard grew up in North Dakota, where his family owned cattle ranches, he has been a vegan since 1980. In 1975, he graduated from Macalester College in St. Paul, Minnesota. He earned his MD from George Washington University School of Medicine, Washington, D.C., in 1980 and trained as a psychiatrist. Barnard serves as an adjunct associate professor of medicine at George

Washington University School of Medicine. He is the founder and president of the Physicians Committee for Responsible Medicine (PCRM), head of the Washington Center for Clinical Research, and the editor-in-chief of the *Nutrition Guide for Clinicians*. The Cancer Project, which Barnard founded in 1991, is dedicated to educating the public about the role of diet in cancer prevention and treatment.

The goal of the PCRM, which Barnard established in 1985, is to educate the public and the medical profession about the health benefits of exercise and low-fat vegan diets. PCRM also campaigns for higher ethical standards in biomedical research and alternatives to the use of healthy animals as experimental models for human disorders. Barnard opposes the use of animals for experimentation and testing on ethical and practical grounds. According to Barnard, the consumption of meat and dairy products is a key factor in the rising epidemic of heart disease and obesity in the United States. Therefore, adopting a vegan lifestyle benefits both humans and the animals that most Americans now consume. While recognizing Barnard's contributions to educating the public about the importance of diet and nutrition, critics have objected to his classification of meat, cheese, sugar, and chocolate as addictive substances.

Although very few Americans follow a strict vegan lifestyle, Barnard's books on nutrition and health have sold millions of copies. These books include *The Power of Your Plate* (1990); *Food for Life: How the New Four Food Groups Can Save Your Life* (1994); *Foods That Fight Pain* (1998); *Foods That Cause You to Lose Weight* (1999); *Turn Off the Fat Genes* (2001); and *Dr. Neal Barnard's Program for Reversing Diabetes* (2007). In addition to his popular books, Barnard has published many articles in major scientific and medical journals. According to Barnard, his research proves that type 2 diabetics who follow a low-fat vegan diet can reduce blood sugar, improve insulin sensitivity, and eliminate or reduce the need for medication.

See also Alternative and Holistic Medicine; Animal Rights and Animal Welfare; Antivivisection; Ethical Vegetarianism; Physiological Benefits; Reform; Veganism.

Further Reading

Barnard, Neal, M.D., Physicians Committee for Responsible Medicine (PCRM). http://www.nealbarnard.org/.

Physicians Committee for Responsible Medicine (PCRM). http://www.pcrm.org.

Walters, Kerry S., and Lisa Portmess, eds. *Ethical Vegetarianism: From Pythagoras to Peter Singer.* Albany: State University of New York Press, 1999.

Lois N. Magner

BATTLE CREEK SANITARIUM

Battle Creek Sanitarium was a vegetarian health resort in Battle Creek, Michigan. Under the leadership of John Harvey Kellogg, physician-in-chief from 1876 to 1943, the sanitarium became internationally renowned and attracted many prominent guests.

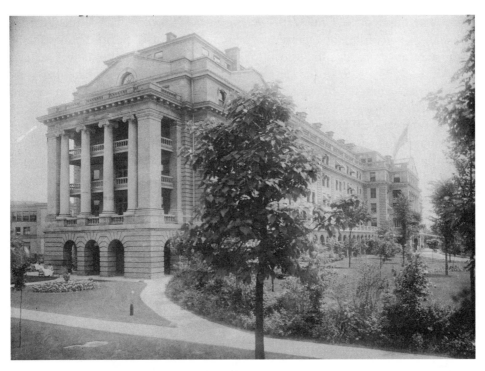

Battle Creek Sanitarium. (Courtesy of the Library of Congress)

Battle Creek Sanitarium began in 1866 as the Western Health Reform Institute, founded by Seventh-day Adventist leaders as a convalescent home compatible with the tenets of their faith, including abstinence from meat, coffee, and tea. In 1876, Kellogg, an Adventist, became superintendent. He aimed to expand the small institute into a popular scientific facility devoted to "biologic living." He renamed it the Medical and Surgical Sanitarium, commonly called Battle Creek Sanitarium or simply "the San," and in 1878, he opened a new 200-patient building. Kellogg also took over editorship of the institute's magazine, the *Health Reformer,* renaming it *Good Health* in 1879, and he established training schools for nurses, cooks, and health missionaries. The sanitarium gradually separated from the Adventists, and Kellogg was disfellowshipped in 1907.

The sanitarium offered a variety of fashionable treatments, including hydropathy, massage, light therapy, electrotherapy, and radium therapy; Kellogg also performed surgeries. Rest and exercise, unrestrictive clothing, sexual restraint, regular enemas, and healthful food, however, were central to Kellogg's program. In lectures and books published by the sanitarium presses, Kellogg promoted the ethical, evolutionary, and especially physiological advantages of vegetarianism. He advocated an unspiced, low-fat, low-protein vegetarian diet rich in whole grains to prevent "autointoxication" by waste in the colon. The sanitarium's laboratories lent him scientific support, and sanitarium dietician Lenna Frances

Cooper cofounded the American Dietetic Association in 1917. With the help of Kellogg's wife, Ella, the facility's test kitchen developed health foods such as granola, caramel cereal coffee substitute, peanut butter, meat alternatives including Nuttose and Protose, and, later, soy milk. In 1894, Kellogg patented Granose flakes, the first flaked cereal, and the sanitarium soon served a corn version as well. The new cereals grew immensely popular, and imitators flooded Battle Creek in the early 20th century. The sanitarium already sold food products, but the demand was so great that Will Keith Kellogg, John Harvey's brother, sanitarium business manager, and fellow food innovator, created the Battle Creek Toasted Corn Flake Company in 1906 and expanded it into a cereal giant.

Fire destroyed the sanitarium building in 1902, but a new facility opened the following year. A 1928 addition brought the total patient capacity to well over 1,000. Two years later, Kellogg opened the Miami-Battle Creek Sanitarium in Florida. In 1933, however, Battle Creek Sanitarium went into receivership, and it was reorganized in 1938. The building was sold to the federal government in 1942. Kellogg died in 1943, and the institution came back under Adventist control in the late 1950s. It survived as a mental health and addiction center before joining the Battle Creek Health System in 1993.

See also Alternative and Holistic Medicine; Consumer Products; Kellogg, John Harvey; Reform; Religious Beliefs and Practices; Seventh-day Adventists.

Further Reading

Carson, Gerald. *Cornflake Crusade.* Toronto: Rinehart, 1957.

Fee, Elizabeth, and Theodore M. Brown. "John Harvey Kellogg, MD: Health Reformer and Antismoking Crusader." *American Journal of Public Health* 92 (2002): 935.

Schwarz, Richard W. *John Harvey Kellogg, M.D.* Berrien Springs, MI: Andrews University Press, 1970.

Caroline Lieffers

BAUR, GENE (1962~)

Gene Baur (formerly Gene Bauston) is the cofounder and president of Farm Sanctuary, the largest farm animal rescue and refuge in the United States. He is also a vegan activist and the best-selling author of *Farm Sanctuary: Changing Hearts and Minds about Animals and Food,* a history of Farm Sanctuary that was released in 2008.

Baur was born in Los Angeles, California, the oldest of six siblings. He graduated from Loyola High School in 1980 and graduated from California State University, Northridge, in 1985, with a bachelor's degree in sociology. During the summer of 1985, he worked for Greenpeace in Chicago, where he met Lorri Houston, with whom he would later found Farm Sanctuary. Baur additionally earned a master's degree in agricultural economics from Cornell University's College of Agriculture and Life Sciences.

In August 1986, Baur and Houston toured Lancaster, Pennsylvania, stock-yards together. Lancaster Stockyards, which incorporated in 1895, was one of the oldest animal-handling facilities in the United States until it closed in 2006. Surveying piles of animal carcasses, Baur and Houston encountered a six-month-old sheep that was still alive. They put her in their van and drove to a veterinarian for assistance. The sheep, which they named Hilda, survived the ordeal. In the following months, many other downed animals were found and rescued in the stockyards, leading Baur and Houston officially to found Farm Sanctuary in Watkins Glen, New York. In 1993, a second Farm Sanctuary location was established in Orland, California.

During its first five years of operation, Farm Sanctuary was sustained by Baur's and others' efforts selling vegetarian hotdogs at Grateful Dead shows. Baur and his crew traveled with the band in the same van that had been used to rescue Hilda the sheep. Over time, Baur's efforts persuaded a local fur farmer to get out of fox breeding and take up vegetable farming. Residents in the sanctuary's area also successfully convinced fast food chain Burger King to offer a veggie burger on their menu. Eventually, the sandwich was enough of a success that it was of-fered at chain locations across the country.

Baur, as part of his work with the sanctuary and in cooperation with organiza-tions like the Humane Society of the United States, has worked to pass animal welfare legislation. Several states, including Arizona and California, have passed legislation that requires humane confinement systems for farm animals. Califor-nia has also banned foie gras, a fatty liver food product produced by force-feeding geese and ducks. Anti-foie gras campaigns in cities like Chicago and New York have also been headed up and funded by Farm Sanctuary. Farm Sanctuary has been one of the largest organizations rescuing stranded and trapped animals after Ohio tornados in 2000, Hurricane Katrina in 2005, and Iowa floods in 2008.

See also Activism and Protests; Animal Rights and Animal Welfare; Ethical Vegetarianism; Houston, Lorri; Policy; Reform; Veganism.

Further Reading

Baur, Gene. *Farm Sanctuary: Changing Hearts and Minds about Animals and Food*. New York: Simon and Schuster, 2008.
Shevelow, Kathryn. *For the Love of Animals: The Rise of the Animal Protection Movement*. New York: Henry Holt, 2008.

Brittany Shoot

BIBLE AND BIBLICAL ARGUMENTS

The Bible is a key source of teaching for Jews and Christians on many ethical topics including food and eating. Yet biblical texts suggest a range of attitudes to meat, and their contexts are very different from those of today. The Bible does not absolutely require its readers to become vegetarian, although it sometimes commends abstention from meat as a spiritual discipline. Moreover, it presents meat as the most problematic human food. The New Testament urges both vegetarians and meat eaters to respond flexibly to the shifting social, religious, and missionary contexts in which meat is eaten or declined.

The book of Genesis presents an ambivalent view of meat eating that persists through the Bible. At the creation, God gave to humankind as food "every plant yielding seed that is upon the face of all the earth, and every tree with seed in its fruit" (Gen. 1:29). But after the Flood, God tells humans that "every moving thing that lives shall be food for you," thus allowing them to eat meat (Gen. 9:3). This permission can be regarded either as a positive command to eat meat or as a divine concession to human weakness.

Meat continues to be regarded as the most questionable food in the human diet. Noah and his sons are told not to eat flesh unless its blood has been drained (Gen. 9:4). As a result, rules are developed about how land animals should be slaughtered; moreover, the flesh of carrion or of animals killed by other animals cannot be eaten (Lev. 17:10–16). Another set of regulations concerns the avoidance of the unclean species preserved by Noah during the Flood (Gen. 7:8). Various birds are listed as unclean, mostly birds of prey and those inhabiting water environments (Lev. 11:13–19, Deut. 14:11–20). Land animals and fish are identified by inclusion. The marks of a clean land animal are that it has a split hoof and chews the cud, while a clean fish must possess both fins and scales (Lev. 11:2–12, Deut. 14:3–10). All other animals and birds are unclean.

For animals, Genesis clearly prescribes vegetarianism. At the creation, God gave to them "every green plant for food" (Gen. 1:30) and did not subsequently amend this provision. Predatory and scavenging animals are classed as unclean for human consumption. They possess claws, not a hoof, and do not chew the cud, which is a digestive process found only in animals with plant-based diets.

Vegetarianism is presented positively in the book of Daniel. In exile in Babylon, Daniel and his companions are given vegetables to eat instead of meat and appear "better and fatter than all the young men who had been eating the royal rations," gaining knowledge, skill, and wisdom (Dan. 1). Furthermore, in Isaiah's vision, predators are presented living peaceably with their former prey and with children (Isa. 11:6–9).

In the New Testament, rules for meat eating are debated by Jewish and non-Jewish Christians. Jesus drove the traders selling cattle and sheep and their money changers out of the temple, where animal sacrifice was a significant business (John 2:14–16) but later cooked and ate fish with his disciples (Luke 24:36–43, John 21:9–13). The Jerusalem Council instructed all Christians to "abstain from what has been sacrificed to idols and from blood and from what is strangled" (Acts 15:29), reaffirming that some Jewish abstinence rules applied not only to Jews but to all human beings (for example, Gen. 9:15–17, Lev. 17:10–16).

In the writings of Paul, the correct approach to eating with people with different dietary codes is discussed at length. In Rome, some of the meat sold originated from sacrifice, meaning that a Christian could not be sure where any specific piece of meat came from. Paul advises Christians to "eat whatever is sold in the meat market without raising any question on the ground of conscience" unless they know that a particular piece of meat is a product of sacrifice (1 Cor. 10:23–33). This is to prevent others passing negative judgments on Christian dietary freedoms, which would hinder the spread of the Christian gospel and the making of new converts (Rom. 14:13–23). Also, by eating meat that had been sacrificed to idols, an established Christian might encourage a weak Christian or potential Christian who had not developed sufficient strength of faith to consume this meat, too, and thereby lapse into paganism.

Drawing on these texts and traditions, Jews and Christians have formulated several arguments in support of vegetarianism. First, meat eating was not part of God's original creation. Humans should choose not to eat meat in order to restore the harmony of this good creation. Second, meat eating was permitted only after sacrifice at the temple. Following the temple's destruction, sacrifices can no longer be made, and meat may therefore no longer be eaten. Third, abstention also expresses mourning for the temple. In diaspora contexts where the source of meat and its method of killing and preparation cannot be verified, vegetarianism is the best way to maintain purity. A fourth argument is that hygiene issues and diseases are associated with meat, and if alternative foods are easily available, meat is best avoided. Fifth, God ultimately wills a world of peace and harmony, and humans should promote these values by not eating meat. One final argument posits that God appoints humans as stewards of the natural world. As good stewards, Jews and Christians should oppose meat consumption based on the notion that current high levels of meat eating are ecologically unsustainable and need to be reduced greatly.

Another common Christian biblical argument for vegetarianism is that because there is no evidence that Jesus ate red meat or poultry regularly, such meat should be avoided whenever possible. In general, Christian arguments have contributed to biblical interpretation by taking Old Testament witnesses seriously and questioning the assumption that Jesus made a complete break with the Jewish law.

See also African Hebrew Israelites; Bible Christians, English; Bible Christians, Philadelphia; Colonies, Communal Societies, and Utopias; Religious Beliefs and Practices; Seventh-day Adventists; Shakers, The.

Further Reading

Grumett, David and Rachel Muers. *Theology on the Menu: Asceticism, Meat and Christian Diet.* New York: Routledge, 2010.

Jewish Veg: Our Diet as Kiddush Hashem. http://www.jewishveg.com.

Sears, David. *The Vision of Eden: Animal Welfare and Vegetarianism in Jewish Law and Mysticism.* Spring Valley, NY: Orot, 2003.

Webb, Stephen. *Good Eating: The Bible, Diet and the Proper Love of Animals.* Grand Rapids, MI: Brazos, 2001.

David Grumett

BIBLE CHRISTIANS, ENGLISH

The English Bible Christian Church was founded by Rev. William Cowherd (1763–1816) in Salford, England, in 1809. The church combined a literal interpretation of the Bible with rationales for abstention from meat and an embrace of other social reform movements, especially temperance. The church eventually established chapels at Ancoats and Hulme, both in Manchester, and contributed to the formation of the Vegetarian Society, the United Kingdom's first national organization to promote abstention from meat, which still exists today.

Cowherd was trained as a minister in the Church of England but quickly became attracted to theologian Emanuel Swedenborg's teachings. Cowherd withdrew from the Church of England and joined a Swedenborgian congregation in 1793, where he also became a pastor. He embraced a radical notion of vegetarianism that had been put forth in some of Swedenborg's writings but did not become a central tenet of that denomination. Cowherd believed that the command in Genesis to act as stewards to animals meant that Christians should care for them and not indulge in eating them. He combined these injunctions with other biblical teachings that advocated moderation in all aspects of life and with the Swedenborgian emphasis on the practical aspects of Christianity.

Cowherd's theology also embraced the notion that the central tenet in Christianity should be "peace on earth, and good will towards all men." To achieve that goal, the abuse and inhumane treatment of animals that was common at the time needed to be eradicated. While he did not claim that animals had souls, their treatment reflected a human's relation to creation. Finally, Cowherd's doctrine embraced the notion of self-denial as a means toward focusing on one's own spirituality and relationship with the divine.

Although deeply influenced by Swedenborgianism and impressed by its focus on rationality and science, Cowherd left the church in 1809 because the theology was too rigid for him. He went on to found his own church in Salford. The Bible Christian Church found its adherents among Swedenborgians and other religious dissenters. To join the church, members had to sign a pledge that committed them to a vegetable diet and abstention from alcohol. Many working-class people were interested in the Bible Christians' doctrines, but because of the demand for temperance and vegetarianism, they did not join in numbers as great as those from more middling backgrounds.

The church in Salford grew, and chapels were opened in Manchester a few years after the denomination's founding. These chapels at Ancoats and Hulme grew slowly but provided several migrants for the group that moved to Philadelphia. In 1817, a group of Bible Christians, led by Rev. William Metcalfe (1788–1862), left Bristol and moved to Philadelphia, where they founded the Philadelphia Bible Christian Church. Metcalfe later went on to assist with the founding of the American Vegetarian Society in 1850.

Bible Christianity was attractive to industrial workers, in part because Cowherd and his successor, Rev. Joseph Brotherton, did not charge pew rents and maintained an open burial ground. Because it was a rapidly growing industrial region, Salford and Manchester became home to a diverse group of people, with specific economic and spiritual needs. Cowherd and the Bible Christians attempted to fill some of those needs and provided a forum for people who were interested in alternative religious structures as well as those who were interested in health reforms. In addition, Cowherd was known among poor people for making good soup that he would share with those who otherwise might not be able to feed themselves. The Bible Christians' poor relief focused on their commitment to providing healthful vegetarian fare to the poor and indigent. This tendency became well known among the more vulnerable people of Salford, although very few of them pledged to become full vegetarians and joined the church.

Cowherd died in 1816, and the church's leadership was taken over by Brotherton, who continued Cowherd's combination of pastoral leadership and vegetarian advocacy. Brotherton also became Salford's first member of Parliament in 1832. Brotherton was originally a Swedenborgian, and he and his wife, Martha, joined the Bible Christian Church shortly after its founding. The Brothertons both advocated vegetarianism and teetotalism in various pamphlets. Martha Brotherton's *Vegetable Cookery, A New System of Vegetable Cookery,* published in 1812, was one of the earliest vegetarian cookbooks. Joseph Brotherton also published several of the earliest tracts on teetotalism.

In 1847, the Bible Christians' advocacy bore fruit in the form of the organization of the Vegetarian Society, which was dedicated to raising interest in dietary reform and to the study of the health and social benefits of following a vegetarian lifestyle. James Simpson, another member of the Bible Christian Church, was elected the society's first president. The Bible Christians were actively involved in the new Vegetarian Society and attracted prominent vegetarians to the secular group, although they did not always gain converts. The Vegetarian Society grew in prominence, and several local chapters were formed in England, most often in industrial or port centers, where they attracted working-class radicals and reformers as well as middle-class reformers and health advocates. In 1851, an international conference was held, with people from the Philadelphia Bible Christian Church and other American and European vegetarians in attendance.

The Vegetarian Society's success coincided with the Bible Christian Church's fall from prominence. The two chapels at Ancoats and Hulme closed during the latter half of the 19th century. By 1930, membership in the church at Salford had declined significantly, and the church voted to merge with a Unitarian congregation in Pendleton. The Vegetarian Society began to participate in the 1880s with other groups from around the world. These came together and formed the International Vegetarian Union in 1908, which still exists today.

See also Alternative and Holistic Medicine; American Vegetarian Society; Bible and Biblical Arguments; Bible Christians, Philadelphia; Cookbooks; Metcalfe, Rev. William; Reform; Religious Beliefs and Practices; Vegetarian Society of America.

Further Reading

Antrobus, Derek. *A Guiltless Feast: The Salford Bible Christian Church and the Rise of the Modern Vegetarian Movement.* Salford, UK: City of Salford, Education and Leisure, 1997.

Forward, Charles W. *Fifty Years of Food Reform: A History of the Vegetarian Movement in England.* London: Ideal Publishing Union, 1898.

Gregory, James. *Of Victorians and Vegetarians: The Vegetarian Movement in Nineteenth-Century Britain.* London: Tauris, 2007.

International Vegetarian Union. http://www.ivu.org/history.

Metcalfe, William. *Out of the Clouds: Into the Light. With a Memoir by His Son, Reverend Joseph Metcalfe.* Philadelphia: J.B. Lippincott, 1872.

The Philadelphia Bible Christian Church. *The History of the Philadelphia Bible-Christian Church, for the First Century of Its Existence, 1817 to 1917.* Philadelphia: J.B. Lippincott, 1922.

Walters, Kerry S., and Lisa Portmess, eds. *Religious Vegetarianism: From Hesiod to the Dalai Lama.* Albany: State University of New York Press, 2001.

Gwynne K. Langley Rivers

BIBLE CHRISTIANS, PHILADELPHIA

The Philadelphia Bible Christian Church was founded in 1817. The church was an offshoot of the English Bible Christian Church that was founded by Rev. William Cowherd in 1809. Members believed in a literal interpretation of the Bible that emphasized practical aspects of living, including the requirement that members abstain from animal food and alcohol. The church gained some prominence in the mid-19th century because of its ties to the American Vegetarian Society and members' involvement with other reform movements at the time.

The first pastor of the Philadelphia Bible Christian Church was Rev. William Metcalfe (1788–1862). Metcalfe joined the Bible Christian Church at Salford, in Manchester, England, after having been a member of a Swedenborgian congregation. Swedish theologian Emanuel Swedenborg believed that Christians could move from a material existence to a spiritual existence, and that this entailed taking practical steps while on earth. These steps included embracing peace, avoiding eating animal foods, and practicing charity. Metcalfe was attracted to the rationalism of Swedenborgian Christianity and became an ordained minister and active in the New Church at Keighly in Yorkshire. Through this association, he met Cowherd, the founder of the Bible Christian Church. Metcalfe became a member of the church and signed the required pledge to give up meat and alcohol on September 1, 1809. Cowherd persuaded Metcalfe that eating meat was not biblically sanctioned and, in addition, was detrimental to one's health. During this time, Metcalfe moved to Salford and took a leading role in the Bible Christian Church.

After Cowherd's death in 1816, Metcalfe planned to immigrate to the United States, where he believed the Bible Christian doctrine would be well received. A group of two ministers, including Metcalfe, and 20 adults and their children arrived in Philadelphia in June 1817. There, they bought a building for their new church and began to attract converts from among various individuals interested in dietary reform and attracted to the doctrines of Swedenborg and Cowherd. The Bible Christians believed that Jesus had been a vegetarian and used scriptural passages that invoked an expanded notion of stewardship and abstention to substantiate their claim.

Because of their radical notions regarding food and spirituality, the Bible Christians were attacked in the Philadelphia press during their first years in their new city. To win converts to their church as well as to promote vegetarianism, many of the church's activities centered on food. Most services or educational meetings were followed by teas and meals of simple vegetarian fare. These menus and occasionally recipes were published in their official documents, a tradition that was continued by the American Vegetarian Society, the first national organization to promote abstention from meat in the United States. The church struggled initially to find converts and a place within Philadelphia but eventually bought a building on Third Street and Girard Avenue, which served as their home from 1823 to 1890. They later moved headquarters to Park Avenue, and the church there lasted from 1891 until 1916.

The Bible Christians quickly became involved in the reform efforts of the early republic. Some of these included abolitionism, dress reform, and health reform. They found kindred spirits in other prominent American vegetarians, including William A. Alcott, Bronson Alcott, and Sylvester Graham, who, while supportive of their efforts, did not join the church. The prominence of these allies and the receptivity of some groups of reformers to the vegetarian creed helped the church to grow, if not in membership, at least in prominence. While their English counterparts were able to set up chapels in other cities, the Philadelphia Bible Christians focused more on vegetarian advocacy than they did on religious evangelism and conversion. The church remained local, and most of their followers lived in the greater Philadelphia area.

In 1850, Metcalfe and other prominent Bible Christians, and Rev. James Clarke helped to establish the American Vegetarian Society. William A. Alcott was elected as its first president and served in this office until his death in 1859. The society was modeled on the English Vegetarian Society that was also founded by Bible Christians. They were dedicated to informing Americans about vegetarianism and promoting it as a more healthful alternative to the national diet. The society was successful, and on its behalf, as well as on behalf of the church, Metcalfe traveled back to England in 1851 to attend the annual meeting of the Vegetarian Society there.

During this encounter, the idea of creating a vegetarian settlement was first broached. This effort possibly served to inspire the creation of the non-sectarian joint-stock Vegetarian Kansas Emigration Company, which bought land along the Neosho River in Kansas in order to create a vegetarian community there. The founders' goal was to develop a community that would serve as a model society. The city would demonstrate the viability of the vegetarian way of life and would also promote other alternative health practices, including hydropathy. The company was led by Henry S. Clubb (pastor of the Philadelphia congregation from

1875 or 1876 until 1921), and in 1856 the group attempted to establish their community in Kansas. Due to problems with malaria and the contest between proslavery and antislavery forces, the experiment was plagued with problems and shortages of labor. The venture failed after a few months, and many settlers moved back east after the experiment was over.

During its midcentury heyday, the church was active in establishing a physiological society and an institution for the care of the sick, which was discontinued in 1861. A Ladies Aid Society was also active beginning in 1863; their work focused on helping the poor and visiting the sick, though their initial role was to aid Union soldiers during the Civil War. The church dwindled in membership and influence through the first two decades of the 20th century, mostly due to the deaths of the founding and early members. Their Park Avenue church building was sold to the Third Church of Christ, Scientist in 1916, but members continued to meet in Rev. Clubb's home in Philadelphia until the pastor's death in 1921.

See also Alcott, William A.; Alternative and Holistic Medicine; American Vegetarian Society; Bible and Biblical Arguments; Bible Christians, English; Clubb, Henry S.; Metcalfe, Rev. William; Reform; Religious Beliefs and Practices; Vegetarian Society of America.

Further Reading

Anderson, Michael W. "Field of Forgotten Dreams: The Ill-Fated Vegetarian Colony in Kansas." *Kansas Heritage* 7, no. 3 (Autumn 1999), 13–16.

Davis, Miriam Colt. *Went to Kansas; Being a Thrilling Account of an Ill-Fated Expedition.* Watertown, NY: L. Ingalls, 1862.

International Vegetarian Union. http://www.ivu.org/history.

Metcalfe, William. *Bible Testimony on Abstinence from the Flesh of Animals as Food.* Philadelphia: J. Metcalfe, 1840.

Metcalfe, William. *Out of the Clouds: Into the Light. With a Memoir by His Son, Reverend Joseph Metcalfe.* Philadelphia: J.B. Lippincott, 1872.

The Philadelphia Bible Christian Church. *The History of the Philadelphia Bible-Christian Church, for the First Century of Its Existence, 1817 to 1917.* Philadelphia: J.B. Lippincott, 1922. http://www.ivu.org/history/usa19/history_of_bible_christian_church.pdf.

Gwynne K. Langley Rivers

CHILDBEARING AND INFANT FEEDING

Pregnant women have long been bombarded with advice about what types of food to eat, and what not to eat, to ensure the health of the growing fetus as well as to reduce morning sickness or cravings. Likewise, the diet of a breast-feeding mother has a direct impact on the content of the milk ingested by her infant. Vegetarian mothers and babies frequently have faced extra scrutiny in cultures where vegetarianism has not been the norm.

During the 19th century, the benefits of a meatless diet for both pregnant and lactating women were sometimes debated, with some doctors recommending that pregnant women consider a vegetarian diet to encourage "soft bones" and an easy labor. A perhaps surprising number of books, both by doctors and self-appointed experts, discouraged the consumption, or at least the excessive consumption, of meat during pregnancy or while nursing. Women were frequently warned away from excesses of all types, including strong flavor and texture, and steered instead toward a fruit- and vegetable-heavy diet. It was an era of rigid gender roles and expectations that spilled over into the material realm, so it is perhaps not surprising that the "masculine" nature of meat would be considered a potential threat to a woman engaging in the uniquely feminine experience of pregnancy and breast-feeding.

By the 20th century, an increasing number of nonvegetarian doctors were addressing the concerns of vegetarian mothers. In 1919, Johns Hopkins obstetrician J. Morris Slemons published *The Prospective Mother: A Handbook for Women during Pregnancy*. While not fully supportive of vegetarianism, Slemons reassured his readers that vegetarian mothers need not worry. "There is no diet specifically adapted to the state of pregnancy; the prospective mother may usually exercise the same freedom as anyone else in the selection of food," he wrote, continuing on to acknowledge that a vegetarian diet was safe for pregnant and nursing mothers alike. Nonvegetarian women were encouraged to eat only very small quantities of meat.

For much of human history, the issue of infant feeding revolved around whether a child was breast-fed by its mother or by a wet nurse. In 1762, Jean-Jacque Rousseau's *Émile, or On Education* (1979) encouraged women to nurse their own children, as well as recommending that lactating women eschew meat. "The milk of herbivorous females is sweeter and healthier than that of carnivores," he wrote.

By the dawn of the 20th century, the introduction of infant formulas and the rise of a domestic science-based approach to diet had shifted the discussion of the proper feeding of infants from "who" to "how." Eugene Christian and Molly Griswold Christian's influential *250 Meatless Menus and Recipes,* published in 1910, was representative of an increasingly scientific 20th-century approach to diet and the adoption of vegetarianism for health, and not moral, reasons. They believed that meat had high levels of "toxic poisons" and recommended that pregnant and nursing women follow a lacto-ovo vegetarian diet, reminding them that their prenatal diet could "leave [the food's] imprint upon the embryonic being and can wield a powerful influence over its future destiny."

A return to ethics-based vegetarianism blossomed in the 1960s and 1970s. *Nature's Children,* by Juliette de Baïrcli Levy, is representative of the genre of vegetarian parenting advice popular at the time. She advocated a "natural," mostly vegan diet, with an emphasis on raw foods, suggesting that it would help to prevent a "heavy-boned" fetus and potential delivery problems as well as nourish the breast-feeding mother and her infant.

By the 1960s, many medical authorities were acknowledging the existence of vegan and vegetarian diets for pregnant and lactating women. In 1974, in response to public demand, the National Academy of Sciences' Food and Nutrition Board produced a pamphlet on the topic of vegetarian families. While not enthusiastically embracing vegetarianism, it did acknowledge that vegetarian diets could be safe and nutritious for pregnant women and young children. The government and most medical practitioners were far more wary of vegan diets, warning mothers of the risks of permanent physical or neurological damage that could result from prenatal or infant vitamin or protein deficiencies. In 1998, Benjamin Spock's sixth edition of the best-selling *Baby and Child Care* departed from earlier editions and advocated that nursing mothers eat a vegetarian diet. Among other things, Spock believed that pesticides and chemicals are found in high concentrations in meat and could make their way into breast milk.

See also Alternative and Holistic Medicine; Backlash; Cookbooks; Domestic Science and Scientific Eating; Ethical Vegetarianism; Family Dynamics; Physiological Benefits; Social Acceptance.

Further Reading

Christian, Eugene, and Molly Griswold Christian, *250 Meatless Menus and Recipes.* New York: Mollie Griswold Christian, 1910.

Iacobbo, Karen, and Michael Iacobbo. *Vegetarian America: A History.* Westport, CT: Praeger, 2004.

de Baïracli Levy, Juliette. *Nature's Children.* Rev. ed. Woodstock, NY: Ash Tree Publishing, 2007.

Rousseau, Jean-Jacque. *Émile, or On Education.* Translated by Alan Bloom. New York: Basic Books, 1979.

Slemons, J. Morris. *The Prospective Mother: A Handbook for Women during Pregnancy.* New York and London: D. Appleton and Company, 1919.

Stuart, Tristram. *The Bloodless Revolution: A Cultural History of Vegetarianism from 1600 to Modern Times.* New York: W.W. Norton, 2007.

Cedar Phillips

CHILDREARING

Society's understanding of the appropriate diet for children has evolved over time and has often been imbued with a meaning that encompasses food for both physical and spiritual growth. While adult vegetarians have also been concerned with the relationship between character and diet, and between diet and health, the issue gained additional significance in the context of children. Decisions made about a child's life or diet were believed to have lasting implications for lifelong character and health, and parents throughout time have worried about making the right—or wrong—decisions.

English philosopher and physician John Locke's influential *Thoughts Concerning Education,* published in 1692, advocated a vegetarian diet for children. "Flesh should be forborne as long as he is in coats, or at least till he is two or three years old," wrote Locke, suggesting that a flesh-free diet would lead to better teeth, less disease, and "lay the foundations of a healthy and strong constitution." While vegetarianism was not the norm for most of Locke's contemporaries, an increasing number of people were familiar with the concept of vegetarianism, and Locke's suggestions would have raised few eyebrows.

In 1762, Jean-Jacque Rousseau's controversial *Émile, or On Education,* also encouraged parents to raise their children on a vegetarian diet. He argued that a taste for meat was not natural and was forced on children by adults. While, like Locke, he believed meat to be unhealthy for children, he also was a staunch believer in the relationship between a vegetarian diet and a higher moral order, suggesting, among other things, that "great eaters of meat are in general more cruel and ferocious than other men."

One of the most significant figures in the 19th-century vegetarianism movement was Sylvester Graham. In 1833, the Orphan Asylum of Albany, New York, implemented the Graham diet for its young residents. In 1836, doctors reported that the orphanage's children were healthier than ever. While not embraced by the general public as evidence of the value of a vegetarian diet for children, vegetarian advocates hailed it as proof that a strict vegetarian, indeed nearly vegan, diet was both physically and morally optimal for children. Graham's teachings were to also greatly influence Bronson Alcott, who, together with Charles Lane, in 1843 helped to found a short-lived utopian community in Massachusetts named Fruitlands. Fruitlands' residents, including children, lived a strictly vegan life, which was later lampooned by Alcott's daughter, Louisa May Alcott, in her short story "Transcendental Wild Oats."

By the mid-19th century, American vegetarian feminists had begun to link vegetarianism with women's rights, as well as with women's roles as mothers and caregivers. "If females would study the laws of health, they would be convinced of its truth, and be themselves blessed, and their children, by the adoption of a pure vegetable diet," wrote Anne Denton in 1852 in the *American Vegetarian and Health Journal.* She thought women should be "benevolent" and that preparing and eating meat violated the laws of nature. Denton and others believed vegetarianism to be a duty directly benefiting the woman as well as her children.

During the later 19th century vegetarian advocates actively highlighted both the moral and the health benefits of raising vegetarian children. *Food, Home and Garden,* the publication of the Vegetarian Society of America, regularly featured articles reassuring parents that the choice to raise vegetarian or vegan children was a smart one. In 1898, for example, T.R. Allinson wrote glowingly of the higher achievements of vegetarian children, claiming that eating meat diverted valuable energy and engendered acquisitiveness and a disregard for others. Vegetarian children, in contrast, were "full of life, fun, and mischief" and would "grow up an intelligent citizen and a humane citizen," as well as study better, think more clearly, and have milder tempers than their meat-eating peers. For those parents not convinced purely by the intellectual and spiritual claims, the publication also included letters praising the economic benefits of vegetarian childrearing.

Early 20th-century vegetarian parents were increasingly influenced by scientific eating, with leaders such as Eugene Christian and Molly Griswold Christian, authors of *250 Meatless Menus and Recipes* (1910), providing details on child-specific nutritional needs. The Christians, like many of their contemporaries, warned parents of the dangers of the uric acid and "toxic poisons" found in meat and instead advocated a vegetarian diet similar to that of an adult but with the addition of great carbohydrates to help provide for growth and "material for the extra mental work and worry" of school.

The 1960s and 1970s once again brought the moral aspects of vegetarian childrearing to the forefront. *Nature's Children,* by Juliette de Baïrcli Levy (1970), was typical of the time. Like others before her, she believed humans to be natural vegetarians. She also warned parents of the dangers of being a "diet fanatic" and suggested that children have some say regarding becoming vegetarian or vegan, with the caveat that parents should ask the children to think through the moral implications, in particular the impact on animals, of choosing a nonvegetarian diet.

By this time nonvegetarian doctors were increasingly addressing the concerns of both vegetarian and vegan parents. Penelope Leach's *Babyhood,* first published in 1974 and updated in 1983, included several pages relating to vegetarian, vegan, and even fruitarian diets. Sympathetic to the wishes of parents to balance personal beliefs with optimal health for their children, she suggested that parents with strong convictions and a highly restrictive diet talk to a doctor before the baby was weaned. While Leach warned against the extremes of raw and fruit-based diets and warned vegan parents to be vigilant about protein sources, she was respectful of parental beliefs and offered hope that an early consultation would allow the needs of the growing child to be met without compromising the parents' beliefs.

The world's most famous children's doctor, vegetarian or otherwise, however, was Benjamin Spock. *Dr. Spock's Baby and Child Care,* one of the best-selling books of all times, reaching tens of millions of parents since its first publication in 1946, long advocated a childhood diet that incorporated meat. His views radically changed in the 1990s, however, and the book's sixth edition, published in 1998, encouraged parents to raise children as vegetarians and to eliminate milk and dairy products after age two. Vegetarian children have stronger bones and are "less likely to develop weight problems, diabetes, high blood pressure, or some kinds of cancer," wrote Spock; he also believed there to be fewer food safety concerns with vegetarian diets. Particularly controversial was his stance on dairy, which he believed to be unnatural in weaned children and adults, high in saturated fat, and potentially aggravating to health problems such as asthma and eczema, among other issues.

See also Childbearing and Infant Feeding; Colonies, Communal Societies, and Utopias; Domestic Science and Scientific Eating; Ecofeminism; Graham, Sylvester; Physiological Benefits; Reform; Social Acceptance.

Further Reading

Iacobbo, Karen, and Michael Iacobbo. *Vegetarian America: A History.* Westport, CT: Praeger, 2004.

Rousseau, Jean-Jacques. *Émile. Or, On Education.* Translated by Alan Bloom. New York: Basic Books, 1979.

Stuart, Tristram. *The Bloodless Revolution: A Cultural History of Vegetarianism from 1600 to Modern Times.* New York: W.W. Norton, 2007.

Cedar Phillips

CHINA

The history of vegetarianism in China is complex and extends back through history to ancient legends that record, for example, that Fu Xi, the first prophet-king, was vegetarian. Confucius, a key figure in the history of the Tao, converted to vegetarianism. During the Han dynasty in the third century BC, Buddhist missionaries from India arrived in China and promoted their vegetarian religion. In the 20th century the ruling Communist Party in China acted to suppress religion and traditions influenced by Taoist, Confucian, and Buddhist teachings during the Cultural Revolution of 1966 to 1976. Antireligious sentiment in the doctrines of Chinese Communism has continued to make the Chinese government suspicious of vegetarian organizations, a stance presumably exacerbated by the strong links between the historical religions of China and vegetarian practice. This bureaucratic prejudice led to initial difficulties in forming a vegetarian society in China in 2005 to join the Asian Vegetarian Union and affiliate with the International Vegetarian Union. However, initial government opposition was eventually overcome, and the organization was formed and officially sanctioned.

In terms of the historical legacy of the Cultural Revolution and vegetarianism, poverty and deprivation in much of rural China continue to this day, and vegetarianism of a sort, motivated not by religion, politics, or philosophy but by poverty and the unavailability and expense of meat, is fairly common. In contrast, recent economic growth has led to increases in meat consumption among China's increasingly affluent urban population. Meat, because of its scarcity, has gained status as a luxury, even a delicacy. However, this increase in meat consumption has led to a decline in health and increasing incidence of obesity, diabetes, and heart disease. Health concerns have thus led to a backlash against new dietary habits, and Western fast food franchises in particular, leading some to turn to vegetarianism out of fitness and health concerns.

Beliefs and Conditions   In China, religious conviction is often a motivation for the dedicated vegetarian. Particularly strong is the Buddhist tradition; however, the other side of the religious aspect to Chinese vegetarianism is that Christian communities are sometimes opposed to vegetarianism because of its association with other faiths, as the association between vegetarianism and faith is so strong. Even for those who are not religious or vegetarian, however, there are many traditions in Chinese culture with a vegetarian flavor to them. For example, a popular custom is that the first meal of the New Year be vegetarian, since having the first act of the New Year be the taking of life is considered by some to be bad luck. In addition, among militant ideological vegetarians in China, there is a pervasive rhetoric that eating meat is unhealthy, perhaps unnatural, and also to some extent a Western practice, particularly when the practice is carried to perceived excess, linked increasingly to Western diet–related illnesses. The other side of the negative connotations of meat eating, in Chinese vegetarian thinking, is the assertion that vegetarianism is innately linked to a peaceful, nonviolent personal philosophy and even to a more tranquil or spiritual mindset. This assumption, though present among non-Buddhist Chinese vegetarians, is probably linked to China's ancient Buddhist traditions.

Vegetarian Practices   The traditional Chinese diet is not vegetarian but has many aspects that are favorable for the introduction of vegetarian and vegan practices. Two examples of this are the traditional consumption of tofu and other soybean products, including soy milk, and the absence of a strong tradition of dairy products. In urban China, vegetarian restaurants and health food stores are becoming increasingly common, and there is increased availability of vegetarian food products in supermarkets. In the cities, the young generation of China's educated, urban elite, particularly students, is a demographic in which politically or health-motivated vegetarianism is gaining a foothold.

Matthew Winston

CHRISTIANITY, INFLUENCES OF

The relationship between vegetarianism and Christianity is long-standing and multifaceted and stretches back to some of the earliest strands in the biblical material. In Genesis 1:29–30, humans and animals are given a vegetarian diet. The significance of this cannot be overstated because the authors of Genesis were not themselves vegetarian, or pacifists, or opposed to capital punishment. Despite their own involvement in violence, they believed that God had originally created a peaceful, nonviolent world and that human wickedness had disrupted God's plan. Thus, the permission to eat meat appears in Genesis 9:3 after the Fall and the Flood, when humans had departed from the divine plan.

Even when the permission to eat meat is given, it entails a condition that the blood of the animal should not be consumed (Gen. 9:4). As blood was identified with the very life of the victim, it implies, however paradoxically, that although the animal may be used, its life should not be misappropriated or claimed as being owned. The Hebrews were still uneasy with the practice of killing, and hence Isaiah 11:1–9 envisages a time when the lion will lie down with the lamb and universal harmony will be restored, both between humans and animals and between animals themselves.

Jesus and Vegetarianism   In the canonical gospels, Jesus is depicted as eating fish and assisting in the capture and killing of fish. There are no precise accounts of Jesus eating meat. It is unclear whether Jesus ate lamb at the Passover, which would have been traditional, because the gospels disagree as to whether the last supper was also a Passover meal. An early noncanonical work called the Gospel of the Ebionites ("Ebionite" is derived from the Hebrew term for "the poor") implies that Jesus was a vegetarian and also rejected animal sacrifice. Although no copies of this gospel are extant, its existence is known because it was attacked as heretical by Bishop Epiphanius in the fourth century.

St. Paul criticizes vegetarians, maintaining that "the weak man [of faith] eats only vegetables" (Rom. 14:1–2). The context appears to be the legitimacy of eating meat offered in sacrifices to idols, though that may have masked a deeper discussion about the propriety of eating meat. It is unclear why there would have been any Christian vegetarians at all in AD 60, when Paul wrote his letter to the Roman church, if Jesus himself was a meat eater. The puzzle is increased when it is appreciated that James, the brother of Jesus, who was also head of the Jerusalem church, was reportedly a vegetarian, which raises currently unanswerable questions about Jesus's family history, their food preferences, and the nature of their possible abstention.

Continuing Vegetarian Tradition   Although vegetarianism never became mainstream Christian practice, there is evidence that it was never entirely lost to Christian consciousness. The "Religion of the Light," as the first Christian church in China has been called, adopted a vegetarian diet, influenced, it seems, by Ebionite beliefs. It lasted from AD 781 until the collapse of the Tang dynasty in 906 or 907. Moreover, peaceful, even vegetarian motifs can be found in a range of apocryphal Christian literature, such as the fourth-century Acts of Philip. In addition, many Christian saints, such as St. Marcian and St. John of Egypt, appear to have adopted a vegetarian diet, although mainly, it appears, for ascetic reasons.

The 19th century saw the rebirth of Christian vegetarianism with the creation of the Bible Christian Church by William Cowherd in England (and later by William Metcalfe in the United States), which lasted from 1809 to 1932. In obedience to Genesis 1, it made vegetarianism compulsory among its members. In 1847, Joseph Brotherton, then pastor of the church, presided over the meeting that inaugurated the Vegetarian Society of the United Kingdom.

Theological Grounds for Vegetarianism Although vegetarianism has been a minority position within Christianity, there are four cogent doctrinal and theological grounds for advocating a vegetarian diet. The first concerns the value of God-given life. According to theistic belief, God is the Creator of all things and all life has value—what is created is loved by the Creator. The prologue to St. John's gospel (1:4) states that "in him was life," meaning that all life has its origin in the logos. Biblical insights underpin the special or intrinsic value of sentient animal life. The land animals, for example, are created on the same day of creation as humans (the sixth day), thereby symbolizing a special closeness between humans and animals (Gen. 1:24–25).

It follows that because animals belong to God, have value to God, and live for God, their needless destruction is sinful. Even the Catholic catechism (1994), while maintaining that it is legitimate to kill for food, still accepts that it is "contrary to human dignity to cause animals to suffer or die needlessly." A great deal hangs on the word "needlessly." In years past it may have been necessary to eat animals to survive—it may even be necessary in some remote regions of the world today—but almost all people can now live happy and healthy lives without recourse to flesh products, so meat eating clearly fails the necessity test. Where humans are free to do otherwise, there is a moral obligation to live free of killing.

Generosity and Nonviolence The second consideration concerns the moral exemplar of Jesus. His ministry involved active concern for the disadvantaged: He healed the sick, associated with lepers, and washed the dirty feet of his disciples. Strikingly, in Matthew 26:42–45, Jesus identifies his own self, and thereby God's own cause, with those who are hungry, thirsty, and held captive in prison. Thus, it can be stated that the "Jesus-shaped ethic" consists of "a paradigm of inclusive moral generosity," one that privileges the poor, the weak, and the vulnerable. Christians can validly claim that following Jesus today requires living out this generosity toward an even wider circle of vulnerable subjects. Christian vegetarianism can thus be seen as a practical outworking of the life of generosity and service glimpsed in Jesus.

The third consideration relates to the centrality of nonviolence. It is now widely accepted that Jesus was an exponent of nonviolence, and especially nonretaliation. Indeed, loving—not just one's neighbors but also one's enemies—is one of the distinguishing marks of the ethical teaching of Jesus. The early church was almost entirely pacifist in practice, with members refusing even to serve as magistrates and soldiers. Given this teaching and example, it is perhaps surprising that Christians have not championed the cause of nonviolence toward animals more strongly. Christians today can argue that living out nonviolence toward other creatures is wholly in accord with the spirit of Jesus.

The Peaceable Kingdom The final ground relates to the eschatological (future-oriented) nature of Christian hope. Isaiah's vision of a peaceable kingdom was not lost in the New Testament. St. Paul writes of how the whole creation is in a state of childbirth awaiting the freedom of the sons of God (Rom. 8:18–24); in Ephesians 1:9–10 and Colossians 1:15–20, "all things" are to be redeemed in Christ, who makes peace by the blood of the cross. There is to be a cosmic redemption of suffering that also includes animal life. Such a perspective is confirmed by the prayer that Jesus taught his disciples that God's will "be done, on earth as it is in heaven" (Matt. 6:10–11).

Given that eschatological orientation, it follows that living without killing is a proper anticipation of the redeemed life that is promised in Christ. Indeed, one theological critic of vegetarianism, the theologian Karl Barth, has argued that vegetarianism represents a "wanton anticipation of the new aeon for which we hope." Ironically, that very objection also supplies the theological basis for vegetarianism, because seeking to approximate or anticipate the kingdom is Jesus's own teaching.

A theology based on following the spirit of Jesus should naturally favor vegetarianism as one example of practical discipleship. To the objection that Jesus himself was perhaps not a vegetarian, the answer can be given that to follow Jesus is to be open to an ever-widening circle of obligation that is progressively inclusive. What Jesus does is to set in time and space a model of moral obligation that can only be properly and fully filled out by the Spirit in subsequent generations. In the light of these considerations, and the growth of Christian animal advocacy since the 1970s, it is highly likely that vegetarianism will figure more prominently as an issue of moral and theological issue in the 21st century than ever before.

See also Bible and Biblical Arguments; Religious Beliefs and Practices.

Further Reading

Barth, Karl. *Church Dogmatics*, Vol. III, pt. 4. Edinburgh: T. & T. Clark, 1961, n. 255–56.

Eisenmann, Robert. *James, the Brother of Jesus: Recovering the True History of Early Christianity: The Cup of the Lord.* London Faber & Faber, 1997.

Jones, Deborah M. *The School of Compassion: A Roman Catholic Theology of Animals.* Leominster, UK: Gracewing, 2009.

Linzey, Andrew. *Animal Theology.* Chicago: University of Illinois Press, 1994.

Linzey, Andrew. *Christianity and the Rights of Animals.* New York: Crossroad, 1987.

Linzey, Andrew. *Creatures of the Same God: Explorations in Animal Theology.* New York: Lantern Books, 2009.

Linzey, Andrew, and Tom Regan, eds. *Animals and Christianity: A Book of Readings.* Eugene, OR: Wpif and Stock, 2007.

Linzey, Andrew, and Dorothy Yamamoto, eds. *Animals on the Agenda: Questions about Animals for Theology and Ethics.* Chicago: University of Illinois Press, 1998.

Roberts, Holly. *Vegetarian Christian Saints.* New York: Anjeli, 2004.

Andrew Linzey

CLUBB, HENRY S. (1827–1921)

Henry S. Clubb was a British-born health and social reformer whose work in the United States helped support the growth of organized vegetarianism. Born in Colchester, England, Clubb was exposed to the benefits of a meatless diet during his formative years. Clubb was raised in the Swedenborgian Church, formed of followers of the 18th-century, vegetarian, spiritualist theologian Emanuel Swedenborg. As a young man Clubb was drawn to a variety of reform causes, leaving his job in 1842 as a postal clerk to live at London's Alcott House, an experiment in communal living that promoted ideas of gender and labor equality, transcendental education, and dietary reform.

Upon Alcott House's closing in 1844, Clubb became involved with London's growing vegetarian community, serving as the secretary to James Simpson, the first president of the Vegetarian Society. By 1849, Clubb was named editor of the *Vegetarian Messenger,* the society's newsletter. Clubb's relationship with Simpson eventually led to religious conversion. In 1850 Clubb was baptized in the Bible Christian Church, which preached the moral and physical advantages of a meatless diet, emphasizing that religion could be best understood through concerted text study.

In 1853, Clubb immigrated to the United States where he started working as a shorthand reporter for the *New York Tribune.* Clubb focused his writings on abolitionism, attempting to humanize slaves and describing the harsh conditions and mistreatment endemic to plantation life. At the same time, Clubb was also an early member of the American Vegetarian Society (AVS), the first national vegetarian organization in the United States. In August 1853, Clubb delivered an address to the AVS's annual meeting, a practice that he would repeat at future meetings. Clubb's focus on slavery and his deep dedication to vegetarianism led to the establishment of a vegetarian colony on the banks of the Neosho River in Kansas in 1855. The colony was a short-lived utopian experiment in communal living aimed at encouraging dietary reform while also attempting to limit the spread of slavery into Kansas.

Following the failure of the colony, Clubb served as a captain in the Union army during the Civil War. After getting discharged from service, Clubb moved to Michigan, where he founded the *Grand Haven Herald* newspaper and served as a state senator from 1873 until 1874. In 1876 Clubb reconnected with the Bible Christian Church in Philadelphia and became the group's minister. In addition to his pulpit role, Clubb worked as an active advocate for vegetarianism, founding and serving as the first president of the Vegetarian Society of America in 1886. In this role, Clubb edited the group's monthly newsletter *Food, Home and Garden* and its successor, the *Vegetarian Magazine.* The Philadelphia-based Vegetarian Society served as a national unifying force for American vegetarians during the Gilded Age, organizing lectures, publishing cookbooks, and selling a variety of vegetarian food products. Further, Clubb organized the International Vegetarian Congress at Chicago's Columbian Exposition in 1893 and wrote a "History of Vegetarianism" that appeared in the *Vegetarian Magazine* throughout 1909. Clubb remained the leader of the Philadelphia Bible Christian Church and Vegetarian Society of America until his death in 1921.

See also American Vegetarian Society; Bible Christians, English; Bible Christians, Philadelphia; Colonies, Communal Societies, and Utopias; Metcalfe, Rev. William; Reform.

Further Reading

Davis, Miriam Colt. *Went to Kansas; Being a Thrilling Account of an Ill-Fated Expedition.* Watertown, NY: L. Ingalls, 1862.

Fogarty, Robert S. *All Things New: American Communes and Utopian Movements, 1860–1914.* Chicago: University of Chicago Press, 1990.

Gregory, James. *Of Victorians and Vegetarians: The Vegetarian Movement in Nineteenth-Century Britain.* London: Tauris, 2007.

The Philadelphia Bible Christian Church. *History of the Philadelphia Bible-Christian Church for the First Century of Its Existence from 1817 to 1917.* Philadelphia: J. B. Lippincott, 1922. www.ivu.org/history/usa19/history_of_bible_christian_church.pdf.

Spencer, Colin. *Vegetarianism: A History.* New York: Four Walls Eight Windows, 2000.

Adam D. Shprintzen

COLONIES, COMMUNAL SOCIETIES, AND UTOPIAS

The 19th and 20th centuries witnessed an explosion of interest in communalism and utopianism. Throughout the United States, France, and Great Britain, communes espousing a wide range of social, economic, religious, and political reforms created alternative models for living and working. In many cases, these utopias also offered new models of eating. As far back as Thomas More's *Utopia* (1515), proponents of ideal communal societies had suggested that the slaughter of animals and the cooking and ingestion of meat threatened social and individual tranquility. Throughout the 19th and 20th centuries, utopian communities and colonies implemented a variety of meatless diets.

The most famous 19th-century vegetarian utopia, Bronson Alcott's (1799–1888) Massachusetts commune Fruitlands (1843–1844), placed a vegetarian diet at the absolute center of its social ethic. The Fruitlands residents championed vegetarianism for a variety of reasons, including health, animal rights, aesthetics, and a sense of austerity. Based on transcendentalist ideals, Alcott, cousin of well-known food reformer William A. Alcott, extended the rights of spiritual freedom to include animals and forbade the use of animals for not only food but also labor. Most scholars argue that, given the lack of mechanized methods of farming, Fruitlands' refusal to employ animal labor directly led to its failure as an agricultural colony.

Though less well known than Fruitlands, the Vegetarian Kansas Emigration Company (1855–1857) and Octagon Settlement Company (1856–1857), both founded and led by Henry S. Clubb (1827–1921), similarly aimed to create communal societies predicated on vegetarian ideals. Under the auspices of these two companies several dozen families attempted to create model utopias in the Kansas frontier, with almost a hundred persons involved at the peak of the two companies. The Vegetarian Company explicitly embraced vegetarianism for reasons of health and morality, whereas the Octagon Company embraced a sense of temperance that discouraged meat eating. Mismanagement, Indian raids, and a series of natural disasters led to both companies' failures within a year of their arrival in Kansas. In many cases, the utopian-minded, mostly urban transplants simply had no experience growing enough food to supply their needs. Clubb later became pastor of the vegetarian Philadelphia Bible Christian Church, a post he held from 1876 until shortly before his death, and he was the first president of the Vegetarian Society of America.

Numerous other utopias also experimented with vegetarianism. Colonies predicated on the social and economic principles of Robert Owen (1771–1858), who espoused a form of socialism, often included vegetarianism among their principles. These include the Owenite groups of Concordium (1838–1850) in Richmond, England, and the Skaneateles Community (1843–1846) near Mottville, New York. Few of these groups lasted longer than a few decades, though their demises owed more to their failures to sustain a functional socialism than to their vegetarianism.

Older communal societies also began to adopt vegetarianism during the early 19th century as well. Most notably this included the United Society of Believers, better known as the Shakers, a group of religious communes predicated on the prophetic leadership of their 18th-century founder, Ann Lee. Having already supported such utopian ideals as gender equality—including celibacy—and shared labor, during the 1820s and 1830s, several Shaker communities adopted vegetarianism as a method of self-control, bodily mastery, and health reform.

In some cases, individual members of communal societies engaged in vegetarianism, but they did not succeed in formalizing their diet as a permanent part of the utopian society. For example, at Brook Farm (1841–1846), the transcendentalist commune outside of Boston, a small faction of self-proclaimed Grahamites—proponents of Sylvester Graham's meatless regimen—instigated vegetarian practices at the commune. Their particular view of diet, however, did not take hold among the other residents of Brook Farm. Similarly, though several individual proponents of Fourierism, the communal social model championed by Charles Fourier (1772–1837), also upheld vegetarianism, no Fourierist communes (or Phalanxes, as they were called) adopted vegetarianism as a foundation for their community.

Several notable communal groups practiced vegetarianism during the early and mid-20th century. Many of these groups upheld vegetarianism in keeping with specific religious views. The House of David (1903–), founded by Benjamin Franklin Purnell (1861–1927) along the Lake Michigan shore in Benton Harbor, Michigan, has practiced vegetarianism alongside other practices that Purnell considered conducive to "wholeness of body." Residents of the House of David have believed that they lived in the end times, and in preparation for the return of Christ, they have preached the need to keep the body whole. This includes not only vegetarianism but also abstinence from alcohol and sex, as well as refusing to cut their hair. The group continues to exist, though with fewer than a dozen members.

Many of the religious utopias practicing vegetarianism developed out of Seventh-day Adventism, a religious tradition that has historically valued abstention from meat. The Mt. Carmel Branch Davidian community in Waco, Texas (1935–1993), infamous because of its fiery demise during a confrontation with the U.S. government, espoused vegetarianism during most of its history. The smaller Davidian Seventh-day Adventist Association (1983–), unassociated with the Waco group, continues to practice vegetarianism at its community in Exeter, Missouri.

In the 1960s there was a renewed interest in both religious and secular communal experiments, some of them espousing vegetarianism. The rise of the counterculture in the United States and western Europe led to a wider interest in Hinduism, Buddhism, Jainism, and Sikhism—Asian religious traditions that historically have valued vegetarianism. Intentional communities espousing beliefs rooted in these religious traditions often practiced vegetarianism. Foremost of these communes, the Hindu-inspired West Virginia Hare Krishna community of New Vrindaban (1968–) and the California Buddhist commune of Tassajara Zen Mountain Center (1966–) both insist on vegetarian practice in their communities, as do numerous other similar but smaller and shorter-lived groups.

Most notable of all the nonsectarian 20th-century vegetarian communes, the self-declared agricultural utopia known simply as the Farm (Summertown, Tennessee, 1971–) placed vegetarianism at the center of its ideology. Fusing elements drawn from the hippie counterculture including drugs, free love, Asian religions, parapsychology, and holistic health, from its beginnings the Farm considered vegetarianism a necessary foundation for social and environmental justice. The community organizers required potential members to abstain from consuming meat. The Farm continues to operate today, though it now functions as a cooperative rather than a true commune.

While the Farm placed vegetarianism at its center, many of the communes of the 1960s and 1970s experimented with vegetarianism, and most of them hosted individual vegetarians or groups of vegetarians. The topic of growing and eating food has been noted to be the most common topic of conversation at most of these communes, but few adopted strict vegetarianism. Groups such as Packer Corner Farm, better known as Total Loss Farm, the pseudonym used to describe the group in a member's popular memoir, experimented with vegetarianism and included a significant number of vegetarians as members but did not itself uphold the practice as a requirement for entrance into the community. Other communes in the 1960s and 1970s followed a similar pattern.

The history of communes and utopias is replete with vegetarian experiments and experimenters. One reason for this is that such groups intended to call into question wider social norms and offer new alternatives. Some of the explicitly vegetarian utopias operated as "cities upon the hill" meant to demonstrate the validity of new forms of social, political, and economic organization. Others upheld separatism, placing their hopes in a pure new community rather than reforming society. Numerous colonies did not formally adopt vegetarianism but included vegetarians or briefly experimented with vegetarian practice. In all cases, such groups challenged existing social norms and offered what they believed to be better alternatives. Eating is a central practice for all human beings and human communities. It is natural, then, that utopian societies looked to reform this necessary biological and social practice in keeping with the ideals of a more perfect society.

See also Alternative and Holistic Medicine; Bible Christians, Philadelphia; Clubb, Henry S.; Eastern Religions, Influences of; Ethical Vegetarianism; Europe; Family Dynamics; France; Graham, Sylvester; Physiological Benefits; Reform; Religious Beliefs and Practices; Seventh-day Adventists; Shakers, The; Transcendentalism; United Kingdom; Vegetarian Society of America.

Further Reading

The Fellowship for Intentional Community. "Intentional Communities." http://fic.ic.org/.

Francis, Richard. "Circumstances and Salvation: The Ideology of the Fruitlands Utopia." *American Quarterly* 25, no. 2 (May 1973): 202–34.

Harrison, J.F.C. *Robert Owen and the Owenites in Britain and America: The Quest for the New Moral Order.* London: Routledge and Kegan Paul, 1969.

Madden, Etta M., and Martha L. Finch, eds. *Eating in Eden: Food and American Utopias.* Lincoln: University of Nebraska Press, 2006.

Miller, Timothy. *The Quest for Utopia in Twentieth Century America.* Vol. 1, *1900–1960.* Syracuse, NY: Syracuse University Press, 1998.

Miller, Timothy. *The 60s Communes: Hippies and Beyond.* Syracuse, NY: Syracuse University Press, 1999.

Pitzer, Donald E., ed. *America's Communal Utopias.* Chapel Hill: University of North Carolina Press, 1997.

Benjamin E. Zeller

CONSUMER PRODUCTS

For many vegetarians, the choice to abstain from animal products extends beyond food and includes consideration of a wide range of consumer goods. Especially for ethical vegetarians and vegans, the avoidance or minimization of animal products influences, if not pervades, many consumer choices. As such, the world of consumer products exists as a site of vegetarian engagement, where good information acts as a basis of ethical choice that manifests itself through economics. In this way the vegetarian understands that every consumer choice has a discrete force that, over a lifetime of such choices, produces a palpable net effect: Boycotting cruel products and purchasing cruelty-free products instead sends a message via the marketplace with every purchase.

The seemingly endless array of consumer products available can appear, at first, daunting. A robust vegetarian understands, though, that the central rubric of animal-ethical relations is about necessity. When alternatives to animal-derived products exist, and it is within one's power to use them, then it is unnecessary to produce cruelty—and therefore ethically laudable to avoid products that do so.

For most vegetarians, the same practice of reading food labels applies to negotiating the field of consumer goods. Indeed, the recent rampant commercialization of vegetarian foods and meat substitutes by large corporations like Kellogg (Morningstar Farms, Gardenburger, Worthington) and Kraft/Philip Morris (Boca) requires careful label reading and moral deliberation; one can question whether to support a corporation that profits both from animal use and from its abstention. Similarly, understanding even a little about the everyday things that one uses proves essential to avoiding cruelty in its myriad forms and to manifesting ethical relationships within the world.

Besides food, another important area of concern in the realm of consumer products is the cosmetic industry. Ranging from toiletries to cosmetics, cosmetic products pose two distinct problems for vegetarians who wish to minimize their use of animal-derived products. First, many cosmetics are produced using animal-derived ingredients, including gelatin, whey, beeswax and royal jelly, lanolin, silk extract, fat-derived stearic acids, and ambergris, among others. Second, though the practice has in recent years, especially outside of the United States, declined, many mainstream companies use live-animal testing as a method of product safety assurance. In most cases, the antiquated—and questionable, experimentally and practically—LD_{50} test is used, where the dosages of subject chemicals are increased until 50 percent of the sample population is killed. In both cases, due in large part to consumer desire for cruelty-free products, corporations are increasingly labeling consumer goods as both "cruelty-free"—meaning without animal ingredients or testing—and "no animal testing." In the case of animal testing alone, however, much ambiguity remains, as corporations may use this label if the finished product was not tested on animals, even if the product's ingredients were, making the cruelty-free label misleading.

In terms of fashion, some vegetarians reject clothing that incorporates materials harvested through a process that harms or kills animals, such as leather, fur, wool, and feathers. Though some argue that the use of leather might be morally allowable because the animal was going to be killed for meat, in fact many cows are killed outright for leather. Further, and more compellingly, any practice that makes the killing of animals profitable perpetuates acts of cruelty. Clothing made from animal products, even if no animals are killed, such as wool, cashmere, angora, collected feathers, and silk, is eschewed because the industrialized practices involved in making these materials are cruel in the same way that factory farming harms chickens raised for eggs and cows used as milk machines.

Many other consumer products are problematic for vegetarians. For example, automobile and furniture manufacturers use leather extensively for upholstery and accents. Some guitars are made using hide-based glues as well as harvested mother-of-pearl inlays. Jewelers secure pearls by destroying oysters, while numerous dyes, like cochineal, result from crushed insect exoskeletons. In many cases, alternatives exist, for example, cloth instead of leather car seats. Where there are no alternatives, consumers must decide whether they need that product. In the end, consumers will make these choices based on their level of commitment to a vegetarian lifestyle.

Until a dramatic change in global attitude toward animal-derived products and testing occurs, the modern world of consumer products will remain a complex landscape, replete with missing, partial, shifting, or simply incorrect information. Practically speaking, unless people produce all of the items they would need in a lifetime, at this point there is no way to ensure a cruelty-free option in every consumer choice. Nonetheless, for those interested in diminishing animal abuses in the world, the effort needed to make cruelty-free choices remains minimal. In the same way, those committed to vegetarianism as merely a dietary practice need only to come to terms with what food products to avoid, a learning curve that in a short time is overcome and internalized, to the point where these choices become second nature.

To this end, a number of third-party organizations have made it their mission to supply good information to aid ethical consumers. Using these resources assists vegetarians in reducing their effect on nonhuman animals. Some of these organizations, such as the Coalition for Consumer Information on Cosmetics and People for the Ethical Treatment of Animals, administer cruelty-free certification programs that investigate a company's manufacturing and testing practices, supporting consumer empowerment by providing obvious labeling, and disseminate guides listing cruelty-free products and companies. At the same time, some companies seeking cruelty-free certification may do so for a number of reasons other

---

"Top Ten Vegetarian Convenience Foods"

In one of her latest works, activist and scholar Carol J. Adams and her coauthor Patti Breitman provide the following list of "Top Ten Vegetarian Convenience Foods":

1. Instant hummus.
2. Canned beans.
3. Vegetable broth. (Canned or powder that you add to water . . .).
4. Canned organic tomatoes: diced and whole, seasoned (Mexican and Italian), and stewed.
5. Instant mashed potatoes. Use them to thicken soups or bind a veggie burger.
6. Frozen vegetables.
7. Instant beans. Add water and you have refried beans or black beans.
8. Curry paste. Add to sautéed veggies and lentils and voila! instant curry.
9. Tomato sauce in jar.
10. Salad dressings.

Source: Carol J. Adams and Patti Breitman. *How to Eat Like a Vegetarian Even If You Never Want to Be One: More Than 250 Shortcuts, Strategies, and Simple Solutions.* New York: Lantern Books, 2008.

than ethical ones. As with developments in the organic foods market, profits are to be made from consumers of cruelty-free products.

Reading labels and remaining vigilant about manufacturing and sourcing practices on one's own—through label reading, press reviews, and direct corporate contact—continues to be a useful, common practice. Given this, many vegetarians invoke an animal-ethical version of the precautionary principle, which dictates that where information remains elusive one ought merely to abstain from that product, at least until useful information comes to light.

Products with animal-derived ingredients and products that were cruelly tested on animals predominate. This situation continues to be an impetus for animal rights activism for many. However, the consumer market also supplies a wide variety of cruelty-free choices to provide comfort, convenience, and aesthetic pleasure in a vegetarian lifestyle.

See also Activism and Protests; Advertising; Antivivisection; Battle Creek Sanitarium; Ethical Vegetarianism; Health Food Stores and Food Cooperatives; Kellogg, John Harvey; Newkirk, Ingrid; Organic Foods and Technology; Pacheco, Alex; People for the Ethical Treatment of Animals; Policy; Veganism.

Further Reading

Caring Consumer: A Guide to Kind Living. http://www.caringconsumer.com.
Coalition for Consumer Information on Cosmetics. http://leapingbunny.org.
Stepaniak, Joanne. *The Vegan Sourcebook*. 2nd ed. Los Angeles: Lowell House, 2000.

Tom Hertweck

COOKBOOKS

Until recently, most vegetarian cookbooks were as much about a philosophy of life as they were a collection of recipes. In many cases the promotion of the reasons for a vegetarian diet was just as important as, if not more so than, the recipes themselves; the authors' reasons for advocating vegetarianism ran the gamut from concern for animals to religious reasons to health concerns. By the 21st century, vegetarian cookbooks were increasingly found on the shelves of both vegetarian and omnivore households, with most modern vegetarian cookbooks written for an audience of both committed vegetarians and vegans and those who simply like to eat that way on occasion.

Thomas Tryon's *A Bill of Fare of Seventy Five Noble Dishes,* published in Britain in 1691, is credited with being the first vegetarian cookbook. Tryon wrote on many topics, but he had a particularly strong interest in issues relating to health and diet. He advocated a vegetarian diet for humanitarian reasons as well as for his belief that moral benefits came from self-denial.

While meatless recipes were included in popular 18th-century cookbooks, it was not until the 19th century that the next round of notable vegetarian

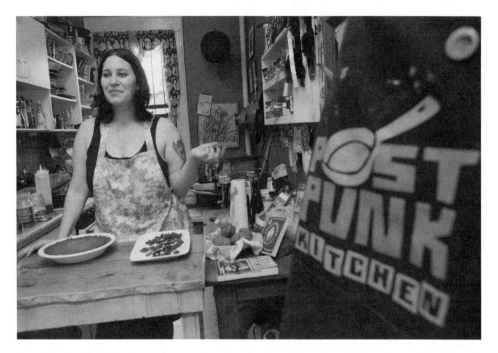

Isa Chandra Moskowitz prepares her vegan chocolate pie recipe at her apartment in Brooklyn, New York, 2007. Moskowitz is author of *Vegan with a Vengeance, Vegan Cupcakes Take Over the World,* and *Veganomicon.* (AP Photo/Diane Bondareff)

cookbooks emerged. Thanks in part to new printing processes and the resulting ready availability and lower cost of books and literature, vegetarianism as a movement began to spread to a broader audience than had been possible in years past. Early vegetarian advocates such as Sylvester Graham and William A. Alcott published widely, as did doctors such as Reuben Mussey. Most of the 19th-century vegetarian writings focused more on the health or philosophical reasons for a vegetarian diet than the food itself. In 1892, a Mrs. Bowdich of London published *New Vegetarian Dishes;* unlike most previous works, Mrs. Bowdich's book concentrated on the gustatory pleasures to be found in vegetarian cooking. The focus on enjoyment and taste was a change from many vegetarian cookbook of the time, many of which advocated a restrictive diet not just in terms of types of food but also in the use of seasonings and bold flavors.

Eugene Christian and Molly Griswold Christian of New York published their cookbook, *250 Meatless Menus and Recipes,* in 1910; like other cookbooks of the time, vegetarian and otherwise, it focused heavily on the science of food. In addition to the recipes, a great deal of space was given to advising readers on the health benefits of a vegetarian diet. Among other reasons to select a vegetarian (although not vegan) diet was to avoid the danger of "toxic poisons" found in meat, because vegetarianism decreased the dangers of overeating (one was advised to cut portion sizes by half due to the purity of a "natural" diet) and because it promoted the thorough chewing of food. While the Christians did see a moral element to vegetarianism, their interest was human health and not a concern for animals.

In contrast to *250 Meatless Menus and Recipes,* Maud Russell Lorraine Sharpe's book, *The Golden Rule Cookbook: Six Hundred Recipes for Meatless Dishes,* published in 1912, focused almost entirely on the moral reasons to embrace a vegan diet. Unlike many vegetarian cookbooks, *The Golden Rule Cookbook* also has no interest in providing recipes for fake meat. Readers are advised that the main reasons to become vegan include both a concern for cruelty against animals and the prevention of the degradation of the men, women, and children working in slaughterhouses. The recipes and kitchen advice themselves are fairly typical of contemporary cookbooks, minus the meat, but thanks to plentiful quotes from famous historical figures about the reasons not to eat meat, it would be difficult for a reader to forget that Sharpe believed that the primary purpose of a vegetarian diet was for ethical, not health, reasons.

Another wave of significant vegetarian cookbooks came in the 1970s. In 1972, Anna Thomas's landmark book *The Vegetarian Epicure* was published. Like most earlier vegetarian cookbook writers, she wrote extensively on the reasons to eat a vegetarian diet. Chief among those was the belief that it was inhumane to kill animals for food, but she also wrote of concerns regarding processed foods and chemical additions, as well as about the growth hormones often found in meat. Thomas also put vegetarianism in a larger environmental perspective, raising concerns that the only way to sustain the Earth's growing population was through a vegetarian diet. Finally, in the spirit of Mrs. Bowdich's *New Vegetarian Dishes,* Thomas appreciated good food and believed that the ethical elements of a vegetarian diet enhanced the overall enjoyment of the food itself.

Another significant 20th-century vegetarian cookbook was *Laurel's Kitchen: A Handbook for Vegetarian Cookery and Nutrition,* authored by Laurel Robertson, Carol Flinders, and Bronwen Godfrey, published in 1976. The book's cover advertised it as "America's first complete guide to cooking delicious natural foods." There was a heavy emphasis on nutrition, in addition to the food itself, but the nutritional information was not provided at the expense of taste.

The *Moosewood Cookbook* is another classic, written by Mollie Katzen and published in 1977. Both its format and its recipes made vegetarian cooking accessible and approachable to those new to the concept of meatless cooking. The *Moosewood Cookbook* is one of top-selling cookbooks of all time, arguably the most popular vegetarian cookbook ever published, and it introduced millions of readers to vegetarian cuisine. It remains a kitchen staple, and Katzen has been inducted into the James Beard Foundation's Cookbook Hall of Fame.

Deborah Madison, author of *The Savory Way* (1990), *The Greens Cookbook* (1987), and *Vegetarian Cooking for Everyone* (1997), among other books, further helped bring vegetarian cooking into mainstream America, eschewing the counterculture elements of the cuisine's past and establishing vegetarian recipes as something everyone could enjoy. She continues to write and has become involved with the slow food movement, which seems to be the next frontier in the evolution of vegetarian cookbooks.

Sample Menus for Early 20th-Century Vegetarians

Spring Menu

Breakfast

Russet (sweet) orange

Hominy grits

Malted milk

Grated nuts

Luncheon

New peas

Dandelion

Egg bread

Nut butter

Rice pudding

Dinner

Cream of pea soup

Omelet rolled in grated nuts and cream

Rice Southern style

Brussels sprouts

Nuts, steamed raisins

Cream cheese

Fall Menu

Breakfast

Melon or plums

Potato cakes

Coddled egg

Chocolate (hot cocoa)

Luncheon

Black bean soup

Cabbage

Sliced tomatoes

Corn hoe cake

Figs and nuts

Dinner

Potato chowder

Salted almonds

Celery

Stuffed peppers

Winter squash

Oat cake

Cheese

Nuts

Raisins

Source: Eugene Christian. *Meatless and Wheatless Menu.* New York: A. A. Knopf, 1917, pp. 14 and 65.

Today, there has been an explosion of vegan cookbook options, catering to the newly health-conscious and appealing to young people who are embracing alternative and ethical lifestyles. These books also appeal to the adventuresome who want to try new cooking techniques and new foods. The titles are pitched at diverse audiences as well, for example, postpunks with *Vegan with a Vengeance* (2005), African Americans with *Vegan Soul Kitchen: Fresh, Healthy, and Creative African-American Cuisine* (2009), trend followers with *The Vegan Mediterranean Cookbook* (2001), and hipsters with *The Urban Vegan: 250 Simple, Sumptuous Recipes from Street Cart Favorites to Haute Cuisine* (2010).

See also Activism and Protests; Alcott, William A.; Alternative and Holistic Medicine; Domestic Science and Scientific Eating; Ethical Vegetarianism; Graham, Sylvester; Katzen, Mollie; Physiological Benefits; Reform; Social Acceptance; World Hunger.

Further Reading

O'Connell, Anne. *Early Vegetarian Recipes.* Devon, UK: Prospect Books, 2008.
Spencer, Colin. *Vegetarianism: A History.* Cambridge, MA: Da Capo, 2004.

Cedar Phillips

DINSHAH, H. JAY (1933–2000)

H. Jay Dinshah was the founder of the American Vegan Society and a lifelong advocate for compassionate, nonviolent living. He was a frequent guest speaker whose portfolio included speaking engagements in 19 countries as well as a prolific author of dozens of journal articles and brochures promoting vegan lifestyle choices.

Dinshah, the sixth of eight children, was raised a lacto-vegetarian in Malaga, New Jersey. His father, Dinshah P. Ghadiali, was a physician and inventor who became a vegetarian after being diagnosed with tuberculosis in the 1920s. Dinshah often pointed to his father's improved health and longevity when discussing the health benefits of vegetarian or vegan life choices.

Dinshah's interest in vegetarian living began to expand when he was in his twenties. In 1956, he began to correspond with members of the Vegan Society in England. Heavily influenced by their literature reporting the atrocities perpetrated on animals in the process of obtaining milk products, eggs, and leather, Dinshah made the choice to become a vegan and began a lifetime crusade against animal-cruelty practices. In 1960, he established the American Vegan Society, providing a voice for both vegetarian and vegan causes. In the same year, he married Freya Smith, whose parents were active in the English Vegan Society. Together, they became the driving force behind the vegan movement in the United States. In 1961, they organized a coast-to-coast crusade for veganism that in 1965 expanded to include Canada. Beginning in 1969, they held seminars at the Suncrest Educreational Center in Malaga, headquarters of the American Vegan Society.

From 1960 to 2000, Dinshah served as the president of the American Vegan Society and editor of its publication, *Ahimsa*. As the journalistic voice of the American Vegan Society, *Ahimsa* remained in publication until Dinshah's death in 2000, when the journal changed its name to *American Vegan*, in an effort to attract a more mainstream audience. The concept of ahimsa is still central to the vegan philosophy, and the journal retains the motto, "Ahimsa lights the way." *Ahimsa* is a

Sanskrit word meaning nonkilling and nonharming. Dinshah defined the essence of ahimsa in an anagram:

Abstinence from animal products
Harmlessness with reverence for life
Integrity of thought, word, and deed
Mastery over oneself
Service to humanity, nature, and creation
Advancement of understanding and truth

Rather than connoting a passive adherence to the idea of nonviolence, ahimsa refers to dynamic harmlessness, a concept that Dinshah advanced through his writing and speaking.

In 1974, Dinshah formed the North American Vegetarian Society and helped to promote the development of vegan societies across the United States. He was one of the key organizers of the 1975 World Vegetarian Congress, which was held in Orono, Maine, and sponsored by the International Vegetarian Union. Throughout his life, Dinshah was a leader in the field of vegetarianism and veganism. He held offices in the International Vegetarian Union, Vegan Society, North American Vegetarian Society, American Natural Hygiene Society, and Vegetarian Union of North America. His publications include *Out of the Jungle* (1967), *Here's Harmlessness* (1964), and *Health Can Be Harmless* (1987).

See also Activism and Protests; Ahimsa; Animal Rights and Animal Welfare; Consumer Products; Ethical Vegetarianism; Periodicals; Physiological Benefits; Reform; United Kingdom; Veganism; Vegetarianism, Types of.

Further Reading

American Vegan Society: Founder, H. Jay Dinshah. http://www.americanvegan.org/founder.htm.
Dinshah, H. Jay. "AHIMSA's On the Spot Illustrated Report of the First Latin-American Vegetarian Congress." *Ahimsa,* March–April 1973.
Hagenmayer, S. Joseph. "H. Jay Dinshah, 66, Vegan Society Leader." *Philadelphia Inquirer,* June 15, 2000. http://www.vegsource.com/articles/dinshah_inquirer.htm.
International Vegetarian Union. "Famous Vegetarians—H. Jay Dinshah (1933–2000)." http://www.ivu.org/people/politics/dinshah.html.
Miner, Judy. "H. Jay Dinshah, 1933–2000. In Memoriam." *International Vegetarian Union,* 8, no. 3 (Summer 2000). http://www.ivu.org/vuna/news/news201/jayobit.html.
Stepaniak, Joanne. "In Memoriam, H. Jay Dinshah." http://www.vegsource.com/articles/dinshah.htm.

Lisa Hudgins

DOMESTIC SCIENCE AND SCIENTIFIC EATING

The scientific approach to eating roared onto the scene in the late 19th century and came into its own in the first decades of the 20th century. This approach to diet focused primarily on the scientific properties of eating, including attention to the nutritional content of the food itself as well as factors such as the role of chewing, the combinations of foods, temperature, and serving size, among other things. Vegetarianism flourished in this climate, with increasing numbers of adherents advocating various specialized forms of vegetarian diets. Domestic science–inspired vegetarians often had little interest in the spiritual or moral arguments for their food choices and instead focused on the scientific and health reasons to forgo meat and other animal products. The combination of the "right" foods and related elements was attributed with almost-miraculous powers to heal ailments of all sorts, as well as prevent future maladies.

During the 1840s and 1850s, German scientists began to break down foods into the categories of carbohydrates, fats, minerals, protein, and water. The chemical composition of food took on great importance and shifted discussions of food and health away from the topic of quantity and refocused it on the chemical makeup of the food consumed. Chemist Wilbur Atwater led the way in the United States and believed that poor people could benefit greatly by switching from an expensive meat-based diet to one consisting of cheaper but equally efficient foods. Atwater believed vegetarianism (but not veganism) to be safe and argued that Americans could benefit by replacing much of the meat in their diets with alternative protein sources. Despite attempts by Atwater and colleagues such as Mary Hinman Abel, Ellen Richards (the "mother of home economics"), and Edward Atkinson, scientific eating, vegetarian or otherwise, never fully caught on with the poorest members of society.

The rise of domestic science as a field was greatly influenced by the increasing numbers of women entering colleges and universities in the 1870s. Women with an interest in the sciences faced limited career and educational opportunities; one of the few open pathways for women to pursue their interests was to apply them to a gendered space—in this case the female realm of the home and of the family kitchen. These new female domestic scientists took the new scientific research and turned it to the kitchen table. This approach was not without its detractors. Scientific eating, after all, had little to do with the pleasures of food.

Ella Eaton Kellogg and her husband, John Harvey Kellogg, were on the forefront of vegetarian domestic science. The two met at a Seventh-day Adventist sanitarium that John Kellogg ran at that time and married in 1879. Together, they focused on exploring and publicizing the relationship between diet and health. Ella Kellogg's *Science in the Kitchen,* published in 1893, was a result of the couple's endeavors to develop a scientifically based vegetarian diet that was easy to prepare, palatable, and, above all, healthy. She went on to found the Battle Creek Sanitarium School of Home Economics, which further spread the ideals of domestic science and of vegetarian-based scientific eating to a broader audience.

Vegetarianism, including domestic science–influenced vegetarianism, became an increasingly visible presence in American life during the first decades of the 20th century and influenced even those who were not vegetarian. Dora Roper, the nonvegetarian author of the 1914 book *Scientific Feeding,* provided a vegetarian-specific supplement for her book as well as integrating vegetarian arguments inside the main text. Like her contemporaries, Roper used a language devoid of emotions and taste to discuss "feeding." She believed that the elimination of certain types of foods, the "correct chemical food combinations" (both within recipes as well as within the framework of the larger meal), and the appropriate preparation techniques would prevent malnutrition, stave off disease, cure insanity, and diminish "criminal tendencies." Like most domestic scientists, Roper saw food as something that is to be mastered, not enjoyed. While she did not actively argue for vegetarian diet, she warned readers against eating meat in great quantities, stressing quality over quantity. She also warned of food safety issues from refrigerated storage of meat and of "forced and improper feeding of animals" and claimed that animal products—meat, eggs, and dairy—from force-fed animals should be avoided.

During World War I, the U.S. government validated the arguments of the vegetarian and vegetarian-supportive domestic scientists when the Food Administration began to actively promote the replacement of meat and meat-derived products, including lard, with vegetarian alternatives. Extensive publicity campaigns, education efforts, and outreach efforts made forgoing meat, or at least consuming less of it, a patriotic act that required no sacrifice of health. While government attempts to change eating habits or encourage a scientific approach to nutrition were not entirely successful, they did help to firmly root the concept of nutrition in American minds.

The discovery of vitamins, starting with vitamin B in 1911, was a late development in the move toward scientific eating. While scientists and nutritionists had been focusing on the different categories of food, the tendency was to treat all carbohydrates or all proteins as equal. This had, in part, helped the embrace of vegetarianism, as it treated meat as no different from other protein sources. Discovery of vitamins' existence did not mean that scientists could yet measure specific amounts of a given vitamin in food or create or package vitamins in pill form. The increasing knowledge of vitamins made it simultaneously easier both for vegetarians to defend their diet as complete and nutritionally sound and for detractors to point to perceived vitamin deficiencies they argued could be adequately filled only by eating meat.

The domestic science and scientific eating revolution of the late 19th and early 20th century has left its mark. While many people today highly value the taste and appearance of food, the science behind eating continues to play an important role in American life, and the belief in the power of a highly prescriptive diet to work miracles persists. Scientific advances seem to have shown that vegetarian diets are sound, although there continue to be arguments over what type of vegetarian diet is best and, depending on one's viewpoint, which meats or animal products are to be embraced or avoided in the name of science.

See also Battle Creek Sanitarium; Cookbooks; Kellogg, John Harvey; Physiological Benefits; Reform; Seventh-day Adventists; Social Acceptance.

Further Reading

Elias, Megan J. *Stir It Up: Home Economics in American Culture.* Philadelphia: University of Pennsylvania Press, 2008.

Iacobbo, Karen, and Michael Iacobbo. *Vegetarian America: A History.* Westport, CT: Praeger, 2004.

Kellogg, Ella Eaton. *Science in the Kitchen.* Chicago: Modern Medicine, 1893.

Levenstein, Harvey. *Revolution at the Table: The Transformation of the American Diet.* Berkeley: University of California Press, 2003.

Cedar Phillips

EASTERN RELIGIONS, INFLUENCES OF

Hindu, Jain, Buddhist, and to some extent Taoist traditions have helped to shape vegetarian thinking and practices in the West and have broadened their cultural base. As historical events have brought diverse peoples into contact, and as literacy, international commerce and travel, immigration, and other trends have accelerated over the past two centuries, strong interest has developed in other cultures, customs, languages, and cuisines, as well as in alternative lifestyles, conceptions of health, and dietary regimes.

Hinduism, the most ancient of the world's major religions, yields several foundations for vegetarianism. The Vedas are considered the oldest and most authoritative Hindu scriptures. According to Vedic teachings, continued later in the Upanishads, all creatures manifest the same life force and therefore merit equal care and compassion. The soul embodied in living things, whether human or nonhuman, is to be venerated without distinction, and as kindness toward animals yields kindness toward humans, it must be carefully cultivated. Other Hindu texts—the *Ramayana* and the *Mahabharata* (which includes the *Bhagavad Gita*)— promote vegetarian diets. The *Bhagavad Gita* prescribes that fruits, vegetables, grains, nuts, and dairy products are appropriate devotional offerings, and those who make such offerings prior to eating are specially blessed. Because respect, kindness, and compassion must be shown to kindred living beings, the idea of nonviolent behavior toward animals naturally follows.

Additional reasons for adopting vegetarianism are also found within Hinduism and, to some extent, Sikhism, another religion originating in India. A main reason is that caring for animals creates good karma (cosmic consequences of one's actions) as one journeys toward spiritual purity and self-betterment. This helps a person to avoid bad karma in this life (eating an animal that has suffered greatly and/or is a reincarnated human) or the next life (having a miserable existence, becoming an animal that is food for humans or for the kinds of animals one has eaten in this life). Clearly, Hinduism's ethical teachings and sense of spiritual kinship, which resonate with Western traditions and movements of thought, have had an impact, while other doctrines, concerning offerings to gods and karmic consequences, have not. Hinduism's influence in the West has been enhanced by the International Society for Krishna Consciousness (Hare Krishna movement) and the activities of gurus with significant followings.

Jainism, dating from sixth-century BC India, also embraced the doctrines of karma, reincarnation (cycles of rebirth), the possession of souls by other creatures, and liberation of the human soul by means of right conduct and ritual. Beyond this, Jainism is alone among the world's religions in featuring resolute dedication to the principle of nonviolence, also known as *ahimsa,* or nonharm. The Jain way of life seeks to avoid causing harm to any living thing, and because there are gradations of souls throughout nature, this entails adherents' eating as little as is minimally necessary, forgoing honey (an animal product), root vegetables (which host abundant microorganisms), or any fruits that may contain insects. The image of Jains wearing masks and sweeping their pathway in order to prevent breathing in or stepping on tiny life-forms is fairly well known. Any occupation that might cause animal suffering, even indirectly, is off-limits. Jain practices that show kindness, concern, and abstinence from causing harm are sometimes held to be self-motivated, prompted by an interest in one's own future spiritual destiny. This is true but only in part, because believers also understand that personal good depends on, and is even constituted in part by, the good brought about in other lives with which they are interrelated. Jain communities in the West are growing, with an estimated 100,000 faithful in North America and 25,000 in England at present.

Interdependency is likewise very close to the heart of Buddhism, which sees it as an essential feature of existence for both living and nonliving things. The origin of Buddhism can be more accurately dated, since its founding figure, Siddhartha Gautama, an Indian prince, lived approximately 563–483 BC. Central to Buddhism is the idea of suffering as universal, meaning not continuous but unavoidable. Suffering is caused by desire, and to eliminate desire is the path of human betterment. Freedom from desire is achieved by overcoming attachment to things, including material goods, aided by the realization that whatever exists, including oneself, is impermanent. Therefore, clinging to life, possessions, other persons, and objects of desire is pointless. The separation between oneself and other suffering beings is illusory, as all are connected. Hence, Buddhism enjoins against causing harm and strongly promotes compassion. For many Buddhists this translates, in part, into vegetarianism, because the rearing and killing of animals for food causes pain and the ultimate harm of a violent end, the slaughter. Buddhism has been popularized in the West by the Dalai Lama, spiritual leader of Tibet, and by the Vietnamese monk, Zen master, and peace activist Thich Nhat Hanh, among others.

Taoism (or Daoism), a Chinese system of thought that probably dates from the sixth century BC, has attracted much attention in the West. This outlook, conveyed in the *Daodejing* (*Tao Te Ching*) and *Zhuangzi* (*Chuang-tzu*), is not as explicitly applicable to dietary matters as are Hinduism, Jainism, and Buddhism. But with its emphasis on noninterference with nature, living in simplicity and peacefulness, and actions showing kindness, humility, and nondomination, many regard it as favoring vegetarianism.

The idea of nonviolence has spread globally through the teachings of Mohandas Gandhi (1869–1948), a lawyer, spiritual leader, and central figure in the liberation of India from British colonial rule. Gandhi was the architect of the kind of strategic, courageous, and committed nonviolence that energized the American civil rights movement of the 1950s and 1960s and many subsequent movements for political change around the world. Drawing inspiration from several sources—including Hinduism, Jainism, Christianity, and the writings of Russian novelist Leo Tolstoy, American essayist and proponent of civil disobedience Henry David Thoreau, and English philosopher Henry Salt—Gandhi affirmed the morally superior power of truth and nonviolence, even in the face of violence against oneself, and the principle of causing no harm by acts, thoughts, or words. In Gandhi's view, nonviolence makes vegetarianism obligatory both as an expression of reverence for creation and unity with all life-forms and as the path of least harm or peacefulness.

With the exception of Jains, not all adherents of the Eastern belief systems are vegetarians, and sometimes there are cases where the killing of animals is thought justified, such as in self-defense or to avoid starvation. However, paramount is that killing can never be done thoughtlessly or when alternatives such as other food sources are readily available.

See also Activism and Protests; Ahimsa; Animal Rights and Animal Welfare; Asia; Ethical Vegetarianism; Gandhi, Mohandas; India; Jainism; Meat and Violence; Reform; Religious Beliefs and Practices; Salt, Henry S.; Transcendentalism; Vegetarians and Vegans, Celebrity; Vegetarians and Vegans, Noted.

Further Reading

Chapple, Christopher K. *Nonviolence to Animals, Earth, and Self in Asian Traditions.* Albany: State University of New York Press, 1993.
Fox, Michael Allen. *Deep Vegetarianism.* Philadelphia: Temple University Press, 1999.
Gandhi, Mohandas Karamchand. *The Moral Basis of Vegetarianism.* Compiled by R. K. Prabhu. Ahmedabad, India: Navajivan, 1959.
Walters, Kerry S., and Lisa Portmess, eds. *Religious Vegetarianism: From Hesiod to the Dalai Lama.* Albany: State University of New York Press, 2001.

Michael Allen Fox

ECOFEMINISM

Ecofeminism, which emerged in the 1970s and 1980s, asserts that all forms of oppression, from racism to sexism to classism to speciesism, are connected.

There is no one orthodox ecofeminism, but rather there are myriad ecofeminisms; the intersection of feminist and environmental practices, theories, and activisms defines its overarching position. Ecofeminism tends to challenge structures rather than individuals, though certainly individuals are held responsible for acts within its cultural critique. Just as ecofeminism is not monolithic, ecofeminists approach the topic and practice of vegetarianism from varied positions.

A foundational ecofeminist claim is that patriarchal structures incorporate dualistic hierarchies in order to reinforce their dominance: mind/body, human/animal, male/female, culture/nature, black/white. It has been posited that all of these binaries must be dismantled, or humanity and nature as a whole will remain "divided against itself." To understand the complexities of these positions, it is helpful to consider several different approaches including the starting point of feminist vegetarianism, the move to an ecofeminist vegetarian ethic, and the various critiques of these positions from within ecofeminism.

Feminist vegetarianism is the starting point for ecofeminist vegetarian theories. Carol Adams's seminal 1990 work, *The Sexual Politics of Meat: A Feminist-Vegetarian Critical Theory*, begins with the claim that "people with power have always eaten meat" (26). She continues by describing the interwoven cultural positions of meat eating and masculinity, as well as the presentation of women's bodies as pieces of meat to be consumed. Her theory of the absent referent is central to this argument. Adams states that "a dead body replaces the live animal." As a result, they (animals) "are absent from the act of eating meat because they have been transformed into food" (40). Language is central to this process as, for example, a cow becomes a steak or a pig becomes bacon. In a similar way, patriarchal societies, through language and structure, construct the male as the norm and the female as the other who is similarly the absent referent.

The ecofeminist vegetarian ethic moves beyond the connection between female humans and other animals to the oppression of the planet as a whole. First, it does so by uncovering and critiquing meat production in the contemporary world. Over the course of the 20th century, meat production shifted from a local, small-scale practice to an industrial, large-scale practice. Confined animal feeding operations (CAFOs), the designation for these factory farms, not only harm animals on a massive scale unequaled before in human history but also have a detrimental impact on the environment as a whole. In the United States alone, over 10 billion animals were killed for food in 2007 (the U.S. Department of Agriculture provides daily slaughter figures). In addition, a 2006 United Nations report stated that livestock operations generated 18 percent of all anthropogenic greenhouse gas emissions, surpassing emissions from the transportation sector. What one eats even more than what one drives affects the earth's climate. These global impacts of meat eating, along with the ethical implications of the massive suffering that occurs as part of the CAFO system, provide a basic foundation for an ecofeminist vegetarian position. Choosing a vegetarian diet is an obvious move into solidarity with other animals, oppressed humans, and the planet as a whole. Such a practice manifests a general ecofeminist ethic of care.

A second ecofeminist vegetarian turn is influenced by its focus on embodiment. Ecofeminists critique the lack of attention to bodies in most Western philosophical, political, and economic systems. Indeed, not only are bodies ignored but they are also degraded or abused, while minds or intellects are elevated and praised. This denial of embodiment has a particularly powerful impact on women's and animals' bodies. Both are viewed as cheap sources of labor and reproduction. The masculine power structure emphasizes mind over matter; therefore, certain bodies are expendable. Animals' bodies in the food-production system are the cheapest and most expendable of all.

Several scholars and activists have critiqued the underlying assumption of ecofeminism—that the oppression of women and the oppression of nature are transcultural and transhistorical. For example, it has been pointed out that women and nature are not associated in Chinese society, but women are still in an inferior social position. Similarly, it has been suggested that ecofeminism tends to ignore cultural, ethnic, and racial differences when it links women and animals, as well as when it links other forms of oppression. Others point to a cultural imperialism inherent in the primarily Western call for vegetarianism. In some cultures, meat eating has not been the norm for most humans. In other cultures, traditional hunting practices are often viewed as balancing species in the ecosystem. From all of these perspectives the primarily Western approach to ecofeminism has been challenged.

Many ecofeminists continue to call for a holistic examination of how food is raised, distributed, and culturally defined, even while they recognize that the traditional ecofeminist analysis is influenced by Western philosophical and cultural systems. As the American diet of meat eating, and along with it the industrial systems of mass production, are exported to other parts of the world, ecofeminists continue to point to the interconnected nature of environmental degradation, animal suffering, and bodies—those of women and those of other-than-human animals. From this perspective, vegetarianism is a necessary embodiment of philosophical, moral, and activist positions.

See also Activism and Protests; Agribusiness; Animal Rights and Animal Welfare; Ethical Vegetarianism; Global Warming; Meat and Violence; Reform.

Further Reading

Adams, Carol J. *The Sexual Politics of Meat: A Feminist-Vegetarian Critical Theory.* New York: Continuum, 1990.

Gaard, Greta, ed. *Ecofeminism: Women, Animals, Nature.* Philadelphia: Temple University Press, 1993.

Griffin, Susan. *Woman and Nature: The Roaring Inside Her.* San Francisco: Harper & Row, 1978.

Haraway, Donna. *Modest_Witness@Second_Millennium. FemaleMan Meets OncoMouse.* New York: Routledge, 1997.

Laura Hobgood-Oster

ETHICAL VEGETARIANISM

Ethical vegetarianism began in the West with the Orphic and Pythagorean traditions in ancient Greece. Both of these sects told of an original Golden Age in which human beings lived in peace with the gods and other animals in a paradise similar to the Garden of Eden. They also taught a doctrine of reincarnation that influenced Plato and is similar to that of the Hindu, Buddhist, and Jain traditions of cyclic existence. According to the Neoplatonic philosopher Porphyry, warfare between humans and greed for possessions first entered society with the slaughtering of animals for food. By abstaining from animal food, Pythagoreans and Neoplatonists believed that they could free themselves from sin and achieve divine wisdom. This early Greek vegetarianism was not merely mystery-oriented or cultic: Killing animals for food was held to constitute real harm to other creatures in addition to its role in fostering vengeful attitudes toward other humans. Other classical writers, such as Seneca, Plutarch, Ovid, and Diogenes, either practiced vegetarianism or expressed vegetarian sympathies as a means of stemming cruelty and selfishness in the moral life.

In contrast, the Judeo-Christian tradition largely advocated humane husbandry and slaughter rather than ethical vegetarianism, but exemplars in both Jewish and Christian traditions have been vegetarian dating from ancient times. Samson and Daniel practiced vegetarianism, and John the Baptist, a sort of divine hunter-gatherer, practiced something similar. The scriptural tradition—referred to as the Nazarite vow (Num. 6)—required abstinence from intoxicants and prohibited cutting the hair and beard. While this vow may not have required vegetarianism, abstinence from meat seems to be practiced by many biblical characters associated with it. This tradition influenced Orthodox Judaism and Rastafarianism, and some adherents of both groups practice vegetarianism as a more strict form of dietary regulation that avoids unscriptural harm to animals. While these groups have religious and political dimensions, ethical concerns clearly play a part in their motivations.

Modern Western vegetarianism began with the utilitarian movement in philosophy in the 18th and 19th centuries, which taught that human aims can be judged based on the "greatest happiness" principle. Founders like Jeremy Bentham and John Stuart Mill taught that those actions can be judged good that maximize the pleasure and minimize the harm to the greatest number of creatures. These founding figures included nonhuman animals in the moral calculus because the animals could experience pleasure and pain, regardless of the question of animal sentience. Utilitarianism, most basically, states that those actions will be morally correct that promote the good for the greatest number of individuals, where "individuals" is defined as those beings capable of experiencing pleasure and pain. In addition to concern for animals, many social reform efforts stemmed from utilitarianism, including animal welfare, child welfare, and education for women, followed later by women's suffrage. In the United States, many of these causes were championed by Henry Bergh, founder of the American Society for the Prevention of Cruelty to Animals and the New York Society for the Prevention of Cruelty to Children.

Beginning in the 1970s, philosophers such as Peter Singer and Tom Regan revived utilitarianism and provoked serious philosophical interest in the question of animal suffering in medical research, factory farming, and the fur trade. At the same time, the New Age movement brought Hindu and Buddhist ideas into mainstream American consciousness. Eastern philosophies appeared to some Americans as an antidote to the materialism and traditionalism that had allowed both the ravages of the Vietnam War and the denial of civil rights to African Americans. Growing health consciousness also influenced the cultural milieu, and more and more Americans began meditating, exercising, and eating vegetarian as part of an overall cruelty-free lifestyle.

In the East, vegetarianism has much more pervasive and long-standing traditions. Jain vegetarianism reaches back to its founder, Vardhamana Mahavira, in the 500s BC and is probably the most austere form of all practices of *ahimsa,* or nonharming. Jains eat only plant food whose harvesting does not entail the destruction of the plant; hence, even root vegetables are not eaten. Some sects of Jainism in India still wear ritual masks to keep from unconsciously inhaling microscopic organisms. Jain monastics are encouraged to watch where they step and avoid disturbing the soil, lest they unwittingly kill or disturb an insect or earthworm.

Among Buddhists worldwide, ahimsa is an important value, although not as pervasive as one might think. The climate of Tibet, for example, did not lend itself to the cultivation of vegetables, and monks and laity in Tibet and the Tibetan diaspora of Vajrayāna often do eat meat. Refraining from eating meat is also a question of the degree of religious observance and the degree of Westernization in any of the schools of Buddhism, in a way that is analogous to Jews and Muslims who occasionally eat pork products.

Of the religions originating in India, the many branches of *Sanātana Dharma,* or Hinduism, perhaps have the claim to the oldest practice of vegetarianism, although Jainism may be at least partially responsible for that reform. The earliest Brahmanic sacrifices did involve the sacrifice of animals, and some goddess-based worshippers still sacrifice animals today. Among Hindu vegetarians, milk products are generally allowed, because they are considered a gift from the cow, the beloved docile animal associated with Lord Śiva and other deities.

Today, the choice for ethical vegetarianism in the West is influenced by a variety of considerations. While numbers are difficult to obtain and vary widely, according to the Vegetarian Resource Group, between 2 and 6 percent of all American adults practice some version of vegetarianism. In addition to the intrinsic wrong of harming living creatures, some vegetarians cite the need to conserve world resources like land and water as reasons to eat a plant-based diet. The scientific consensus has also shifted away from the view that animals are mere automata, and a variety of studies now confirm that other animals, ranging from rats to monkeys to insects to whales, have emotions, preferences, and other faculties that can be considered thinking. Even among people who still eat meat, some show a willingness to reduce their intake of animal products and abstain from at least some forms of animal exploitation, such as the consumption of veal and foie gras.

Vegetarians, however, differ from each other in their eating preferences almost as much as they differ from meat eaters. Vegans, who eat no meat, dairy, or eggs and avoid all animal-based products, argue that the egg and dairy industries are just as abusive as other factory farming operations. Vegans cite the fact that the dairy and meat industries are not separate industries at all, as most of the beef consumed in the United States comes from spent dairy cows. Dairy- and egg-eating (lacto-/ovo-) vegetarians believe that the harm caused by eating dairy and eggs is less than that caused by eating flesh and is therefore more permissible. Vegetarians can find allies in those with similar concerns, as in the raw food, slow food, and macrobiotic movements.

For most Americans, the group People for the Ethical Treatment of Animals (PETA) automatically springs to mind at the mention of vegetarianism or veganism. The group, founded in 1980, has had a long string of campaign victories, including elimination of animal testing from the automotive industry and many cosmetics companies. In the near-absence of federal oversight over animal cruelty, PETA plays an important role in pressuring companies and governments to abide by anticruelty legislation already on the books. PETA has come under attack, however, from feminists and other sympathizers because of its ad campaigns that have been held to demean women. Its street-level actions have also been targeted as unnecessarily shocking and radical. PETA supporters counter that such demonstrations help to capture the attention of a media-saturated culture and bring the message closer to the point of origin, for example, the laboratory, fast food restaurant, or department store.

PETA's official stance against all human use of animals in entertainment, food, and experimentation is not shared by all organizations in the humane movement. While PETA is certainly the most visible and well-known animal activist organization in the United States, many organizations work for the protection of animals from a broad spectrum of views, including welfare-oriented perspectives. Organizations like Farm Animal Reform Movement (FARM) and the Humane Farming Association, though they may encourage vegetarianism, also appeal to meat eaters by advocating for a return to more traditional farming methods. This approach allows for the possibility that meat eating is not unethical as such, but care should be taken to ensure that the animal has freedom of movement and healthy living conditions in accordance with the needs of its species.

Ethical vegetarians, vegan or not, remain a minority faced with the enormous task of opposing the many traditional uses of animals. Evidence suggests, however, that attitudes toward animals have begun to change over the past few decades. Many law schools now have concentrations in animal issues, states and cities have passed anticruelty legislation, and the popular media abound with news stories about animal sentience. Ethical vegetarians may not convince large numbers of meat eaters to change their diets in the coming years, but they will continue to serve as a conscientious voice against widespread animal cruelty.

See also Activism and Protests; Agribusiness; Ahimsa; Animal Rights and Animal Welfare; Antivivisection; Eastern Religions, Influences of; Global Warming; Jainism; Meatless Diets before Vegetarianism; Organic Foods and Technology; People for the Ethical Treatment of Animals; Reform; Religious Beliefs and Practices; Singer, Peter; Veganism; Vegetarianism, Types of; World Hunger.

Further Reading

Bekoff, Marc. *Animals Matter: A Biologist Explains Why We Should Treat Animals with Compassion and Respect.* New York: Shambhala, 2007.

Farm Animal Reform Movement (FARM). www.farmusa.org.

Feuerstein, George. *The Deeper Dimension of Yoga: Theory and Practice.* Boston: Shambhala, 2003.

Humane Farming Association. www.hfa.org.

People for the Ethical Treatment of Animals (PETA). www.peta.org.

Singer, Peter. *Animal Liberation.* New York: Harper, 2001.

Stuart, Tristram. *The Bloodless Revolution: A Cultural History of Vegetarianism from 1600 to Modern Times.* New York: W.W. Norton, 2007.

Vegetarian Resource Group. http://www.vrg.org/index.htm.

Walters, Kerry S., and Lisa Portmess, eds. *Religious Vegetarianism: From Hesiod to the Dalai Lama.* Albany: State University of New York Press, 2001.

David Dillard-Wright

ETHNIC AND RACIAL GROUPS, U.S.

For many ethnic groups in the United States, vegetarian and plant-based diets are actually closer to the traditional dietary practices of their recent cultural ancestors. Due to a variety of historical and socioeconomic circumstances over the last several centuries, however, high levels of meat consumption have become the norm among these U.S. minority populations. With the increase in meat and dairy consumption, several American minority groups have seen a parallel and disproportionate rise in related chronic ailments and disease. This has prompted many to return to vegetarian or plant-based diets for the purposes of improving health.

A number of Native American groups can be looked at as early examples of this dietary transition. Before the arrival of European settlers, most Native Americans survived predominantly on a vast array of agricultural crops and grains like melons, root vegetables, beans, and corn. With the introduction of horses by the Spanish in the 1500s and, later, guns by European American settlers, many Native American groups gave up their agricultural lifestyle and began to focus on hunting. As range animals went extinct and geographic and economic marginalization of Native Americans continued into the 20th century, these communities lost access to high-quality fruits and vegetables. While some Native Americans have retained or rediscovered plant-based diets in the late 20th and early 21st centuries, often as a means to treat chronic health maladies, there is currently not a widespread vegetarian movement among Native Americans. Traditional Native American staples like blue corn, amaranth, and sweet potatoes remain popular vegetarian options and serve as a testament to the enduring influence of Native American agriculture on the vegetarian lifestyle in the United States.

The Latino population has undergone a similar transformation in more recent years. While meat plays a role in the dietary traditions, rice, beans, tortillas, tropical fruits, and vegetables have historically been the culinary centerpieces. Today, Latinos have one of the lowest fruit and vegetable intakes of any American ethnic group. As chronic diseases like obesity, diabetes, and hypertension have run rampant in the Latino community, there have been a number of efforts to communicate the value of a plant-based diet to Latinos. For instance, People for the Ethical Treatment of Animals (PETA) maintains a Spanish-language Web site with information and resources tailored to the Latino community. As demand has risen, items like soy chorizo and tofu tacos have been made available in some grocery stores and restaurants. The Latino community can claim several notable vegetarians as well, including Mexican American farmworker and nonviolence activist Cesar Chavez and his niece, Camila Chavez.

Over the last several centuries, African American culinary practices have followed a parallel path to those of Native Americans and Latinos, although the vegetarian movement in the African American community appears to be significantly stronger. The diet of early African American slaves consisted mainly of organically grown vegetables along with scant amounts of undesirable meat scraps that were given to them by their slave masters. Eventually, however, meat became a focal point of African American "soul food." In recognition of growing African American health disparities, several influential African Americans of the 1960s and 1970s wrote about the benefits of vegetarianism and natural health. Nation of Islam leader Elijah Muhammad urged his followers to pursue a vegetarian diet that was free from processed and refined foods. Popular comedian and social activist Dick Gregory also railed against contemporary soul food in his writings and commentaries, as he espoused the benefits of his raw food diet.

A number of entrepreneurs, celebrity advocates, and other members of the African American community have worked to spread the word on the positive value of vegetarianism. While concerns for animal welfare and the environmental implications of meat production have played a role in these efforts, the movement for vegetarianism in the African American community is fundamentally about the improvement of health. Several vegan soul food cookbooks have been published, and successful vegetarian soul food restaurants in Atlanta, Washington, D.C., Chicago, Los Angeles, and elsewhere serve up vegan versions of soul food dishes. Community-based nonprofit organizations like the Black Vegetarian Society of Georgia provide resources to African Americans who are interested in switching to a plant-based diet and host events and lectures that promote holistic health. Similar organizations exist in Texas, New York, and North Carolina. Notable African American thinkers and celebrities—including the late Coretta Scott King and her son Dexter King, Alice Walker, Prince and Russell Simmons—have been outspoken in their commitment to vegetarianism. In addition, several online communities for African American vegetarians provide an outlet for discussion, the sharing of vegetarian recipes, and professional and social networking.

Other American ethnic and religious groups have strong vegetarian communities as well. Throughout the county, Asian and Indian vegetarian restaurants proliferate, their ethnic grocery stores provide a variety of vegetarian options, and countless Asian and Indian cookbooks and recipes cater to the vegetarian diet. Considering the role of animal sacrifice and meat eating in Islamic culture, Muslims would seem unlikely vegetarians. Many Muslim Americans, however, have pointed to the incompatibility between Islamic *halal* dietary practices and factory farming and have opted to become vegetarians in response.

Jewish Americans are another notable ethnic group with a vibrant and active vegetarian community. Advocates argue that vegetarian diets are in line with the most important biblical commandments, which include the protection of human health, compassion for animals, preservation of the environment, conservation of resources, the provision of charity to hungry people, and the pursuit of peace. The Jewish Vegetarians of North America (JVNA) is one prominent organization working in this area. Their Web site (JewishVeg.com) serves as a major reference point on the connections between Judaism and vegetarianism and provides practical advice on Jewish vegetarian activism. The Jewish Vegetarians of North America also produced a documentary, *A Sacred Duty,* which focuses on how Jewish teachings and vegetarianism can help address global environmental dilemmas. Another active organization is Jews for Animal Rights, founded by Roberta Kalechofsky. Kalechofsky operates Micah Publications, which publishes books on Judaism and vegetarian life. In recent years, a number of Jewish vegetarian voices and communities have emerged on the Internet, which has allowed for greater information exchange and community-building among Jewish American vegetarians as well as Jews in Israel and abroad.

See also Africa; Eastern Religions, Influences of; Global Warming; India; Jainism; Physiological Benefits; Religious Beliefs and Practices; Vegetarians and Vegans, Celebrity; Vegetarians and Vegans, Noted; World Hunger.

Further Reading

Gregory, Dick. *Dick Gregory's Natural Diet for Folks Who Eat.* New York: Harper & Row, 1973.

Laws, Rita. "Native Americans and Vegetarianism." *Vegetarian Journal* (September 1994): http://www.ivu.org/history/native_americans.html.

Schwartz, Richard. *Judaism and Vegetarianism.* New York: Lantern Books, 2001.

Garrett Broad

EUROPE

Europe is the cradle of modern vegetarianism. Although the word "vegetarianism" was coined only in 1847 in England by the founding of the Vegetarian Society, vegetarian ideas about health, animal ethics, and food economy were shaped from the late 17th century on. Support for vegetarianism gained momentum in the 19th and 20th centuries, spread to other parts of the world, namely, the United States, and influenced current food debates and practices.

The origins of vegetarianism in the early modern period are, first, classical vegetarian texts, surfacing due to the general resurgence of the study of classical sources. Second, increasing world trade brought knowledge about other cultures, notably India, which adheres to the doctrine of *ahimsa,* nonviolence to all living creatures. Third, debates about the nature of man throughout Europe—and consequentially the significance and meanings of diet—were boosted by emerging scientific developments. These old, faraway, and new ideas blended with elements from the Christian tradition: ascesis, good stewardship of creation, and the image of paradise as vegetarian utopia. Since the late 17th century, a continuous vegetarian cultural tradition can be traced, making Leonardo da Vinci's ethical vegetarianism foremost proof of the human's exceptional status.

Motives for meat abstinence were from the beginning often an integral part of a radical political agenda of pacifism and egalitarianism, as in the case of the Englishman Roger Crab (1621–1680), author of *The English Hermite,* and his followers. The Eastern influence is clear in the work and life of another Englishman, Thomas Tryon (1634–1703). In his *An East-Indian Brackmanny or Heathen-Philosopher, and a French Gentleman* (1683), the Brahmin is morally victorious over the European, largely because of his respect for all animal life. From Tryon on, vegetarianism would be part and parcel of animal rights, though not necessarily the other way around.

This ethical and cultural critical content of vegetarianism became invariably connected to ideas about health, longevity, and the proper food for humankind. The classical ideal of a sober lifestyle, distinguished by virtues like temperance and self-control, perfectly fit a herbivorous diet, as meat was associated with luxury and overindulgence. The supposedly anatomical concordance between humans and fruit-eating animals, with their similar teeth and guts, gave weight to this belief. Revived by the French philosopher and priest Pierre Gassendi (1592–1655), the construction of humans as frugivorous creatures was invigorated by 18th-century science: If the plant-eating orangutan was nearest to *Homo sapiens,* so the argument went, the latter was presumably also herbivorous in nature. Widespread as these and related ideas became, without an ethical impetus they seldom gave rise to strict vegetarianism. Influential temperance writers from Luigi Cornaro (1467–1566) to Christian Wilhelm Hufeland (1762–1836) warned against meat eating but did not ban it.

The growth of scientific knowledge helped to spread ideas about vegetarianism. It contributed to an attack on scriptural truths, which in turn made a belief in a personal God give way to more pantheistic beliefs or, in some cases, to atheism. As a result, not only the biblical justification for meat eating evaporated—opening up possibilities for vegetarian beliefs—but also nature gained more prominence as an object of reverence, as a moral compass, and as a site where the good, the true, and the beautiful were inextricably united. Already reflected in Jean-Jacques Rousseau's ideals of a vegetarian education, this was elaborated in the oeuvre of the French writer Jacques-Henri Bernandin de Saint-Pierre (1737–1814). John Frank Newton's *The Return to Nature* (1811) is also a case in point, as is *A Vindication of Natural Diet* (1813) by Newton's famous associate, the romantic poet Percy Bysshe Shelley.

Shelley also testified to the ongoing revolutionary appeal of vegetarianism. Earlier attempts, notably by the Scottish revolutionary John Oswald, to found a vegetarian society by expanding the French ideals of *liberté, égalité,* and *fraternité* toward the whole animal kingdom had failed miserably. But for some, like the French philosopher Jean-Antoine Gleïzès (1773–1843), the terror and bloodshed into which the French Revolution had descended only underlined the need for a true and complete regeneration of the human race: Society had to be radically changed by naturalizing it. For similar reasons, revolution and vegetarianism continued to travel together in the 19th century, exemplified by such different revolutionaries as the leading figure of the German revolution of 1848, Gustav von Struve (1805–1870); protagonists of the Paris Commune in 1871 like the anarchists Élysée Reclus (1830–1905) and Louise Michel (1830–1905); and the famous Russian prophet of individual life reform, Leo Tolstoy (1828–1910).

With industrialization and urbanization accelerating, the attraction of a return to nature to solve social disruptions and woes associated with modernity increased steadily. In England, where these developments hit first, interest in vegetarianism was not just confined to radical circles but also blossomed, understandably, in movements turning against Enlightenment reason and its consequences. Originating from the Methodist Church, whose founder, John Wesley, lived as a vegetarian, and the New Church, based on the teachings of the Swedish mystic Emanuel Swedenborg, who discouraged meat eating, the Bible Christian Church was founded in 1809 and its congregation had to take a vow to abstain from meat. It was from this Bible Christian Church that the Vegetarian Society was founded in 1847; it is still in existence as the Vegetarian Society of the United Kingdom. Vegetarianism started to become institutionalized to different degrees throughout Europe.

The first German vegetarian society also had religious roots, albeit rationalistic and liberal in kind. The leader of the Free Religious Movement in Nordhausen, the Reverend Edward Baltzer (1814–1887), began his Verein für naturgemässe Lebensführung in 1866. Through it, he preached vegetarianism, equating it with a new, secular religion, with some success. Other societies sprang up, and in the next decades vegetarianism became a key ingredient in a new bodily culture, celebrating the outdoors, sunbathing, sport, nudity, chastity, pureness, and strength. This appeal of bodily health as armor against the decadence, alienation, degeneration, and fatigue of which contemporary culture was accused would remain popular and suited different ideologies, from socialism to Nazism.

Vegetarians in the rest of Europe soon organized as well. Vegetarian societies were founded in Austria-Hungary (in Vienna in 1878, Budapest in 1884, and Prague in 1891), France (1879), Switzerland (1880), the Netherlands (1894), Sweden (1895), Denmark (1896), Belgium (1897), Italy (1899), and Russia (1901). In addition, vegetarianism was exported to colonies. Vegetarian societies were

WITHDRAWN
COLORADO SPRINGS, COLORADO LIBRARY

established in New Zealand (1882), Australia (1886), India (1889), and the Dutch East Indies (1920s). In Europe around the turn of the 20th century, tens of vegetarian health clinics, dozens of vegetarian colonies (notably Eden in Oranienburg and Monte Verità in Ascona), and hundreds of vegetarian restaurants were established. Knowledge began to travel fast and to reach mass audiences. Vegetarian cookbooks were published, new techniques used, and recipes invented, some of which went mainstream, such as Bircher Benner's muesli or the practice of eating raw vegetables. Nevertheless, although popular in circles of theosophists, feminists, Christian-anarchists, Fabians, and the like, vegetarianism was restricted to a tiny percentage of the European population and mainly found in the middle and upper classes.

Much of vegetarian dietary theories were often dismissed as pseudoscience, but from 1900 on the orthodox medical community had to reluctantly accept that a vegetarian diet could indeed be healthy. Modern food science, emerging in the mid- to late 19th century, had put a strong emphasis on animal proteins and fats, considering vegetables and fruit as mere decoration. But after the discovery of vitamins, plant-based diets were reevaluated, although seldom recommended. Yet World War I put the merits of vegetarianism in the forefront. With the import of animal feed becoming difficult if not impossible due to the Allied naval blockade, agriculture had to focus on crops rather than livestock so as to adequately feed the population. Some countries, such as Denmark and the Netherlands, turned into half-vegetarian states by 1917 and succeeded in preventing starvation. In Germany, in contrast, food shortages resulting from farms left unattended by farmers sent to war led to widespread hunger and suffering. Although highly exaggerated, there was some truth in the view held by some that the Germans were defeated, in part, by a lack of sufficient food and other supplies.

This economic principle of vegetarianism—eating low on the food chain is generally more efficient than growing crops for livestock to eat—proved even more important during World War II, but ironically, the war destroyed much of prewar vegetarian culture and hopes. Postwar reconstruction gave rise to an unprecedented intensification and industrialization of animal production. If meatless meals were associated with war, hunger, and misery, daily meat consumption became the epitome of prosperity.

Vegetarianism gained momentum again in the era following the Vietnam War. This happened mainly in the slipstream of the countercultural movement of young people in western Europe who were revolting against the establishment. Out of the desire to show solidarity, vegetarian economics became a key argument in debates about fighting hunger in developing countries. And following the rise of an environmental consciousness in the 1970s, concerns grew strong about the destructive impact of animal production in terms of deforestation, loss of biodiversity, pollution, use of antibiotics, and the spread of contagious diseases. In recent years, as climate change began to dominate the environmental debate, animal production was found to be the single largest contributor to greenhouse gas emissions. Furthermore, in an ever-expanding world of concrete and plastic, "naturalness" was again to be cherished. To fill the rapidly growing void created by secularization, a renewed search began for other forms of spirituality, tailored to the New Age, and meat consumption usually did not fit well in the longed-for cosmic harmony.

The public discovery of how animals were kept in industrial farming systems was arguably the single biggest factor for Europeans to stop eating meat. Alarmed by events like the publication of Ruth Harrison's *Animal Machines* (published in Britain in 1964 and immediately translated into several foreign languages, including Danish, German, and Dutch), advocacy groups formed and campaigned for humane farming methods and vegetarian lifestyles. Outbreaks of pandemics in the 1990s and 2000s, such as mad cow disease, foot and mouth disease, swine fever, and avian flu, also boosted this movement. Substantial as it became, large differences remained between countries, between west and east, north and south, urban and rural, female and male, and so on. And in no European country did vegetarians exceed 5 percent of the population by 2010.

See also Activism and Protests; Agribusiness; Ahimsa; Bible and Biblical Arguments; Cookbooks; Eastern Religions, Influences of; Ethical Vegetarianism; France; Germany; Global Warming; Netherlands, The; Organic Foods and Technology; Physiological Benefits; Reform; Religious Beliefs and Practices; Shelley, Percy Bysshe; United Kingdom; Vegetarian Society of the United Kingdom; World Hunger; World Wars in England.

Further Reading

Crossley, Ceri. *Consumable Metaphors: Attitudes towards Animals and Vegetarianism in Nineteenth-Century France.* Oxford: Peter Lang, 2005.

History of the International Vegetarian Union. www.ivu.org/history.

Meyer-Renschhausen, Elisabeth, and Albert Wirz. "Dietetics, Health Reform and Social Order: Vegetarianism as a Moral Physiology: The Example of Maximilian Bircher-Benner (1867–1939)." *Medical History* 43 (1999): 323–41.

Spencer, Colin. *Vegetarianism: A History.* 2nd ed. London: Grub Street, 2000.

Stuart, Tristram. *The Bloodless Revolution: Radical Vegetarians and the Discovery of India.* London: HarperPress, 2006.

Dirk-Jan Verdonk

FAMILY DYNAMICS

With food traditionally at the center of family life, vegetarianism can be a loaded household topic. In the case of an individual, the decision to embrace vegetarianism can separate one from the family. The opposite effect can occur when the entire family is vegetarian; in that case, the family's shared dietary decisions often heighten the sense of a communal family identity.

In recent decades, modern family life increasingly involves balancing hectic schedules, eating on the run, and rarely, if ever, sitting down at the same table to share a common meal. On one hand, the trend of each family member eating a meal in isolation makes it easier for an individual to follow a vegetarian diet; on the flip side, when a family does sit down to share a group meal, there is increased pressure to celebrate the communal aspect of sharing the same meal. A family with some but not all vegetarian members will have to choose whether to provide two different meals, create an all-vegetarian meal (potentially upsetting the nonvegetarians in the family), or provide enough food that all family members, regardless of their dietary restrictions, can be sated.

Food also has great cultural significance during holidays. These are often an opportunity for the extended family to gather. Unless a household is vegetarian for religious reasons shared by the extended family, it is possible that other relatives won't understand or agree with a family's or an individual's decision to eat a vegetarian diet. For some people, the rejection of traditional, meat-based foods, whether an old family recipe or the Thanksgiving turkey, can be seen as a rejection of family itself.

Libraries and bookstores are filled with books for young vegetarians and vegans, offering counseling on how to inform parents—usually presumed to be vigorously against a vegetarian diet—of a decision to become vegetarian, as well as how to handle the practicalities of a vegetarian diet. As vegetarianism increasingly becomes a mainstream dietary option, it seems likely that conversations of this type will become less strained.

Parents of a vegetarian child are usually foremost concerned with nutrition, especially if they themselves are not vegetarians. Other pressing concerns are the fear of difficult mealtimes, with each family member requiring a different meal. Some parents also see the embrace of a vegetarian diet as the rejection of the family's values; they find it difficult not to take their child's decision as a personal attack on their lifestyle or decisions. Other issues arise when vegetarian parents choose to raise a nonvegetarian child; often this choice is made either due to nutritional concerns or because of the desire to let the child make her own decision when older. In either case, parents and children eating different diets can often be difficult, as much for the larger cultural and social issues as for the meal-preparation logistics.

See also Backlash; Childbearing and Infant Feeding; Childrearing; Religious Beliefs and Practices; Social Acceptance.

Further Reading

Adams, Carol J. *Help! My Child Stopped Eating Meat!* New York: Continuum, 2004.
Stepaniak, Joanne, and Vesanto Malina. *Raising Vegetarian Children: A Guide to Good Health and Family Harmony.* Boston: McGraw-Hill, 2003.

Cedar Phillips

FRANCE

Approximately 2 percent of the French population is vegetarian, with the majority of practitioners in the educated middle and upper classes. Understood as a positive choice to govern everyday eating, the deliberate avoidance of animal flesh or all animal foods has been a minority practice in France. Regular abstinence from meat has been a part of the culture for centuries, because of conditions imposed on substantial segments of the population by poverty and due to the historical role of Catholicism as the primary religion. The observance of "lean" days, sanctioned by the Catholic Church, provided a regular reminder of the secondary importance of the flesh in the quest for moral purity. But several factors have mitigated against the development of a pervasive, positive vegetarianism in France. According to the predominant interpretation of biblical precept, to eat meat was to accept the bounty of God, including humans' dominion over other creatures and the earth. Prestige has long attached to meat as the prized result of both hunting and agriculture. The French take pride in a rich gastronomic heritage that favors ingenious inclusiveness in its cuisine. Today, meat plays a central role in the main dishes preferred across the class spectrum, while the culture values harmony, assimilation, and moderation. In this context, vegetarianism can appear as an exceptional if not actually fanatical practice, as it does not conform to the main, omnivorous stream. The motivations of those who have deliberately avoided meat eating form a counterpoint to the main themes in France's food history. Today, most vegetarians in France cite reasons of health and of ethics, related to the modern industrial agricultural system, as the impetus for their dietary choices.

Religious asceticism motivated early instances of the deliberate avoidance of meat in Christian France. Paradoxically, this was equally true for monastic orders that followed the Rule of St. Benedict, which advocated a frugal vegetable diet, and for saintly individuals, and also for some sects considered heretical. Notable ancestors to Christian forms of abstinence include the mystical-philosophical Pythagorean diet of Greek antiquity that extends from the belief in metempsychosis, or the migration of souls from body to body. The dualist conception of the Manicheans, loathed and vilified by St. Augustine, which spread west from Persia during the Roman Empire, posited equal powers of good and evil, the spiritual and the material. A vegetable diet, embraced by the most elect followers of Mani, was thought to enhance spirituality and the possibility of redemption. To avoid doing violence even to plants, these elect could not so much as gather their own food but had to accept alms. By the Middle Ages, the Catholic Church in France had become powerful, wealthy, attached to formal ritual, and strongly hierarchical. It viewed with intolerance practices and ideologies thought to conflict with its own. In the eyes of the church, the Albigeois or Cathars, who disdained marriage, refused to tithe, ate no meat, and avoided the killing of animals in the effort directly to imitate the exemplary lives of Christ and the apostles, were dangerous neo-Manicheans. Cathars, associated especially with the Languedoc region, held that the material world, wealth, and power were incompatible with the religious principle of love. From this perspective, abstention from meat eating was part of the renunciation of the principle of power and the effort to attain unity with that of love. In 1147 the discovery of large numbers of the "heretics" at Albi prompted Pope Eugenius III to charge St. Bernard of Clairvaux with quelling the "rebellion" against the true church. The Albigensian Crusade of 1209–1229 resulted in the massacre of the Cathars and the obliteration of much of the population of southern France, as the original justification for the church's military campaign became entangled with territorial politics and the Inquisition, established in Toulouse in 1229.

Renaissance and early modern debates about the vegetable diet drew not only on religious and philosophical ideas from Greek antiquity and from Christianity but also on contemporary science—medical and anatomical theories—and the observations of travelers abroad in foreign countries. The vegetable diet proved a telling problem in debates to reassess the relationships among the divine, humans, and animals. Following on the Aristotelian notion that animals lack a rational soul, René Descartes (1596–1650) affirmed the superiority of humankind, possessed of a soul and thus connected to the divine. Pierre Gassendi (1592–1655), who developed a rival school of atomistic, Epicurean thought built on the conception that the soul pervaded and inhabited the body, reasoned as well that it may be healthier not to eat animal flesh. Attentive to advances in comparative anatomy, Gassendi observed that human teeth were primarily effective in the grinding action common to herbivores. It would therefore accord with nature to select the vegetable diet instituted by God for the Garden of Eden before the fall from divine grace. François Bernier (1625–1688), a pupil of Gassendi and a member of the medical faculty at Montpellier, traveled to India and saw firsthand the large population of vegetable eaters. For Bernier, Indian notions of abstinence coincided with the revival of western Hippocratic dietetic recommendations, including the appropriate therapeutic balance for addressing sickness.

Some physicians practicing in the late early modern period found further evidence for the positive effects of a vegetable diet in the cases of their own patients, contributing to theories about the original diet of humans. The idea that man has lost touch with nature and was in fact meant to be an herbivore found strong articulation in the writings of doctor and botanist Louis Lémery (1677–1743), who bemoaned the corrupting influence of current custom, understood in opposition to nature. Philippe Hecquet (1661–1737), a physician based in Paris and early associated with the ascetic doctrines of the Jansenist Catholics at the convent at Port-Royal-des-Champs, promoted a "theological medicine" that, similarly, sought to return to original, Christian fare by abstaining from meat. His moral diet would cure social ills, including the lucrative traffic in Lenten dispensations that allowed people to eat meat or eggs on fast days for a price handed over to the church. Borrowing Gassendi's insights from comparative anatomy, Hecquet insisted that meat eating was inefficient as well as unhealthy, immoral, and unnatural. Against the reigning chemical explanation for digestion (the stomach ferments foods through acid), Hecquet posited that a mechanical crushing action transformed ingested food into the desirable smooth, nutritive paste that could be absorbed by the body. Vegetables, according to Hecquet, lent themselves far better to this conversion than fibrous, resistant meat. The sick, in particular, should be encouraged by physicians to abstain from the clogging, putrefying results of eating meat. Medical, as well as moral, arguments for the vegetable diet were clearly defined in France by the early 1700s.

Political overtones distinguish alike 18th-century reflections on the vegetable diet and critiques of the hierarchical, monarchic underpinnings of French society elaborated during the same era. Indeed, the call to return to a "natural" diet now voiced interest in social change and political foment. Novelist and political philosopher Jean-Jacques Rousseau (1712–1778), convinced of humans' herbivorous origins, added notably that female humans, like plant-eating animals, have only a single pair of breasts. Rousseau advocated, at least for other people, a pastoral diet of milk products, vegetables, and grains as the way to achieve physical health and avoid the decadent, corrupting effects of city life including overly sophisticated food. Given the popularity of Rousseau's writings, his dietary recommendations immediately found a wide audience, although how many readers actually followed his prescriptions for food has yet to be established. An admirer of Rousseau, Jacques-Henri Bernardin de Saint-Pierre (1737–1814), gave lasting expression to a similar ideal of living in harmony with nature and also according to the practices of the East, viewed as sagely exemplary, in popular fictions.

Extending the new articulations of human rights to the plight of animals, mathematician and philosopher Pierre-Louis Moreau de Maupertuis (1698–1759) wrote against the killing or injury of animals who presented no threat to human life. Étienne Bonnot de Condillac (1715–1780) argued that animals were sentient creatures possessing a spiritual dimension, while writers including Voltaire (1694–1778) objected to the practice of vivisection that was current in medical and scientific research. Moral, theological, ethical, and political arguments for the vegetable diet found extensions in the reflections of the Physiocrats, who viewed agriculture as the backbone of the country's economic health, and among those worried about how to feed an increasing population. In the early 1770s, flying in the face of old evidence linking the cure for scurvy to the consumption of citrus fruits, the physician and naval administrator Antoine Poissonnier-Desperrières (1722–1793) subjected a shipful of sailors in the French navy to an ill-balanced but inexpensive "vegetal regime." In theory, the rice diet would save them from scurvy while balancing the books for the trans-Atlantic voyage. With chagrin, a critic noted that the regimen only added severe stomach and intestinal upset to the scurvy that afflicted the marines. In the Revolutionary era, the diet of the lower classes, largely meatless due to poverty, and Spartan austerity became signs of political fervor and the desire for social and political change. Among radical Revolutionaries, the creation of the Republican fraternity could logically extend to the enfranchisement of animals.

In the 19th century, groups organized in order to better propound the vegetable diet, newly termed "vegetarian" in English by 1842, with the French neologism *végétarien* appearing in 1873. The intensification of industrial manufacturing, a series of civil and foreign wars, and rapid alternation in political regimes produced in France the broad sense of a crisis in human society. During the social and political reordering in the wake of the Revolution of 1789, Jean-Antoine Gleïzès (1773–1843) developed arguments for a vegetable diet that would finally realize revolutionary ideals while correcting for the excesses and violence of the Terror. His influences include liberal Enlightenment ideals, but the character of his writing is mystical. Gleïzès connected the exultant violence of the revolutionary crowds before the guillotine to the work of butchers and the meat diet. The solution to the present crisis of decline, he thought, would begin with strict adherence to a vegetable diet. The physical, moral, and spiritual regeneration of humankind would follow, along with the recreation in modern times of a social fraternity patterned on ancient Greek ideals. In the social cosmology of Gleïzès, the vegetable diet would replace the Eucharist, imbue humankind with a spark of divine purity, and avoid inflicting human violence on any innocent being capable of suffering. The rejection of Christian and Cartesian dualism in a philosophy such as that of Gleïzès cleared the way to reimagine the relationship between humans and animals.

Following the example set in Britain two decades earlier, a group including the physician Parisot de Cassel founded the French Society for the Protection of Animals (SPA) in 1846. By lobbying, the SPA encouraged the passage of the Grammont Law of 1850, criminalizing acts of cruelty toward domestic animals in public. The issues of animal treatment and the vegetable diet brought to the fore contradictions and conflicts still embedded within the fabric of French society. The aristocratic love of animals, notably dogs and horses, was also associated with the hunt, in which these animals were deployed to facilitate the ritualized killing of still other creatures. The topic of hunting also raised vexed class issues, as elites who controlled land rights had long monopolized access to hunting. It was therefore noteworthy when writer, poet, and politician Alphonse de Lamartine (1790–1869), who loved horses, dogs, and the hunt, gave up hunting on principle, joined the SPA in 1858, and adopted a vegetarian diet. In the 1850s the SPA began to publish a journal about animal protection. Such publications found many supporters among aristocrats and Catholics including the historian Jules Michelet (1798–1874), whose political and religious convictions led him to deplore the cruel treatment of animals—vivisection, bullfighting, hunting, cockfighting, and butterfly collecting—as contrary to the will of God.

In the late 19th through the mid-20th centuries, secular and scientific but also religious forms of vegetarianism offered competing visions of cures for social ills. In this period, the rise in alcoholism, crime, and prostitution and the appearance of new forms of stress, disease, and exhaustion associated with the modern industrial society contributed to the preoccupation with social degeneration. The doctor Hureau de Villeneuve founded the Vegetarian Society of Paris in 1880 to promote this "rational" and "hygienic" diet. The emblematic treatise *Vegetarianism and the Rational Vegetarian Regime* (1891) published by Ernest Bonnejoy (1833–1896) drew especially on the discoveries of Louis Pasteur and the new germ theory of disease. For Bonnejoy, the vegetable diet logically followed from the new scientific understandings of how diet and health interact. His "muscular vegetarianism" would promote health and boost the immune system of individuals, resulting in better public health and the reversal of the decline of the body politic.

Paul Carton (1875–1947) advocated a three-part system of healthy living requiring a vegetable diet, a hygienic program of sun, fresh air, and exercise, and also faith in God and a return to religion. Carton's ideal of good health for all bore superficial similarities to goals of the Third Republic government (1870–1940) and the medical and academic establishment, which also favored national strength and unity. Carton's philosophy diverged in its principles, however, being neither materialist nor secular. Carton's "naturist vegetarianism" appealed to marginal groups at risk of falling behind in the latest shifts from rural to modern, urban life. For those who had little, some consolation, along with economic and health benefits, came from living frugally and abstaining from meat: The practitioner was at least virtuous. The cookbook that Carton first published in 1925 went through many editions, to influence home cooks through the mid-20th century as well as a few restaurant chefs and cooking teachers such as Gilles Daveau. Menus from Carton responded to the standard expectation in France that a meal be served in courses and follow seasonal variation for the choice of ingredients. His diet focuses on fresh vegetables and fruits, grain in familiar forms such as bread and pastry, and large quantities of eggs and cream. Acknowledging the vast reaches of the Republic beyond Europe, Carton included dietary recommendations for French living abroad in the colonies. Aiming for a "pure" and "nontoxic" regimen, one should use local foods as much as possible, adapting them to French preparations and meal structures. By following the hygienic, naturist diet and avoiding traditional physicians, drugs, and foods, everyone could achieve a state of health.

By the early 20th century, recognizing the commonalities with their own cause, women seeking to enter a public sphere shaped by the patriarchal and discriminatory character of French republicanism appropriated arguments for vegetarianism and against cruelty to animals. The teacher, revolutionary, and activist Louise Michel (1830–1905) identified women with animals in order to critique the oppression of both in the social order. The writer Rachilde (Marguerite Vallette-Eymery, 1860–1953), herself a vegetarian, earned a medal from the SPA in 1932 for animal rights activism. Through the two World Wars, differently rationalized philosophies of vegetarianism—anarchist, libertarian, fascist—found their own constituents, presses, and publications.

Today's vegetarianism exists as an alternative and minoritarian, if increasingly popular, choice that differs from mainstream practices. During World War II and early in the Thirty Glorious Years of rebuilding thereafter, a vegetable diet became the default mode of eating for many, due to food shortages and rationing. By the early 1960s, agricultural policies, including farming subsidies instituted by then, resulted in a stable food supply with regular surpluses of meat and dairy products as well as low prices. In consequence, meat consumption increased; meat became the central feature around which any "proper" meal had to be built, and it acquired the heavy symbolic and cultural weight that had long attached to bread. The postwar industrial agricultural system and the consumer economy provide the backdrop against which most vegetarians in France today define their own positions. Vegetarians tend to be health-conscious and highly reflective about diet. They take seriously research such as that on the benefits of the modern Mediterranean diet, consisting primarily of vegetables, fruits, and grains, and on the ills associated with the dietary abundance of affluent nations, from obesity and diabetes to eating disorders having a psychological cause. Today, the decision to adopt a primarily or uniquely vegetable diet reconciles the wish to maintain personal nutrition and health, seen as closely related, with ethical stances on ecology, animal rights, and food access for the less affluent whether at home or abroad.

The full practical realization of the contemporary holistic vegetarian philosophy is at odds with the advice of many physicians in the medical establishment and with the current overall structure of the food economy. The consumer patterns that support a vegetarian diet differ sharply from those in the meat-eating majority. Yet vegetarian culture occupies a niche now solidly constructed in France. Bookstores sell vegetarian cookbooks of all stripes—whether for the sophisticated tastes of the *gourmand*; for the diversified, cosmopolitan palate of the traveler open to exotic (that is, of foreign origin) vegetable foods such as soy milk and tofu; or for the harried parent in need of a quick recipe appropriate for an everyday dinner. Vegetarian and even vegan bistros and restaurants can now be found in large cities, if not small towns and villages, while natural, organic, and vegetarian produce and preprepared foods fill new kinds of chain stores such as Naturalia. Since the early 1990s academicians in disciplines such as sociology and anthropology have become increasingly attentive to vegetarianism as a dietary practice. Media space devoted to vegetarianism increases practically by the day. While vegetarianism in France remains the practice of a relatively small minority, it plays an important role as a leader for the trend to merge considerations of ecology, animal rights, nonviolence, and human health as key contemporary issues for French and also for European society.

Further Reading

Abramson, Julia A. *Food Culture in France.* Westport, CT: Greenwood, 2007.

Abramson, Julia A. "Vegetable Carving: For Your Eyes Only." In *Vegetables: Proceedings of the Oxford Symposium on Food and Cookery 2008*, edited by Susan Friedland. Totnes, UK: Prospect Books, 2009.

Association Végétarienne de France. http://www.vegetarisme.fr/.

Bernier, François. *Voyages de François Bernier, contenant la description des États du Grand-Mogul, de l'Indoustan, du royaume de Kachemire, & c.* 2 vols. Amsterdam: P. Marret, 1709–1710.

Carton, Paul. *La Cuisine simple* (1925). 3rd ed. Paris: Librairie Le François, 1931.

Chanteur, Janine. *Du droit des bêtes à disposer d'elles-mêmes.* Paris: Seuil, 1993.

Condillac, Étienne Bonnot de. *Traité des animaux.* Paris: De Bure, 1755.

Crossley, Ceri. *Consumable Metaphors: Attitudes towards Animals and Vegetarianism in Nineteenth-Century France.* New York: Peter Lang, 2005.

Ferry, Luc. *Le Nouvel ordre écologique.* Paris: Grasset, 1992.

Gleïzès, Jean-Antoine. *Le Christianisme expliqué, ou l'Unité de croyance pour tous les chrétiens.* Paris: Firmin-Didot, 1830

Gleïzès, Jean-Antoine. *Thalysie, ou Système physique et intellectuel de la nature.* Paris: Librairie nationale et étrangère, 1821.

Hecquet, Philippe. *De la Digestion.* Paris: François Fournier, 1712.

Hecquet, Philippe. *Traité des dispenses du Carême.* Paris: François Fournier, 1709.

Leméry, Louis. *Traité des aliments.* Paris: J. B. Cusson and B. Witte, 1702.

Mandelblatt, Bertie. "'On the Excellence of the Vegetable Diet': Scurvy, Antoine Poissonnier-Desperrières's New Naval Diet and French Colonial Science in the Atlantic World." Unpublished manuscript presented as Working Paper No. 09-14 at the International Seminar on the History of the Atlantic World, 1500–1825, at Harvard University, July 2009.

Méry, André. *Les Végétariens. Raisons et sentiments.* Saint-Léger: La Plage, 1998.

Ouédraogo, Aouna P. "Food and the Purification of Society: Dr. Paul Carton and Vegetarianism in Interwar France." *Social History of Medicine* 14, no. 2 (2001): 223–45.

Rousseau, Jean-Jacques. *Émile, ou De l'Éducation* (1762). Paris: Garnier-Flammarion, 1966.

Rousseau, Jean-Jacques. *The First and Second Discourses* (1750 and 1755). Translated by Roger D. Masters and Judith R. Masters. New York: St. Martin's, 1964.

Saint-Pierre, Jacques-Henri Bernardin de. *Paul et Virginie* (1788); *suivi de La Chaumière indienne* (1790). Paris: Nelson, n.d.

Spencer, Colin. *The Heretic's Feast: A History of Vegetarianism.* Hanover, NH: University Press of New England, 1993.

Stuart, Tristram. *The Bloodless Revolution: A Cultural History of Vegetarianism from 1600 to Modern Times.* New York: W.W. Norton, 2007.

Végétariens Magazine (VegMag).

Julia A. Abramson

FRANCIONE, GARY L. (1954–)

Gary L. Francione is an American legal scholar and influential animal rights philosopher. He is distinguished professor of law and Nicholas deB. Katzenbach Scholar of Law and Philosophy at Rutgers School of Law. At Rutgers, with Anna Charlton, he taught the first courses in animal rights law offered as part of a U.S. university's regular academic curriculum. Through his lectures, publications, and Web site (Animal Rights: The Abolitionist Approach), his ideas, including his advocacy of veganism, have become a significant factor in the movement for animal liberation. Francione's thought can be summarized in terms of four key ideas: abolitionism, sentience as the basis for rights, veganism as the moral baseline, and nonviolence.

Abolitionism   At the heart of Francione's conception of animal rights is the demand for the abolition of the status of nonhuman animals as property. To this end, he rejects all so-called animal welfare measures, which seek to ameliorate the living and dying conditions of animals without challenging the alleged right of humans to exploit them. This includes rejecting, on moral and practical grounds, what he calls the "new welfarism": the belief that an eventual end to animal exploitation can be achieved through welfare reforms. New welfarism, Francione asserts, is morally problematic because it involves promoting, at least for the time being, inherently wrongful use of animals. It is also impractical because, for one thing, this approach tends to reassure consumers that exploitation is acceptable so long as animals are treated humanely—the upshot being that welfare reforms may actually make abolition more difficult. Though it is better to inflict less harm than to inflict more harm, Francione's argument is that humans should not be inflicting any unnecessary harm.

Sentience as the Basis for Rights   Francione argues that sentience—the capacity for conscious experience, and in particular the capacity to experience pain or pleasure—is a sufficient condition for having rights. His philosophy rejects the utilitarianism of Peter Singer, and it differs from Tom Regan's animal rights view by making simple sentience the basis of rights. Francione derives the fundamental right of sentient animals not to be treated as mere things directly from the principle of equal consideration, which he says is a logical requirement of any sound moral theory. This principle says that people must treat like cases alike. There are many ways in which animals differ from humans, and this means that animals will not have exactly the same set of rights as humans. But if it is judged that animals (like all humans, regardless of mental abilities) have morally significant interests, then, logically, people must ascribe to animals the same right that humans have not to be treated merely instrumentally. This is to say that all sentient individuals ought to be regarded as persons, or members of the moral community. Giving meaningful content to the belief that the infliction of unnecessary suffering is wrong cannot be squared with animals' current status as property, any more than it can be squared with the practice of human slavery. Neither can people justify depriving sentient creatures of life when there is no need to do so.

Veganism as the Moral Baseline   According to Francione, veganism ought to be viewed as the nonnegotiable moral baseline of the animal rights movement. That is, it ought to be viewed as a morally obligatory expression of respect for the rights of sentient beings, not simply as a means to reduce animal suffering. Vegetarianism that permits the consumption of animal products, including eggs or dairy, in practice condones the exploitation of animals and is incompatible with animal rights. Veganism is more than a matter of diet; it is about trying to eliminate animal exploitation in whatever form it takes. Admittedly, it is impossible, given the centrality of animal products in modern economies, to entirely avoid being implicated in animal exploitation. Nonetheless, says Francione, people should strive to eliminate such exploitation, and a vegan diet is crucial to this endeavor.

Nonviolence   Francione insists that the movement for animal liberation must be resolutely nonviolent if it is to give consistent expression to the ideal of respecting the right of all sentient beings never to be treated as mere means. His views have drawn him to the teachings of Jainism, with its doctrine of *ahimsa,* or nonviolence toward all living beings. Francione's opposition to any violence, whether against persons or property, has proved controversial, with some animal advocates rejecting his principled pacifism for allegedly being politically naïve in the face of institutional power. But Francione holds that, in practice, violence will not diminish the overall supply of animal products; it will only alienate people, giving them an excuse to ignore the message and marginalizing the issue of animal rights. What is needed instead, he says, is creative, nonviolent vegan education to reduce demand for animal products.

See also Ahimsa; Animal Rights and Animal Welfare; Ethical Vegetarianism; Reform; Singer, Peter; Veganism.

Further Reading

Animal Rights: The Abolitionist Approach. http://www.abolitionistapproach.com/.

Francione, Gary L. *Animals as Persons: Essays on the Abolition of Animal Exploitation.* New York: Columbia University Press, 2008.

Francione, Gary L. *Animals, Property, and the Law.* Philadelphia: Temple University Press, 1995.

Francione, Gary L. *Introduction to Animal Rights: Your Child or the Dog?* Philadelphia: Temple University Press, 2000.

Francione, Gary L. *Rain without Thunder: The Ideology of the Animal Rights Movement.* Philadelphia: Temple University Press, 1996.

Francione, Gary L., and Robert Garner. *The Animal Rights Debate: Abolition or Regulation?* New York: Columbia University Press, 2010.

Angus Taylor

G

GANDHI, MOHANDAS (1869–1948)

Mohandas Karamchand Gandhi, popularly known the world over as Mahatma Gandhi or simply Gandhi, was an apostle of peace who practiced and advocated nonviolence and renunciation of prejudice based on institutions such as caste, creed, language, or country. He is best known for his leadership in ousting the British from their control of India. He was vocal about vegetarianism and spoke often of the horror experienced by animals used as food. His concern for animals was exemplified when he said, "The greatness of a nation and its moral progress can be judged by the way its animals are treated."

Originally, Gandhi was vegetarian because of his parents. Karamchand, his father, was a Hindu who practiced Vaishnavism, a sect devoted to Vishnu. His mother, Putlibai, was deeply committed to Jainism. Both religions view nonhuman animals as sacred and oppose eating them, so unlike many other families in their community, his family would not kill the free-living animals who destroyed their crops. As a teenager, however, Gandhi envied stronger boys and believed their claims that bravery and strength came from eating animals. For a year, Gandhi had meat-eating feasts with a friend. Gandhi did not grow taller or stronger, and his remorse over keeping his meat-eating secret from his parents caused him to stop eating meat.

After graduating from high school in 1888, Gandhi decided to become a lawyer and to be educated in London. His caste believed that meat eating was required in England and demanded that he not go. Nonetheless, he took a vow not to eat meat to satisfy his mother and left for England. In his first month, Gandhi read English reformer Henry S. Salt's "A Plea for Vegetarianism" and said that from that reading he was vegetarian by choice rather than tradition, that he no longer envied meat eaters, and that advocating vegetarianism became his mission. While in England, Gandhi joined the London Vegetarian Society, served on its executive committee, and wrote articles for its journal. His parents' religions permitted the consumption of milk, but Gandhi believed that the moral duty was not to live off other animals. He stopped consuming cow and buffalo milk, though he thought that he had to consume goats' milk, which he later termed the tragedy of his life. Otherwise, Gandhi ate no animal products.

Gandhi derived many of his values and principles from ancient Indian scriptures such as the Vedas and the Upanishads. These moral codes—including truth, celibacy, nonviolence, and nonpossessiveness—became Gandhi's dearest principles and shaped his activism, politics, and philosophy throughout the rest of his life. He also believed that people should eat sparingly and fast occasionally.

Unlike other vegetarian activists of his day, such as the well-known Herbert Shelton, Gandhi believed that the moral consequences of vegetarianism should be emphasized, not its physical benefits. Gandhi claimed that people who stopped their vegetarian diets were usually those who became vegetarian for health reasons or because they were suffering from some disease. When health was restored, they would revert to their unhealthful diet. Thus, Gandhi concluded that to remain a vegetarian requires a moral basis. A selfish basis, such as personal health, would not take a person higher along the paths of spiritual evolution; what was required was an altruistic purpose. This was a great discovery in his search for truth.

Gandhi once observed ritual killing of sheep and goats and was shocked at the animals' cries and pools of blood. His friend tried to comfort him by saying that the sheep felt no pain. Gandhi retorted that if the sheep were asked, they would say differently. Finally, Gandhi argued that vegetarians need to be tolerant and adopt a little humility if they want to convert others to vegetarianism: to build the spirit, not the body. His vegetarianism is revered throughout the world and is a source of inspiration for people worldwide. Nearly 500 million people in India are vegetarian.

See also Activism and Protests; Eastern Religions, Influences of; Ethical Vegetarianism; India; Reform; Salt, Henry S.; Social Acceptance; United Kingdom.

Further Reading

Gandhi, Mohandas. "The Moral Basis of Vegetarianism." Speech given before the London Vegetarian Society, November 20, 1931. http://www.ivu.org/news/evu/other/gandhi2.html.

Gandhi, Mohandas Karamchand. *Gandhi: An Autobiography: The Story of My Experiments with Truth.* Boston: Beacon, 1993.

Shankar Narayan and Jerold D. Friedman

GERMANY

Vegetarianism in Germany has the same historical roots as in the United Kingdom and United States. After the fall of the Roman Empire the religiously and ethically motivated demand for meat abstention on the continent survived mostly in Christian monasteries, but its roots go back to Orpheus and Pythagoras. The Catholic church dictated regular fasting days, imposing a strict diet that today would be considered vegan, but later loosened to include dairy products, eggs, and fish. However, as in the rest of Europe, for a large part of the population during the Middle Ages meat was very often simply too costly or not available.

With the onset of the Enlightenment, the ancient vegetarian ideals reemerged among the educated classes. Vegetables, fruits, and herbs were increasingly recommended for therapeutic and moral reasons. The French-Swiss writer and philosopher Jean-Jacques Rousseau (1712–1778) was the primary source and influence for all nature-orientated movements in Western Europe at this time. In his writings, especially the book *Émile* (published in 1762), he worshipped nature in a religious way and presented the unspoiled child as the opposite of the grown-up man degenerated through civilization. The more brutal, unnatural carnivore was opposed to the peace-loving frugivore. Among the German writers of the time, Johann Gottfried Herder (1744–1803) especially embraced Rousseau's ideas. Christoph Wilhelm Hufeland (1762–1836), a friend of Goethe and one of the best-known physicians of his time, reinforced the growing belief in benign mother nature with his lectures on *Makrobiotik oder die Kunst, das menschliche Leben zu verlängern* (Macrobiotic or the Art to Prolong Human Life), which centered not on illness but on the human being as a whole. His ideas are one of the theoretical foundations of the *Lebensreform,* the life reform movement that developed in the second half of the 19th century in Germany and that strongly advocated vegetarianism.

In 1840 Germany lagged 50 years behind England in industrializing, but in 1914 it was the leading industrial state in Europe. This led to rapid urbanization and massive migrations within the country. Subsequently, and as was the case in England, life reform developed as a counter movement to industrialization, espousing the slogan "back to nature." The campaign for a healthy lifestyle included temperance and/or abstinence from alcohol, coffee and meat, as well as animal rights. These anti-industrial social activities often replaced more political ones that had become almost impossible following the revolution of 1848–49.

Of all the pioneers of vegetarianism in Germany, Gustav Struve (1805–1870) is arguably the most important. Having converted to vegetarianism in 1832 after reading Rousseau, Struve went on to write the first vegetarian-themed novel in German, *Mandaras Wanderungen* (Mandara's Travels, 1833), which detailed the travels of a young Indian through Europe who wrote letters home about a Christianity demoralized through meat eating, all the while defending the vegetarian lifestyle of his homeland. In 1868 Struve founded the *Vegetarische Gesellschaft Stuttgart* (Stuttgart Vegetarian Society). With his book *Pflanzenkost—die Grundlage einer neuen Weltanschauung* (Plant Diet—Basis for a New Philosophy of Life, 1869), he gave the movement an important theoretical foundation.

The second founding father of German vegetarianism, Wilhelm Zimmermann (1807–1878), was closely connected to some of the leading hydrotherapists of the time. After a trip to England he published *Der Weg zum Paradies. Oder: Die einzigen und wahren Mittel, das physische und moralische Elend unserer Zeit im Keim zu ersticken und auszurotten* (The Way to Paradise. Or: The Only and True Means to Suppress and Eradicate the Physical and Moral Misery of Our Time, 1843). This in turn convinced the book printer Emil Weilshäuser to join the vegetarian cause and to publish between 1855 and 1861 a wealth of vegetarian literature, including some writings translated from English for the first time, by Sylvester Graham and Charles Lane, among others.

Theodor Hahn (1824–1883), a pharmacist and natural healer who also worked as a hydrotherapist, was converted through Hufeland's *Makrobiotik* and in 1852 started to prescribe his patients a vegetarian diet. In 1865 he published the hugely successful *Praktisches Handbuch der naturgemäßen Heilweise* (Practical Handbook of the Natural Way of Healing). He propagated a holistic approach to human health and a total life reform to solve the social question. His first book, an edited translation of *Vegetable Diet* by the American physician William A. Alcott, *Die naturgemäße Diät—die Diät der Zukunft* (The Natural Diet—The Diet of the Future), was to be the motivation for the theologian, philosopher, and anthropologist Edward Baltzer (1814–1887) to take up vegetarianism in 1866, followed by his family and friends. Subsequently Baltzer wrote effusively on all aspects of vegetarianism, culminating in the four-volume *Die natürliche Lebensweise* (The Natural Way of Living, 1867–1872). Baltzer became the most important theorist and organizer of the German vegetarian movement, actively working for the dissemination of vegetarian and life reform ideas. In 1867 he founded the *Verein für natürliche Lebensweise* (the Society for a Natural Lifestyle), the first vegetarian society in Germany and on the continent, which in 1869 was renamed *Verein für naturgemäße Lebensweise* (True to Nature Lifestyle) and, from 1868 on, he regularly published a newsletter. Similar societies were founded in the following years in a number of cities. On June 7, 1892, the national umbrella organization *Deutscher Vegetarierbund* (German Vegetarian League) formed. It published the *Vegetarische Rundschau* (Vegetarian Magazine), later on *Vegetarische Warte* (Vegetarian Outlook).

Agrarromantik, the romantization of agrarian life, was a part of the life reform movement that led to various attempts to enable the urban population to get in touch with or back to the countryside through cooperative land-ownership. As in England, garden cities (*Gartenstädte*), with garden plots, were built at the edge of large cities. These plots have been known as *Schrebergärten* or *Kleingärten,* named after the physician Daniel Moritz Schreber (1808–1861), a professor from Leipzig. His publications discussed children's health and the social consequences of massive urbanization and he advocated physical exercise in the countryside.

The largest, still-existing garden project is Eden, a settlement dedicated to fruit-growing, founded in 1893 in Oranienburg near Berlin. For the first seven years it was strictly vegetarian, but then relaxed its rules to a more general organic, healthy lifestyle. It produced a whole range of *Reformwaren* (reform products), including fruit and vegetable juices, vegetarian margarine, and *Kraftnahrung* (powerfood), a vegetarian sausage and meat. These products were the first examples of ersatz meat products and are the precursors to today's tofu sausages and the like. These products for the new reformed, healthy, natural lifestyle were sold in Germany in special shops known as *Reformhäuser,* the first of which was founded in 1887. They still exist and are the precursors of the organic stores that augmented them from the late 1980s on.

At the first vegetarian world conference in Dresden in 1908, the International Vegetarian Union (IVU) was formed. The number of vegetarian societies in Germany grew (25 in 1912), but overall membership declined, which was blamed partly on the new Oriental Mazdaznan movement, as well as on new life reform groups such as *Wandervögel, Freideutsche Jugend,* and *Pfadfinder* (hiking and scout movements for young people). Nevertheless the IVU persevered, with sporting events being very popular, particularly races to prove the strength of vegetarian athletes.

The Nazi regime exploited the life reform ideas for its own cause, particularly the vegetarian ideal of a "pure" and thus healthy body. *Körperkultur* (body culture) became an Aryan, neo-pagan cult. Bakers were legally obliged to sell *Vollkornbrot,* wholegrain bread. This push must be seen in the context of preparations for war: Germany was not self-sufficient in the production of fat and protein, so, for instance, the cultivation and use of the hitherto unknown soy beans was heavily propagated. Adolf Hitler regarded pastures for animals as a waste of land that could be put to better use by cultivating potatoes. At the same time, the Nazis were deeply suspicious of the pacifist and sectarian vegetarians. In 1935, the same year Johannes Haussleiter provided a German history of meat abstention in antiquity, *Der Vegetarismus in der Antike,* the *Vegetarierbund* disbanded to avoid being forced into the *Deutsche Gesellschaft für Lebensreform* (German Life Reform Society) founded by the Nazis.

In 1946, after the war, a new start was made with the *Vegetarier-Union Deutschland* (German Vegetarians' Union), which developed into the *Vegetarierbund Deutschland* of today. Its newsletter is called *Natürlich vegetarisch* (Naturally vegetarian) and the association works with young and old to promote vegetarian ideals. The 100th anniversary of the Vegetarian World Conference took place in 2008 in Dresden.

Increasing ethical and ecological concerns as well as fears caused by recent health scares like BSE in 2000 has made vegetarianism attractive once again. Since then, many Germans have apparently felt uncertain about the safety of animal products. Meat consumption had already been declining for the first time since war times to 132 pounds (60kg) per person per year in 1997.

The image, importance, and symbolism of meat have been gradually changing. At the beginning of the 1970s most people still thought of meat as valuable and healthy—a famous marketing slogan used by CMA, a government-related agency marketing German agricultural products, stated that *"Fleisch ist ein Stück Lebenskraft,"* meat is a piece of vitality. But in a poll conducted in 1994, 63 percent of respondents said their first associations with meat were "scandals of all sorts." In a survey conducted in 2001, 26 percent of those asked about what defined a healthy diet responded that it was eating less or no meat.

It is difficult to obtain reliable numbers about active vegetarians, not the least because of the frequent discrepancies between the image people project of themselves and their actual eating practices. A 2006 survey showed that 10 percent of

Germans were vegetarians, but a different type of survey in 2008 reported that 1.6 percent were vegetarians, 1.1 percent ate only raw food, and the percentage was even lower for vegans. Vegetarianism in Germany today is mainly based on concerns about animal rights and welfare, environmental problems, and world hunger, as well as the search for a healthy, life-prolonging diet. This could explain why many self-declared vegetarians feel much less religious about it than the pioneers at the end of the 19th century. Many of them consume dairy products, eggs, and fish and may even occasionally eat meat or eat less of it. Vegetarianism is most common among the well-educated and the affluent, more women (in 2001 13%) than men (3%) are vegetarian, and the percentage of vegetarianism is highest among women between 18 and 24 years of age (16% in 2002).

Up until the 1980s, vegetarians were commonly seen as odd and often had to explain their chosen dietary lifestyle, whereas today vegetarianism is socially more or less accepted. In urban, well-educated circles it is even regarded as morally and ethically superior, which might be the reason for some stars and prominent people to call themselves as vegetarians.

Food and drink manufacturers are increasingly aware of vegetarian consumers. In some cases they have actively changed formulas to avoid using animal-derived ingredients, such as gelatin, so that they can label their products as vegetarian or vegan.

Reformhäuser (health food stores) are still very popular, but younger people mostly shop at *Bioläden* (organic stores). *Bioläden* also tend to offer a wide range of vegetarian and vegan products. But even regular shops, supermarkets, and discounters today cater to that growing group of customers.

More Germans are cooking vegetarian at home and out. Modern vegetarian cookbooks started to appear in the 1980s. Today there are many choices for all kinds of groups, occasions, and cuisines. Until very recently chefs in Germany showed very little creativity in vegetarian cooking and vegetarian options in restaurants amounted to little more than a *Gemüseplatte, wahlweise mit Ei* (vegetable plate, with or without egg). However, with the general trend toward more regional, seasonal, and sustainable food, vegetables are slowly being treated as more than just a *Beilage* (side dish). Vegetarian options are becoming more varied. Today established fast-food outlets offer vegetarian choices, but purely vegetarian restaurants are quite rare, tending mostly to be Indian or Sri Lankan.

Further Reading

Spencer, Colin. *The Heretic's Feast: A History of Vegetarianism.* London: Fourth Estate, 1994.

Stuart, Tristram. *The Bloodless Revolution: A Cultural History of Vegetarianism from 1600 to Modern Times.* New York: W. W. Norton, 2007.

Teuteberg, Hans-Jürgen. "Zur Sozialgeschichte des Vegetarismus." *Vierteljahresschrift für Sozial- und Wirtschaftsgeschichte* 81 (1994): 33–65.

Vegetariar Bund Deutschland. www.vebu.de.

Ursula Heinzelmann

GLOBAL WARMING

Global warming is a phenomenon caused by certain gases in the atmosphere that allow the incoming lower-wavelength solar radiation to enter the atmosphere and that block the outgoing higher-wavelength radiation. This results in an increase in the net temperature of the atmosphere, causing melting of the polar ice caps and other wide-ranging climatic and environmental changes. Carbon dioxide (CO_2), methane, and nitrogen oxides are typical greenhouse gases. The livestock sector plays a significant role in the anthropogenic release of these greenhouse gases. Thus, dietary choices affect global warming.

Energy transformations are prevalent in nature. Energy is conserved (the first law of thermodynamics) and dissipated (the second law of thermodynamics) in all such transformations, which also results in physical and chemical changes of materials. Examples of these chemical changes include the release of hydrocarbons, carbon monoxide and CO_2, water vapor, sulfur dioxide, and nitrogen oxides as residuals in the atmosphere. These residuals pollutants diminish in value over time and become detrimental to the environment.

An incandescent light bulb has an efficiency of about 5 percent. This means that it transforms 95 percent of the energy into wasteful forms while converting only 5 percent of the electrical energy into light energy. Similarly, food energy moves along the food chain from one level to the next. Each jump in the level results in at least a 90 percent loss of energy. In this respect, it is better to consume

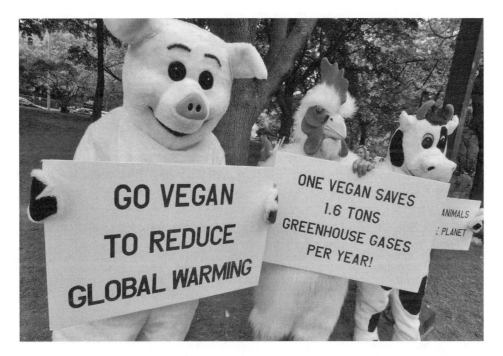

Animal rights activists promote a vegan diet as an answer to global warming, 2007, in Boston. (AP Photo/Lisa Poole)

foods that are lower on the food chain. Thus, dietary habits have serious consequences for the environment, which raises major concerns about the long-term sustainability of the energy-intensive lifestyle.

The livestock industry takes up 70 percent of all agricultural land and covers 30 percent of the planet's land surface, excluding the polar ice caps. The livestock industry contributes up to 7.1 billion tons of greenhouse gases each year to the atmosphere, which accounts for up to 24 percent of the total current greenhouse gas production. This release of greenhouse gases is higher than releases from all forms of transportation combined.

The livestock industry is responsible for 37 percent of anthropogenic methane, 65 percent of anthropogenic nitrous oxide, and 64 percent of anthropogenic ammonia emissions. Acid rain and acidification of ecosystems are substantially increased. Methane is 23 times more potent than CO_2 in its impact on global warming, while nitrous oxide is 296 times more potent than CO_2. Ammonia in the atmosphere causes acid rain, another serious concern to environmentalists.

The daily meat consumption per person in developing countries is about 1.66 ounces (47 grams) versus 7.9 ounces (224 grams) for the developed countries, and Americans consume approximately 12 ounces (340 grams) of meat per day, the highest amount in the world. The food-animal industry in the United States reportedly accounts for about 55 percent of erosion and sedimentation, 37 percent of pesticide use, 50 percent of antibiotic use, and about 33 percent of the nitrogen and phosphorus content in fresh waterways. This results in toxic chemical residues in the food chain and in potable water.

Dietary choices are causing climate changes due to the greenhouse effect, while the greenhouse effect, in turn, causes lower food yields. The relations between

---

Did You Know . . .?

Did you know that the cultivation of livestock for human consumption is responsible for the production of more greenhouse gases than all of the world's automobiles combined? It's true . . The nitrous oxide and methane gases that are released into the atmosphere every day from the millions of cows, pigs, chickens, and other imprisoned farmed animals are the leading cause of global warming. Therefore, saying no to meat is just as important as saying yes to that new hybrid car you've had your eye on. Actually, it is more important.

The Environmental Protection Agency (EPA) has found that nitrous oxide gas is about three hundred times more dangerous and destructive than the carbon dioxide that leaks out of your car.

Source: Ingrid Newkirk. *The PETA Practical Guide to Animal Rights: Simple Acts of Kindness to Help Animals in Trouble.* New York: St. Martin's, 2009, p. 54.

energy, food, health, and the environment have become a complex and multifaceted issue that requires responsible agencies to design appropriate policies accordingly. Therefore, it is thought that future global treaties like the Kyoto Treaty must pay more attention to the livestock issue in relation to the sustainability of the planet for future generations.

See also Agribusiness; Ecofeminism; Ethical Vegetarianism; Organic Foods and Technology; Policy; World Hunger.

Further Reading

Steinfeld, Henning, et al. *Livestock's Long Shadow: Environmental Issues and Options.* Rome: Food and Agriculture Organization of the United Nations, 2006.

Alok Kumar

GRAHAM, SYLVESTER (1794–1851)

Sylvester Graham was a prominent American health and social reformer who helped build an American vegetarian identity as a reform movement in the antebellum period. Born in Suffield, Connecticut, in 1794, Graham became an ordained minister in 1826, three years after dropping out of Amherst College. Having overcome a lengthy illness in the early 1820s, by 1829 Graham began preaching about a variety of reformist ideals throughout Pennsylvania and New Jersey. At the forefront of Graham's speeches were calls for temperance, sexual abstinence, and dietary reform. In 1829, Graham invented what would become known as "Graham bread," made from unsifted flour and free of chemicals such as chlorine.

Attempting to fight the effects of industrialized baked goods, Graham portrayed his bread as a whole wheat–based, healthy alternative, free of chemicals often used to whiten the color of bread. Motivated by the cholera epidemic of 1832, Graham questioned the efficacy of traditional American medical practices such as bloodletting or the use of cathartic purgatives such as arsenic. Linking the cholera outbreak directly to physical overstimulation, Graham intensified his public crusade, launching invectives against corporal stimulants such as sex, alcohol, meat, and spicy foods. In his writings Graham emphasized the study of human physiology, understanding the internal workings of the human body and living accordingly. In 1837 Graham began publishing the *Journal of Health and Longevity,* utilizing the growth of the printed word to promote ideals of temperance, sexual restraint, personal hygiene, and vegetarianism.

Graham's popularity surged during this time as followers—known as Grahamites—began building boardinghouses that followed a vegetarian lifestyle. In addition, recipes using Graham's methodologies began appearing in cookbooks throughout the United States, disseminating his ideas to a wider audience. By the 1840s vegetarianism stood at the forefront of the political consciousness of

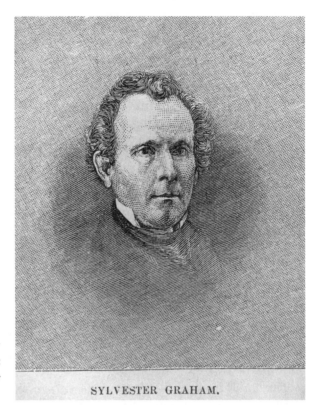

Engraving of Sylvester Graham, from *Harper's* 60 (1880): 190. (Courtesy of the Library of Congress)

SYLVESTER GRAHAM.

Graham and his followers. Partnering with Rev. William Metcalfe and William A. Alcott, Graham helped form the American Vegetarian Society (AVS) in 1850, modeling the organization after the Vegetarian Society started in England three years earlier. Graham would not live to see the growth of the organization, passing away just a year later in 1851. Graham's work as a health advocate, however, established meatless living and personal health care as visible reform movements, connecting personal choices with social reform.

See also Alcott, William A.; Alternative and Holistic Medicine; American Vegetarian Society; Bible Christians, Philadelphia; Metcalfe, Rev. William; Periodicals; Physiological Benefits; Reform; Shakers, The.

Further Reading

Gamber, Wendy. *The Boardinghouse in Nineteenth-Century America*. Baltimore: Johns Hopkins University Press, 2007.

Larkin, Jack. *The Reshaping of Everyday Life: 1790–1840*. New York: Harper Perennial, 1989.

Lefkowitz, Helen Horowitz. *Rereading Sex: Battles over Sexual Knowledge and Suppression in Nineteenth-Century America*. New York: Vintage Books, 2002.

Nissenbaum, Stephen. *Sex, Diet, and Debility in Jacksonian America: Sylvester Graham and Health Reform.* Westport, CT: Greenwood, 1980.

Puskar-Pasewicz, Margaret. "'For the Good of the Whole': Vegetarianism in Nineteenth-Century America." PhD diss., Indiana University, 2003.

Sack, Daniel. *Whitebread Protestants: Food and Religion in American Culture.* New York: Palgrave Macmillan, 2001.

Adam D. Shprintzen

GREGER, MICHAEL (1972–)

Michael Greger is a physician, author, and internationally known vegan nutrition expert who was one of the first to speak out about the risk of bovine spongiform encephalopathy (BSE)—popularly known as mad cow disease—in American cattle populations and its ability to be transmitted to humans who eat beef. Greger discovered the risk of the disease in 1993, three years before it became accepted by the biomedical community, while he was a junior at the Cornell University School of Agriculture. In the same year, he was hired as the chief BSE investigator for Farm Sanctuary, based in Watkins Glen, New York, to speak publicly about mad cow disease. Greger became a vegan after touring a stockyard in Lancaster, Pennsylvania, with a colleague from Farm Sanctuary. He received national attention in 1996 when he was asked to be an expert witness at Oprah Winfrey's defamation trial after the talk show host was sued by a group of cattle ranchers after declaring that she would no longer eat hamburgers. He also had the opportunity to debate publicly the policy director of the National Cattlemen's Beef Association at a Food and Drug Administration conference. In 2001, he became the mad cow coordinator for the Organic Consumers Association while continuing in his position as chief BSE investigator.

Five years after graduating from the Tufts University School of Medicine as a licensed general practitioner specializing in clinical nutrition, Greger launched AtkinsExposed.org in 2004 to counter the meat-heavy, low-carbohydrate Atkins diet weight-loss craze that had swept the nation by providing expert opinions and peer-reviewed scientific studies that condemned the diet as unhealthy and showed the research supporting it to be misleading. The same year, Greger's *Carbophobia! The Scary Truth about America's Low-Carb Craze* was published, further documenting the ineffectiveness of the Atkins diet.

In 2005, Greger became the director of public health and animal agriculture in the farm-animal welfare division of the Humane Society of the United States, where he conducts research on food safety, the public-health threats of industrial factory farming, and the affects on human health of routine practices used in intensive animal agriculture, such using nontherapeutic antibiotics and growth hormones in animals raised for food. This research is then used by the Humane Society to advocate for changes in public policy in the areas of agriculture and nutrition.

A founding member of the American College of Lifestyle Medicine, Greger is also the author of *Heart Failure: Diary of a Third Year Medical Student* (2000) and *Bird Flu: A Virus of Our Own Hatching* (2006) and has produced eight DVDs advocating a plant-based diet. Greger donates all fees and proceeds from the sale of his educational materials and speaking engagements to charity.

See also Agribusiness; Animal Rights and Animal Welfare; Baur, Gene; Houston, Lorri; Physiological Benefits; Organic Foods and Technology; Policy; Reform; Veganism.

Further Reading

Bird Flu: A Virus of Our Own Hatching. Film. University of Wisconsin-Madison, Innovations in Medical Education. http://videos.med.wisc.edu/videoInfo.php?videoid=241.

Greger, Michael. *Bird Flu: A Virus of Our Own Hatching.* New York: Lantern Books, 2006.

Greger, Michael. *Carbophobia! The Scary Truth about America's Low-Carb Craze.* New York: Lantern Books, 2005.

Hebb, Wendy, and Michael Richard. *Back to the Garden: The Real Food Revolution.* Film. Red Door Media, Damariscotta, ME. http://backtothegardenmovie.org/news/?page_id=39.

Michael Greger, M.D. http://www.drgreger.org/.

Mandy Van Deven

HEALTH FOOD STORES AND FOOD COOPERATIVES

Contemporary food cooperatives typically emphasize the sale and promotion of natural and organic food products, often with an emphasis on vegetarian and vegan products, and promote nonhierarchical organization, participatory democracy, and socially responsible consumption in general. Consumer cooperatives, which include food cooperatives, are distinct from worker or producer cooperatives that are owned and democratically operated by workers themselves. Consumer cooperatives are member-owned, democratically governed by member-owners, and operated according to general principles agreed on by the International Cooperative Alliance—an organization of cooperatives worldwide founded in 1895. The seven cooperative principles are open membership, democratic member control (one member, one vote), member economic participation (democratic control over the use of capital, for example), autonomy and independence from political and other partisan organizations, education, cooperation among cooperatives, and concern for the community.

According to the Natural Cooperative Grocers Association, an umbrella association that organizes many food cooperatives in the United States, the average (median) food cooperative was founded in 1975. As of 2009, the National Cooperative Grocers Association has 111 members. It is estimated, however, that there are closer to 300 food cooperatives in the United States.

Consumer cooperatives may vary slightly in their structure and organization. For example, most offer the opportunity for members to voluntarily work at the cooperative, usually a few hours a month, in exchange for a further discount on purchases. A smaller number of consumer cooperatives, however, require that each member-owner complete a set number of work hours as a part of membership. A growing number of consumer cooperatives are using a patronage dividend system where, in lieu of discounts for completing work hours, member-owners receive an annual dividend based on their total purchases. Consumer cooperatives also vary in their management structure. What could be termed "participatory" consumer cooperatives rely on direct democracy in the day-to-day management of the cooperative. The more common "traditional" consumer cooperative elects a board of directors who in turn oversee management. Traditional cooperatives promote a high degree of democracy in addition to the election of the board. For instance, they are likely to hold regular meetings where member-owners may vote on important decisions concerning the cooperative.

Contemporary food cooperatives typically trace their roots back to the organizing principles of the Rochdale Society of Equitable Pioneers established in 1844 in Rochdale, England; these later evolved into the seven cooperative principles. Robert Owen, an early Welsh-born utopian socialist and social reformer, promoted cooperation as a way toward a moral organization of society and economy. The first successful experiment in cooperation, however, took place in Rochdale in the midst of the "hungry forties" (more widely known as the period of the potato famine that devastated Ireland and the Scottish Highlands, in particular). Rochdale, a prominent textile town, had been the site of intense labor conflict as the power loom quickly replaced the work done by handloom weavers. Workers in the Rochdale mills struck unsuccessfully for higher wages. Defeated but not broken, the workers turned to innovative forms of consumption to survive despite low wages and to avoid the corruption of company stores—stores owned and operated by the employer that charged inflated prices and limited other consumer options. The leaders of the Rochdale cooperative, comprising 27 men and 1 woman, were familiar with Owen's work and as such viewed cooperation as an alternative to the exploitation of early industrial capitalism. During 50 years of operation, the Rochdale cooperative grew from the original 28 founders and their families to 12,000 families. The success of Rochdale spread, and by the 1860s there were over 400 consumer cooperatives in England alone.

The first consumer cooperative in the United States that was founded specifically on the Rochdale principles was the short-lived Union Cooperative Association #1 in Philadelphia; it opened in 1864 and closed two years later. The Union Cooperative Association was established to offer quality groceries to workers at fair prices and to improve the overall well-being of American workers. Despite its short life, the cooperative captured the attention of labor leaders, including future members of the Knights of Labor.

The Knights of Labor, initially established in 1869 as a craft union with the goal of uniting both skilled and unskilled workers into one union, became a key proponent of cooperation in the United States. The Knights of Labor adopted cooperation as a mechanism for social change and helped to create hundreds of cooperatives based on the Rochdale model in New England and the Midwest. The relationship between the cooperative movement and organized labor became strained, as the American Federation of Labor, which did not support cooperative development to the same extent as the Knights of Labor, gained in membership and power and the membership of the Knights of Labor declined in the 1890s.

After a number of years of dormancy, the U.S. consumer cooperative movement reemerged in 1916 with the establishment of the Cooperative League of America (now known as the National Cooperative Business Association). James

Peter Warbasse, the founder of the Cooperative League, served as its president from 1916 to 1941. The Cooperative League, based on the Rochdale principles, quickly established itself as the recognized organization of cooperatives in the United States. Warbasse sought to define the American cooperative movement as a viable and evolutionary form of social and economic change, within the context of the social and political unrest that defined America in the World War I and Great Depression eras.

The Great Depression brought cooperation back into the American mainstream. President Franklin D. Roosevelt's administration promoted and helped organize agricultural and urban cooperatives, which were incorporated into the Tennessee Valley Authority and migrant work camps. The administration's clear interest in the use of cooperation as a tool for economic development indicated a high point for cooperatives in the United States. World War II and the economic prosperity that followed, however, led to an end in the federal government's support for cooperation. Some interest in cooperation did continue in the United States based on the growth of credit unions and the use of agricultural cooperatives in Midwestern farming economies, but specific interest in consumer cooperatives declined.

It was not until the 1960s and 1970s that consumer cooperatives experienced revitalization. This new wave of cooperation was not necessarily connected to the labor history of cooperation in Europe and the United States. Instead, it grew out of the antiwar, social democracy, and antipoverty movements of the era. The new wave of cooperators did, however, find inspiration in the Rochdale principles. The principles of cooperation provided the building blocks for these social activists to establish alternatives to hierarchical and capitalist organization, which were viewed as alienating and exploitative. At the same time, the new cooperative movement connected to a growing interest in natural foods, voluntary simplicity, and a broader consumer rights movement. Second-wave cooperatives can best be characterized by a commitment to socially responsible consumption, participatory democracy, and the equitable production and distribution of food.

Many second-wave food cooperatives began as small buying clubs. Such clubs are made up of individuals and families who pool their resources to buy products in bulk at wholesale prices and distribute the goods among themselves. Buying clubs are typically run out of people's homes, churches, or other community locations and require little start-up capital because there is no physical retail space or paid staff. Thus, they provided access to natural and organic foods or tofu and other vegetarian items at a time when these items were not available in traditional supermarkets. Many buying clubs evolved into brick-and-mortar cooperatives as their membership and access to capital grew.

Food cooperatives have played a major role in bringing food politics to the mainstream. Existing food cooperatives, however, face challenges from national organic and natural food retailers—most notably Whole Foods Market—that have taken the formerly unique offerings of the food cooperative to the masses. The emergence of Whole Foods as a major aspect of the organic and natural foods market is forcing food cooperatives to reevaluate their business strategies. Two dominant approaches to dealing with this new challenge have surfaced. Some food cooperatives have emphasized expansion over core cooperative principles in order to better compete with large national retailers like Whole Foods. Other food cooperatives have decided to focus on the principles of cooperation as a way to distinguish themselves from large retailers but maintain their relatively smaller size and inventory. This schism among food cooperatives reflects a larger debate over whether cooperatives are simply an instrumental means to an end or an ideological social movement. It is too early to understand the long-term effect the widespread availability of organic, natural, and vegetarian products will have on second-wave food cooperatives. More data on food cooperatives at the national level are needed before any conclusions may be drawn or predictions made.

See also Activism and Protests; Agribusiness; Colonies, Communal Societies, and Utopias; Consumer Products; Policy; Reform; World Wars in England.

Further Reading

Furlough, Ellen, and Carl Strikwerda, eds. *Consumers against Capitalism?* Lanham, MD: Rowman and Littlefield, 1999.

Leiken, Steve. *The Practical Utopians: American Workers and the Cooperative Movement in the Gilded Age.* Detroit, MI: Wayne State University Press, 2005.

Sekerak, Emil, and Art Danforth. *Consumer Cooperation.* Santa Clara, CA: Consumers Cooperative Publishing Association, 1980.

Williams, Richard C. *The Cooperative Movement: Globalization from Below.* Burlington, VT: Ashgate, 2007.

Joshua L. Carreiro

HOUSTON, LORRI (1959~)

Lorri Houston (formerly Lorri Bauston) initiated the farmed-animal sanctuary movement in the United States in the mid-1980s by cofounding Farm Sanctuary, the first shelter established to rescue and protect farmed animals. Since then, it has become the second-largest farm-animal advocacy group in the world. Houston's work has garnered national media attention to the ways animals are used, and abused, for food production. A native of Madison, Wisconsin, Houston stopped eating meat at 16 years of age when her love for animals prevented her from seeing them as food. She later cut eggs and dairy from her diet to become vegan after becoming involved with the animal rights group Mobilization for Animals in 1981. She has said, in an interview with the author, that not consuming animals is "the single most important way that people can save lives and stop horrendous cruelty" every day.

Houston met Gene Baur during the summer of 1985 while working in Chicago for Greenpeace. The couple married in December 1986 and combined their last names into Bauston. After finding a still-alive sheep left for dead on a stockyard pile and rescuing her, Houston and Baur cofounded the Farm Sanctuary

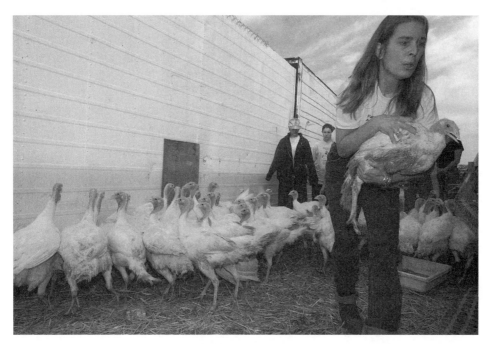

Lorri Houston (formerly Bauston) grabs a turkey in 2001 from a car salvage yard in Wilmington, California. Farm Sanctuary stepped in after a salvage yard owner was ordered to stop a turkey hunt he had organized as a Thanksgiving promotion. Customers who came to buy an auto part could take a turn chasing the turkeys around the yard. If they caught one, they could take the animal home for 25 cents. Farm Sanctuary was allowed to take 150 rescued turkeys to their sanctuary in Orland, California. (AP Photo/Damian Dovarganes)

in 1986 with the mission to save other mistreated farmed animals as well. They fund-raised for the organization by selling tofu hotdogs out of the back of their Volkswagen van at Grateful Dead concerts. While serving as the executive director, president, and chief fund-raiser for 18 years, Houston helped to save over 5,000 animals from the cruel conditions of factory farms, stockyards, and slaughterhouses; provide lifelong care for the rescued animals; conduct research on and raise public awareness about industrialized farming practices; investigate abuses of farmed animals and lead rescue efforts; and promote the creation and enforcement of legislation to protect farm animals. Farm Sanctuary has locations in New York and California, over 50 employees, and thousands of members. It has been used as a model for similar organizations worldwide and holds trainings to provide information on how to effectively open and operate a farm-animal shelter.

After Houston and Baur divorced in 2005, Houston founded Animal Acres, a sanctuary for farm animals and compassionate living center outside of Los Angeles that provides refuge, advocates the prevention of cruelty to farmed animals, and engages in public education and outreach projects. Animal Acres employs "animal ambassadors" who oversee one-on-one human-animal interactions so as to build compassion for cows, pigs, chickens, and other farmed animals. It also enforces anticruelty laws and was instrumental in the establishment of an Animal Cruelty Investigations unit, the first-ever state-incorporated humane enforcement agency devoted exclusively to the protection of farm animals. Animal Acres has attracted the support of many celebrities—including Ellen DeGeneres, Bill Maher, Kim Basinger, Alicia Silverstone, and Ed Begley Jr.—and was featured in the television series *30 Days* and the PBS series *Visiting with Huell Howser.*

See also Activism and Protests; Agribusiness; Baur, Gene; Reform; Veganism.

Further Reading

Baur, Gene. *Farm Sanctuary: Changing Hearts and Minds about Animals and Food.* New York: Touchstone, 2008.

Marcus, Erik. *Vegan: The New Ethics of Eating.* Ithaca, NY: Mcbooks, 2000.

Mandy Van Deven

I

INDIA

India has the world's largest proportion of vegetarians, although, contrary to what many people believe, they constitute a minority of the population. The 2006 *Hindu*-CNN-IBN State of the Nation Survey of nearly 15,000 people in 19 Indian states found that only 31 percent of Indians are lacto-vegetarian (meatless diet that includes dairy but excludes eggs); another 9 percent are lacto-ovo vegetarian (meatless diet that allows both dairy and eggs); and 60 percent of the population eats meat at some time. Very few Indians are vegans.

However, many Indians are de facto vegetarians. Meat is expensive, and most people eat it only on special occasions, something that was true in the Western world until modern times. Even today, many middle-class Indian households eat meat only on weekends. On average, Indians get 92 percent of their calories from vegetable products and only 8 percent from animal products (meat, dairy products, and eggs). While growing affluence has led to a rise in the consumption of animal products, meat and fish consumption is still much less than in the Western world or even in countries with comparable economies, such as Pakistan and China.

The 2006 *Hindu*-CNN-IBN survey found that 21 percent of all households consist of only vegetarian members, which indicates considerable differences even within families. Thirty-four percent of all Indian women are vegetarian, compared with 28 percent of men; 37 percent of people over the age of 55 are vegetarian, compared with 29 percent of people under the age of 25. Those family members who eat meat generally do so outside the home.

There are considerable regional variations. The smallest proportion of vegetarians (2–8 percent) live in coastal states—Andhra Pradesh, Kerala, West Bengal, Tamil Nadu, and Orissa, where seafood is abundant. The highest proportion live in landlocked states: Madhya Pradesh (45% of the population are vegetarian), Uttar Pradesh (33%), Punjab (48%), and Haryana (62%). An exception is the state of Gujarat: Although its coastline is on the Indian Ocean, 45 percent

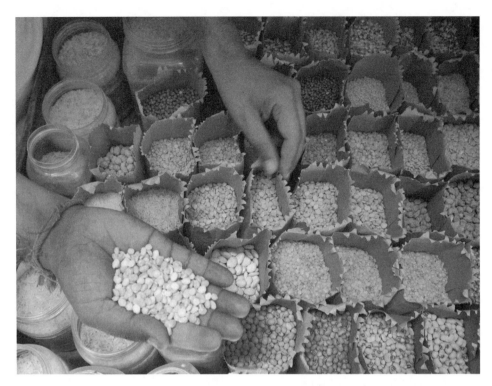

A wide variety of legumes at a market in Ahmedabad, India, 2008. (AP Photo/Ajit Solanki)

of Gujaratis are vegetarians, reflecting the strong influence of Jainism, a religion whose followers are strictly vegetarian.

Religion plays an extremely important role in determining what Indians eat. More than 80 percent of the population is Hindu, but 13.5 percent—138 million— are Muslims, making India the world's second-largest Muslim country after Indonesia. The population also includes 24 million Christians, 19 million Sikhs, 8 million Buddhists (0.8 percent), 4 million Jains; and small communities of Parsis (Zoroastrians), animists, and other religions.

Among Hindus, Brahmins (the priestly caste) are least likely to eat meat. More than 55 percent of Brahmins are vegetarian, although there are regional and individual exceptions: Bengali Brahmins eat fish, for example, while some Kashmiri Brahmins eat goat and mutton. Among other upper castes, 28 percent are vegetarian. Some 3 percent of Indian Muslims report themselves as vegetarians as do 8 percent of Christians.

Background of Vegetarianism Little is known about the food of the subcontinent's early inhabitants. Archaeological and linguistic evidence indicate that their diet featured rice, millet, lentils, gourds, eggplant, banana, coconut, jackfruit, citrus fruits, mangoes, spices (including turmeric, ginger, tamarind, and long pepper), fish, goat, and wild game. By 2500 BC, water buffalo were domesticated in the Indus Valley civilization—a sophisticated urbanized society whose wealth came from agricultural surpluses and trade.

Starting around 2000 BC pastoral small groups of cattle-raising seminomads living between the Caspian and Black seas moved through Central Asia, Persia, and Afghanistan into North India. These Indo-Europeans, sometimes called Aryans, brought with them cattle, horses, the Indo-European language, and religion, which was related to those of classical Greece and Rome.

Moving east and south, they conquered the local people and developed the caste system as a means of maintaining their separation and dominance. There were four main castes (*varnas*): *brahmins,* or priests; *kshatriyas,* the warriors and rulers; *vaisyas,* farmers, traders, and artisans; and *shudras,* serfs and laborers. Outside of the caste system were the "outcastes," who did such "unclean" and distasteful tasks as handling dead bodies and removing garbage. As society became more settled, society was further organized into hundreds of *jatis,* occupational groups, such as weavers, physicians, barbers, physicians, and so on, which eventually became hereditary.

The essence of Indo-Europeans' religion, sometimes called Vedism or Brahmanism, was animal sacrifice, which was seen as the only way of propitiating the all-powerful and capricious gods and other supernatural forces. The rituals accompanying these sacrifices became extremely elaborate and were known only to the Brahmins, who became very powerful as a result. The Indo-Europeans ate the flesh of the sacrificed animals, including beef, and meat was a normal article of diet for all members of society. A guest in ancient India was even called *goghna,* one for whom a cow was killed.

However, as early as 1000 BC some religious texts began to express antipathy to eating beef and killing cows. The reasons were in the main economic: Cows were too useful an asset to be slaughtered, since they provided labor, fuel (dried cow dung is still a common cooking fuel in India), and milk, which yielded yogurt and butter, important items in the Indian diet.

By the sixth century BC a revulsion against eating all meat arose that was associated with new philosophical and religious movements in northern India, one of the wealthiest regions of the world. Agricultural surpluses and a flourishing trade supported the development of towns and cities and the founding of universities that drew students from as far abroad as China. In this environment, people had the time and resources for philosophical speculation and began posing fundamental questions about the meaning of life and the nature of reality. One of the ideas that came into vogue was reincarnation, the idea that people are reborn over and over in many different forms, including animals. A related concept was karma, the belief that every action, good and evil, bears fruit and determines present and future lives. Both reinforced anti-meat-eating sentiments.

Beliefs and Conditions

Buddhism and Jainism In the sixth century BC, two movements, Jainism and Buddhism, emerged in North India. Their founders—Siddhartha Gautama (566–486 BC), later known as the Buddha ("enlightened one"), and Vardhaman (540–468 BC), known as Mahvahira ("great hero")—were born in North India into princely families. Despite differences, both religions posited that the goal of existence is to attain enlightenment and ultimate release from the cycle of rebirths and emphasized the need for kindness to all living creatures.

Gautama Buddha rejected asceticism and preached the middle way to salvation, based on nonviolence, compassion, and moderation in all things, including food. Although Buddhist monasteries were vegetarian, outside of the monasteries, monks, who begged for their food, had to accept anything that was given, even meat or fish, provided that they did not ask for the meat or see or hear the killing of the animal. Laypeople were not expected to follow such a rigorous regime. By the 13th century Buddhism had virtually disappeared in India as its followers and ideas were absorbed into Hinduism. However, missionaries accompanied Indian merchants to Southeast Asia and spread Buddhism throughout Asia.

Jainism is the world's only unconditionally vegetarian religion. Its central concept is *ahimsa,* or noninjury, defined in the *Ācārāṅga Sūtra* in the following way: "All things breathing, all things existing, all things living, all beings whatever, should not be slain or treated with violence or insulted or tortured or driven away." Nowhere do Jain concerns about ahimsa manifest themselves more vigorously than with regard to food. Jains believe that everything in nature has a *jiva,* or soul, and thus must not be killed. All Jains are enjoined from eating meat and meat products, fish, eggs, alcohol, and honey. Itinerant Jain monks and nuns, who survive on food given by laypersons, also avoid fruits and vegetables with seeds, root vegetables, onions and garlic, fresh ginger and turmeric, foods containing yeast, and all buds and sprouts. Laypersons avoid these foods during periods of fasting. Jains do not eat after sunset to avoid inadvertently killing insects. As Jains progress on their spiritual journeys, they limit the kind and number of foods they consume. In general, the old follow more restrictions than the young, and women more than men. Jainism became prevalent in southern and western India. Unlike Buddhism, it was not a missionary religion, so that its presence today is limited to India and the Indian diaspora.

Both Buddhism and Jainism attracted many adherents not only because of their message but also because of their opposition to the powerful priests and the caste system. Caste was not a barrier to those who wanted to be monks or lay followers. It is likely, too, that farmers were happy that their animals were not constantly being used for sacrifices. The spread of these religions was advanced by the political patronage and financial support of wealthy merchants and rulers, most notably the emperor Shoka Ashoka the Great (273–232 BC), who propagated the idea of ahimsa throughout his kingdom and became a vegetarian himself.

India's vegetarian practices were known to the ancient Greeks and may have influenced Pythagoras (b. 580?–506), a contemporary of Buddha and Mahavira, who propagated the idea of transmigration and advocated vegetarianism. There was even a legend that Pythagoras traveled to India.

Hinduism   Under the influence of Jainism and Buddhism, animal sacrifice came to a virtual end among Hindus, although it is still practiced in some places, notably Calcutta's Kali temple and in Nepal. In its place worshippers made offerings of fruits, flowers, vegetables, and coconuts to the image of a deity in a temple.

Most followers of the god Vishnu, called Vaishnavs, which include modern-day followers of the Hare Krishna sect, gave up meat. Brahmin priests followed suit and also became vegetarians.

In the process dietary habits took on caste connotations. Food came to be regarded as either clean (vegetarian) or unclean (nonvegetarian), and meat eating became associated with the lower castes and outcastes, especially in southern and western India, where Jainism was dominant. The Manu Smriti, written down between 200 BC and AD 200, laid down a code of behavior for Hindus that contains many admonitions about food. It states that "there is no greater sinner than that man who . . . seeks to increase the bulk of his own flesh by the flesh of other beings." Manu's Code also prohibits the eating of fish, although some "clean" varieties are allowed in certain rituals. Fish eating even by people who consider themselves vegetarians is still common in West Bengal, where religious texts dating back to the 12th century condone the eating of fish with the exception of those that have no scales or look like snakes, crabs, and tortoises.

Islam   India's second-largest religion, Islam, was brought to India's west coast by Arab traders in the 8th century AD. Starting in the 12th century, invaders from Afghanistan and Central Asia conquered northern India. In 1526 Babar, the ruler of a small Central Asian kingdom, seized the throne in Delhi and founded the Moghul dynasty, which ruled India until 1857. Although Islam does not advocate vegetarianism and even sanctions the eating of meat, followers of the mystical Sufi sect often abstain from meat during periods of retreat and meditation. Under the influence of Sufism and perhaps also for political reasons, the Moghul emperors, notably Akbar (1556–1605), ate meat sparingly and even banned the slaughter of animals at certain times.

Christianity   According to legend, St. Thomas brought Christianity in the first century AD when he landed on the Malabar Coast, now Kerala. The Portuguese, who conquered parts of western India starting in the 15th century, converted people en masse to Roman Catholicism and forced converts to eat meat, especially beef and pork, as a sign that they had given up their heathen ways. However, many Hindus who converted to Christianity retained their social customs, including caste and vegetarianism, and today 8 percent of Indian Christians report themselves as vegetarians.

Ironically, while the Portuguese were forcing Indians to abandon their vegetarianism, Indian vegetarian practices became known to Europeans through travel literature and had considerable impact on Western thinking. Voltaire, among others, praised Hindus' treatment of animals and contrasted it with the Christian practices. Sir Isaac Newton's reading about "Eastern sages" convinced him that mercy to beasts was one of God's first laws, which Europeans were violating.

Sikhism   India's fourth-largest religion, Sikhism, emerged in the 14th century in the Punjab. Its founder, Guru Nanak (1469–1538), was born a Hindu but rejected caste and preached the doctrine of "one God, the Creator, whose name was truth." Under the leadership of his successors, the Sikhs became a distinct community who adopted five distinguishing symbols: the beard, the dagger, an iron bracelet, special underwear, and the turban.

Sikhs do not have to be vegetarian, but they also do not advocate meat eating; many Sikhs avoid meat altogether. Their sacred writings contain passages that indicate concern over the morality of killing animals for food but say that the decision whether to eat meat should be left to the individual. Sikh places of worship include a community kitchen (*langar*) that provides free meals to all worshippers and visitors, even those from other religions. The food served here is always vegetarian, which makes it accessible to people of all faiths.

Yoga The link between diet and spiritual and physical health is a key component of Indian yogic philosophy. Yoga is more than a series of physical postures; it is a philosophy of life that aims at the development of a balance between the body and the mind in order to reunite the individual self with the Absolute or pure consciousness. Diet has an intimate connection with the mind, which is formed out of the subtlest portion of the food. Yogis, students, and all those aspiring to spiritual advancement must eat vegetarian *sattvic* foods that render the mind pure and calm and are conducive to enlightenment and serenity. They include fresh fruits and vegetables, wheat, rice, cow's milk, dry ginger, cucumber, green vegetables, honey, kidney beans, nuts, and seeds. Ghee, or clarified butter, is considered particularly sattvic since it helps to stimulate the healthy flow of fluids throughout the body. Garlic and sometimes onions as well as meat are strictly forbidden.

Vegetarian Practices   In India, 70 percent of average per capita calorie consumption comes from cereals. In northern India, the main cereal is wheat ground into flour and made into bread. In eastern and southern India, the dietary core is rice. Indians prefer rice varieties with long, slender grains that retain their shape when cooked, the best known of which is *basmati*. Much of western India (Rajasthan, part of Gujarat) is barren desert where only millets, sorghum, and other coarse grains grow. In the past, they were made into breads, but today wheat is becoming the standard throughout the country both because it is relatively cheap and abundant and because it has become a symbol of modernity.

Legumes play an important part in the Indian diet in the form of more than 50 varieties of lentils, peas, chickpeas, and beans. In Hindi both the raw ingredients and the boiled dish made from them are called *dal*. Almost all Indians eat dal every day. The combination of grains and lentils provides most of the amino acids the human body needs to stay healthy.

Milk and its products are another important source of protein. In North India milk is drunk by itself or boiled with tea and spices to make *chai*. Yogurt is widely used as a marinade, served as a side dish, or churned to produce butter, which is made into clarified butter, called *ghee*, which is the preferred cooking medium in India for those who can afford it.

In an Indian meal, relatively small amounts of meat, fish, and vegetables—the fringe—are added to enhance the taste and qualities of the main grain. Indigenous vegetables include bitter melon (*karela*), many varieties of squash and gourds, eggplant (*brinjal* or *baingun*), long green beans (*seema*), white radish (*mooli*), and various leafy greens, collectively called *saag*. Potatoes, tomatoes, green peppers, winter squash, corn, okra, and other popular vegetables were introduced by the

Portuguese starting in the late 15th century. Fruits and vegetables are also made into chutneys and pickles that add a contrasting flavor and texture to a meal.

See also Eastern Religions, Influences of; Gandhi, Mohandas; Jainism.

Further Reading

Achaya, K.T. *A Historical Dictionary of Indian Food*. New Delhi: Oxford University Press, 1998

Achaya, K.T. *Indian Food: A Historical Companion*. New Delhi: Oxford University Press, 1994.

Sen, Colleen. *Food Culture in India*. Westport, CT: Greenwood, 2004.

Sen, K.M. *Hinduism*. London: Penguin, 1991.

Stuart, Tristram. *The Bloodless Revolution: A Cultural History of Vegetarianism from 1600 to Modern Times*. New York: W.W. Norton, 2007.

Yadaav, Yogendra, and Sanjay Kumar. "The Food Habits of a Nation." *The Hindu*, August 14, 2006.

Colleen Taylor Sen

INTERNATIONAL VEGETARIAN UNION

The International Vegetarian Union (IVU) is a nonprofit organization founded in 1908 in Dresden, Germany, at the first World Vegetarian Congress. Its membership comprises hundreds of vegetarian and vegan societies from across the globe. The IVU has organized a nomadic World Vegetarian Congress since 1908, usually every two to three years. The IVU is governed by an International Council elected by member societies at each congress. In 2008, the 38th Congress was held in Dresden to celebrate the event's centenary and that of the IVU itself. The IVU's stated aim is to promote vegetarianism throughout the world. The long history and global reach of the IVU are reflected in its Web site, which is one of the most comprehensive sources of information about vegetarianism available.

The formation of the IVU reflected a culture of peaceable internationalism in the vegetarian movement at the time: The 1908 Congress was organized to coincide with the International Esperantist Congress. Many then-prominent vegetarians, including Leo Tolstoy, were enthusiasts for Esperanto, a language created in the late 19th century and designed to foster peaceable international relations through providing a universal and politically neutral form of communication. The 1908 Congress was also a result of international cooperation between the French, British, German, and local Dresden vegetarian societies. Since 1908, the theme of cooperation across geographic and cultural differences, with the ethics of vegetarianism providing a unifying principle, has continued to shape the IVU's history. In 1957, the first congress outside Europe was held, in India. This event provided the impetus for the formation of IVU regions, which are now responsible for organizing regional activities, including congresses, under the IVU ambit. There are currently six IVU regions: Africa; Asia-Pacific; Europe; India, South and West Asia; Latin America and the Caribbean; and North America.

See also Africa; Asia; Ethical Vegetarianism; Europe; France; India; Internet, The; Reform; United Kingdom.

Further Reading

International Vegetarian Union. http://www.ivu.org/.

Matthew Cole

INTERNET, THE

The Internet has enabled suitably skilled and motivated individual vegetarians to make an unexpected and disproportional contribution to the growth of the vegetarian diet worldwide. The origins of the Internet date back to a U.S. Military of Defense project in 1957, but the creation of the World Wide Web in 1991 simplified the way in which information was searched for and retrieved and allowed for the possibility of large numbers of people accessing the Internet. It was not until the mid-1990s, however, that the technology was fully exploited commercially.

Individual vegetarians who were familiar with the Internet were quick to see its potential to provide an international platform for the movement and to offer their services to national vegetarian societies to create and maintain Web sites and later Internet discussion groups. As early as 1994, the Vegetarian Society of the United Kingdom had a Web page that was created by Ben Leamy at the University of East London and hosted by Lindsay Marshall at Newcastle University. Leamy was also responsible for creating Web pages for other vegetarian and animal rights organizations such as Vegetarian International Voice for Animals (VIVA!) and Animal Aid. A Vegetarian Society member, John Davis, added a range of information sheets to the Vegetarian Society's pages in January 1995, and these early pages received 500 page views per month. By the end of the year, the greater availability to the general public of Web browsers had produced 45,000 page views per month for the society. By the following year, this figure had more than doubled to 100,000 page views per month. Davis also created the first European Vegetarian Union (EVU) Web pages in April 1995 and, in November of the same year, the International Vegetarian Union (IVU) Web pages. These Web pages placed vegetarian organizations clearly in the vanguard of what would later be referred to as an information superhighway revolution.

One of the earliest domain name registrations was that of veg.org, created in 1994 by Geraint Edwards and known as the "Vegetarian Pages." This site was also hosted by Lindsay Marshall at Newcastle University. Although this site currently offers little more than links to other organizations, it was for a time the premier source of all the other known vegetarian sites in cyberspace and the home of many early message boards and discussion groups for vegetarians.

People for the Ethical Treatment of Animals (PETA) first registered the domain name peta.org in September 1995, and this site continues to be the most popular vegetarian/animal welfare Web site. PETA has clearly mastered the art of successful vegetarian Web sites and also owns a number of other successful Web sites including goveg.com, petatv.com, peta2.com and peta.de. Another early domain name that is still among the top 20 most popular vegetarian sites on the World Wide Web is vegsource.com, founded in 1996 by Jeff and Sabrina Nelson, who from 1998 have hosted the IVU Web site as well as the Web sites of many other vegetarian organizations. By 2001, vegsource.com was receiving 1.4 million hits a month. Another early adopter of the World Wide Web was Maynard Clark, a Massachusetts Software Council fellow, who, at the turn of the 21st century, created a vegetarian portal at www.vegetarian.org. This site provided information about the Vegetarian Resource Centre (VRC) and offered a wide range of around 100 topical and specialized e-mail groups for vegetarians. The aim of these groups was to provide networking opportunities for vegetarians that went beyond merely a shared diet, with e-mail lists for particular professions, ethnicities, religions, ages, and life stages, such as parenting. These lists were subsequently transferred to the Yahoo groups platform, where many continue to this day.

In 1999, Clark, along with Robert Conrow and T. Colin Campbell, had attempted to establish a supply-chain business called VeggieSeek.com that aimed to make vegan businesses more profitable. This venture was unsuccessful owing to the decline in dot.com funding, and the three principals instead focused their energies on promoting veganism in other ways. Other early sites that remain popular are vrg.org, owned by Charles Stahler and Deborah Wasserman; the Christian vegetarian Web site all-creatures.org; and fatfree.com (now fatfreevegan.com). Many of the successful vegetarian Web sites today were founded in the early days of the Internet by individual vegetarians and are now operated as commercial or not-for-profit sites.

One of the key benefits of the growth of the Internet has been the reduction in isolation for minority groups such as vegetarians. In a survey of 1,249 vegetarians and vegans, recruited via the vegan Web site www.veganvillage.com, that took place twice a year from 2000 to 2003, 82 percent of respondents in June 2003 agreed that the Internet made them feel less isolated, a substantial increase over June 2000 when 54 percent of respondents felt that the Internet had reduced their isolation as a vegetarian or vegan. Ninety-four percent of respondents were using the Internet to search for vegan products, and 67 percent purchased vegan products online, suggesting that vegetarians and vegans were at that time more willing than most consumers to use the Internet to make purchases. This survey also demonstrated that 16 percent of the respondents, almost all of whom were vegetarians or vegans, did not know any other vegans.

The development of the Internet in recent years has seen vegetarians, in common with other Internet users, utilizing film to promote their cause either on campaigning Web sites such as PETA, on youtube.com, or on niche Internet TV stations such as www.veggievision.tv. Specialist online shops continue to spring up and join established online vegetarian retailers such as www.vegetarianshoes.co.uk and www.veganstore.com. Vegetarian campaigning organizations are also increasingly using blogs and social networking sites such as Twitter and Facebook as part of their integrated campaign strategies. Organizations such as the

Vegetarian Society of the United Kingdom plan to integrate their membership database function with far greater facilities for members to interact with the society online. There have been recent moves to create specifically vegetarian social networks such as www.vegppl.com and www.volentia.com, which have the potential, if fully realized, to further reduce the isolation of vegetarians. To date, however, vegetarians seem to have exploited the existing opportunities of the Internet to promote their diet and lifestyle rather than seeking to locate themselves in an exclusive network. As a result there are vegetarian contributions to vegetarian Facebook groups and to Wikipedia, Twitter, and www.meetup.com.

It is possible that the Internet will have a greater impact on vegetarian organizations in the future. The Internet has removed the need for the traditional 19th-century organization of vegetarian and animal welfare societies. There is no requirement to form a group, allocate responsibilities, and raise membership subscriptions for the group to flourish. One person can competently organize a Web site or discussion group for a local organization, and this can be done with minimal or no expense to the organizer. Information on healthy eating for vegetarians and on suitable stores and restaurants worldwide is freely available on Web sites, although there is no guarantee of quality control, and this further lessens the reason for joining a traditional society.

See also Activism and Protests; Animal Rights and Animal Welfare; Consumer Products; Health Food Stores and Food Cooperatives; International Vegetarian Union; People for the Ethical Treatment of Animals; Reform; Restaurants; Social Acceptance; Television and Films; Veganism.

Further Reading

A Bit of Veg Web History, IVU History News. www.ivu.org/news/online/history/html.
Iacobbo, Karen, and Michael Iacobbo. *Vegetarians and Vegans in America Today*. Westport, CT: Praeger, 2006.
The Top One Hundred Veg Related Websites. www.ivu.org/members/weblist.html.
The Vegan Research Panel. www.imaner.net/panel.

Samantha Calvert

J

JAINISM

Jainism is one of the two main Sramanic spiritual traditions, which involve ascetic practices and various forms of worldly renunciation, that originated on the Indian subcontinent. There is historical evidence that the Sramanic tradition is as least as old as the Vedic tradition that gave rise to Hinduism. About 2,500 years ago, the Sramanic tradition split into two groups: Jainism and Buddhism. Although Hinduism and Buddhism promote vegetarianism to some degree, virtually all Jains avoid the consumption of meat, poultry, fish, and eggs.

Jains consider the eating of these animal products as a violation of Ahimsa (Ahinsa), or nonviolence, one of the central tenets of their religion. Jains are forbidden to commit intentional violence against all mobile, multisensed beings. The mammals, birds, and fish that humans regularly consume are, like humans, mobile beings with five senses. The ban against intentional violence is not limited to what a person does directly; it extends to causing others to do violence (Himsa or Hinsa) as well as to approving of the Himsa of others.

Although Jains are permitted to eat plant foods, which involves taking the life of one-sensed immobile beings, Jains recognize that fewer plants are killed if humans eat plants directly rather than feeding them to animals that humans then consume. Animals raised for meat consume more protein than they produce. So the standard Jain diet not only seeks to eliminate violence to animals but also has the effect of minimizing the amount of plants necessary to feed humans. Jains recognize that meat-based agriculture is an ecological disaster, and a central tenet of Jain philosophy involves the obligation of humans to minimize their adverse impact on the environment.

Jains maintain that all sentient beings have equal inherent value as living beings. The proscription against violence against all sentient beings has strong support in Jain scriptures and widely accepted secondary literature. For example, the *Ākārāṅga Sūtra,* states that "all breathing, existing, living, sentient creatures should not be slain, nor treated with violence, nor abused, nor tormented, nor driven away." Acharya Hemachandra, a 12th-century Jain ascetic and scholar, wrote that "[t]hose who eat the meat of other [living beings] in order to satisfy their own flesh, they are definitely murderers [themselves], since without a consumer [there can be] no killer." Some Jain ascetics go so far as to place a small rectangular piece of cloth, called a *muhpattī*, in front of their mouths to avoid injuring insects and other airborne life-forms and use a small whisk broom, called a *rajoharana*, to sweep an area before sitting or walking to avoid any injury to sentient beings.

Although Jains accept that considerations of Ahimsa and ecology mean that humans should not consume the flesh or eggs of animals, many Jains continue to consume dairy products, to wear leather, wool, and silk clothing, and to use dairy products and wool in temple rituals. These animal products, however they are produced, all necessitate the suffering and death of five-sensed beings. For example, animals used in the dairy industry are kept alive longer than animals used for meat, are treated as badly, if not worse, and end up in the same slaughterhouses. There would be no veal industry without the dairy industry. The production of wool, silk, and leather also involves intentional violence and death.

There is, therefore, a tension within Jainism in that although Ahimsa is the central principle of the religion and is interpreted by Jains to require abjuring all flesh and eggs, Jains arguably promote Himsa by consuming and using nonflesh animal products. There are several justifications offered for this use of animal products, the primary one being that milk, ghee (clarified butter), wool, and so forth have been used for centuries and have not been thought to involve violence. But Jainism is a tradition that requires continuing rational examination of moral principles, and it simply cannot be denied that all animal products involve Himsa as an empirical matter.

Some Jains maintain that dairy, wool, and other animal products can be made without Himsa, so they are not inherently objectionable. But this neglects the reality that these animal products involve a great deal of suffering and death, irrespective of where and how they are produced. For example, dairy cows may suffer less on a small family farm than in a large intensive operation, but there is still suffering and death under the most ideal circumstances, and Jain doctrine clearly forbids the intentional infliction of any suffering, distress, or death on a mobile, multisensed being. Others claim that veganism represents an extreme position and that Jainism avoids taking extreme positions. But that view is also inconsistent with the prohibition against inflicting any violence against mobile, multisensed beings.

The sentiment in the Jain community is, however, moving in the direction of veganism. For example, for some years now, Gurudev Chitrabhanu, a former Jain monk who came to the United States in 1971 and who is an important figure in the Jain community worldwide, has been a tireless advocate for veganism, emphasizing that the principle of Ahimsa requires abjuring eating, wearing, or using any animal products. Pravin Shah has, through his extensive work on educational materials for the Federation of Jain Associations in North America, promoted discussion of veganism in many Jain publications. Jain youth, particularly those born in the United States, United Kingdom, and Canada, are increasingly embracing veganism.

See also Ahimsa; Asia; Eastern Religions, Influences of; Ethical Vegetarianism; India; Religious Beliefs and Practices; Veganism.

Further Reading

Ākārāṅga Sūtra, in *The Sacred Books of the East: Vol. 2: Jaina Sutras, Part I.* Translated by Hermann Jacobi; edited by F. Max Müller. Delhi: Motilal Banarsidass, 1989.

Chapple, Christopher K. *Nonviolence to Animals, Earth, and Self in Asian Traditions.* Albany: State University of New York Press, 1993.

Francione, Gary L. "Ahimsa and Veganism," *Jain Digest,* Winter 2009.

Jain, Jagdish Prasad. *Fundamentals of Jainism.* New Delhi: Radiant Publishers, 2005.

Jain, Jyoti Prasad. *Religion and Culture of the Jains,* 5th ed. New Delhi: Bharatiya Jnanpith, 2006.

JAINA Education Committee. *Jain Philosophy and Practice—1 & 2.* Raleigh, NC: JAINA, 2005–2006.

Muniśrī Nyāyavijayajī, *Jaina Darsana.* Translated by Nagin J. Shah as *JAINA Philosophy and Religion.* Delhi: Motilal Banarsidass, 1998.

Shah, Natubhai. *Jainism: The World of Conquerors.* Vols. 1 and 2. Portland, OR: Sussex Academic Press, 1998.

Wiley, Kristi L. *Historical Dictionary of Jainism.* Lanham, MD: Scarecrow, 2004.

The Yogaśāstra of Hemacandra. Translated by Olle Quarnström. Cambridge, MA: Harvard University Press, 2002.

Gary L. Francione

KATZEN, MOLLIE (1950~)

Born in 1950 in Rochester, New York, Mollie Katzen is a cookbook author and artist who was instrumental in the advent of the vegetarian cooking movement with the publication of the *Moosewood Cookbook* in 1977. Katzen is one of the best-selling and most prolific vegetarian authors of the late 20th century and beyond. Katzen was one of the original cooks at the Moosewood Collective in Ithaca, New York, which was started by her brother and five other people in January 1973. Katzen committed to helping out for three months and ended up staying five years. Katzen's interest in writing and art led to her keeping an illustrated recipe journal for years. This morphed into the cookbook.

Prior to the commercial version of the *Moosewood Cookbook,* Katzen turned her recipe journal into a spiral-bound book; the initial 800 copies sold out immediately. Over the next six months, she sold 2,000 more copies. After repeating that the following six months, she finally struck a deal with Ten Speed Press, and the book became a commercial success when published in 1977. The *Moosewood Cookbook* was a breakthrough book due to its large format, hand lettering, illustrations by Katzen, and creative vegetarian recipes. The revised, updated, and lightened-up version of *Moosewood Cookbook* was published in 1992.

Katzen retired from the restaurant around the time of publication of the *Moosewood Cookbook* in 1977 but has continued writing and illustrating cookbooks. Her other books include *The Enchanted Broccoli Forest* (1982), *Vegetable Heaven* (1997), *Moosewood Restaurant New Classics* (2001), and *The Vegetable Dishes I Can't Live Without* (2007). Katzen is also a children's book author. Her latest book, *Get Cooking: 150 Simple Recipes to Get You Started in the Kitchen,* was released in 2009. It was inspired by teaching her children how to do basic cooking once they moved out of the house.

Beyond authoring cookbooks, Katzen has been influential in the nutrition field. She was appointed as a charter member of the Harvard School of Public Health Nutrition Roundtable. She coauthored *Eat, Drink, and Weigh Less* (2007) with Harvard physician Walter Willett. Katzen also works as a consultant to

Harvard University Dining Services and food companies and often staffs booths at trade shows and signs copies of her books.

Since 1995, Katzen has appeared on public television in four different vegetarian shows. Her company, Mollie Katzen Designs, located in northern California, also provides artwork for menus and celebrations. She is still creating artwork and producing it for sale. In 2007, Katzen was inducted into the James Beard Cookbook Hall of Fame as one of its few vegetarian authors.

See also Cookbooks; Policy; Restaurants.

Further Reading

Global Gourmet. http://www.globalgourmet.com/food/egg/egg0798/katzen2.html.
Harvard University Dining Services. http://www.dining.harvard.edu/about_HUDS/katzen. html.
MollieKatzen.com. http://www.molliekatzen.com/.

Jill Nussinow

KELLOGG, JOHN HARVEY (1852–1943)

John Harvey Kellogg was a vegetarian health reformer and physician-in-chief of Battle Creek Sanitarium in Michigan. He wrote and lectured extensively and developed many vegetarian food products. Kellogg was born in 1852 in Tyrone, Michigan, to John Preston Kellogg and Ann Stanley. The family soon joined the Seventh-day Adventist faith, which advocated alternative medical therapies and abstinence from tea, coffee, tobacco, alcohol, and, by the mid-1860s, meat. When Kellogg was four, the family moved to Battle Creek, and in 1864, James and Ellen White, founding members of Adventism and fellow Battle Creek residents, invited the precocious boy to learn the printing trade. Kellogg was captivated by health reform materials, and in 1872 the Whites arranged for him to attend the alternative Hygieo-Therapeutic College in New Jersey. Kellogg also studied conventional medicine at the University of Michigan and Bellevue Hospital, New York, earning his medical degree in 1875. He edited the Adventist *Health Reformer* magazine, renaming it *Good Health* in 1879, and in 1876, he became superintendent of the Western Health Reform Institute, a small Adventist convalescent home established in Battle Creek in 1866. Kellogg renamed it the Battle Creek Sanitarium and in 1878 opened a new 200-patient building.

Under Kellogg's leadership, the sanitarium became a fashionable destination, offering alternative treatments such as hydropathy and light therapy. Kellogg's program of "biologic living," however, centered on rest and exercise, sexual restraint, comfortable clothing, frequent enemas, and healthful food. Although Kellogg was disfellowshipped from the Adventist church in 1907, he continued to believe that vegetarianism held ethical, evolutionary, and especially physiological advantages. To prevent "autointoxication" from colonic waste, the sanitarium served an unspiced, low-fat, low-protein diet rich in fiber and whole grains. Zwieback and yogurt were staples, and the sanitarium's test kitchens developed foods such as granola, caramel cereal coffee substitute, peanut butter, and meat alternatives, including Nuttose and Protose. In 1894, Kellogg patented Granose flakes, the first flaked cereal, and the sanitarium soon served a corn version as well. The cereal business held great potential, and Kellogg's brother and fellow food innovator, Will Keith, created the Battle Creek Toasted Corn Flake Company in 1906. Business interests, however, drove the brothers apart.

In 1879, Kellogg married Ella Eaton, and the two fostered over 40 children. Always energetic, Kellogg often worked 20-hour days. He went on lecture tours, educated sanitarium guests, dictated dozens of books and articles for the sanitarium presses, and performed over 22,000 surgeries. In 1906, Kellogg organized the American Medical Missionary Board, which later became the Race Betterment Foundation, a center for the eugenics movement. He also continued to expand the sanitarium, and he opened Miami-Battle Creek in 1930. The Depression, however, struck Battle Creek Sanitarium hard, and the institution was forced to reorganize. Kellogg died in 1943 at age 91.

See also Alternative and Holistic Medicine; Battle Creek Sanitarium; Consumer Products; Reform; Religious Beliefs and Practices; Seventh-day Adventists.

Further Reading

Fee, Elizabeth, and Theodore M. Brown. "John Harvey Kellogg, MD: Health Reformer and Antismoking Crusader." *American Journal of Public Health* 92 (2002): 935.

Schwarz, Richard W. *John Harvey Kellogg, M.D.* Berrien Springs, MI: Andrews University Press, 1970.

Caroline Lieffers

KINGSFORD, ANNA (1846–1888)

Anna Kingsford was a British physician, writer, social activist, spiritualist, and passionate advocate of vegetarianism. Born Annie Bonus in 1846, she began writing at an early age, publishing her first book, *Beatrice: A Tale of the Early Christians,* in 1863. Other books followed, as did her marriage to Algernon Kingsford in 1867. Rejecting comfortable middle-class domesticity, however, Kingsford quickly became engaged in some of the more controversial social issues of the era, publishing pamphlets like *An Essay on the Admission of Women to the Parliamentary Franchise* in 1868. During the early 1870s she founded and edited the *Ladies Own Paper,* a vehicle for her condemnation of vivisection and support of women's emancipation. Soon embracing vegetarianism as well, Kingsford began giving lectures before the Manchester Vegetarian Society and similar organizations. She was especially critical of much contemporary scientific and medical research, both for its dismissal of the mysteries of human spirituality and for the continued expansion of vivisection in laboratories and classrooms.

In 1874, Kingsford's life and work were shaped by two major events. The first was her introduction to Edward Maitland, a writer and spiritualist who shared Kingsford's progressive philosophies, interest in vegetarianism, and fascination with religion, spirituality, and occultism. Both believed they were endowed with powerful psychic abilities, and they quickly became close friends and frequent collaborators. The second was that Kingsford—having been turned away from British institutions due to her gender—enrolled in medical studies at the University of Paris. She was intent on claiming the rhetoric of science for her own vegetarian and antivivisectionist causes and eager to face her critics armed with the imprimatur of the same scientific establishment from which they asserted their own authority.

By 1880, Kingsford had completed her exams and written her doctoral thesis, an elaborate defense of vegetarianism titled "De l'Alimentation Végétale chez l'Homme." Her faculty readers insisted that she remove a section describing the moral aspects of a meatless diet before they would approve it, however, and after reluctantly doing so Kingsford earned her doctor of medicine degree on July 22, 1880. Upon graduation Kingsford reinstated the section on the ethics of vegetarianism, and her thesis was soon published in English as *The Perfect Way in Diet*. With its systematic presentation of the physiological, anatomical, biochemical, sociological, and evolutionary arguments supporting a fleshless diet and its grounding in contemporary scientific knowledge, Kingsford's book was embraced by vegetarian advocates as a serious work of scholarship that underscored the legitimacy—and even superiority—of a vegetarian diet.

Kingsford's book, lectures, and status as one of the first female physicians in Britain were a boon to the burgeoning vegetarian movement of the 1880s. Yet she remained a controversial figure, since for many, her close association with Maitland and their ongoing explorations of mysticism and occult spirituality often appeared to undermine the scientific credibility of her vegetarian arguments. Kingsford, who had long suffered from asthma and other pulmonary conditions, developed pneumonia late in 1886, and her health began to decline rapidly. She died of tuberculosis on February 22, 1888, at the age of 42.

See also Alternative and Holistic Medicine; Antivivisection; Reform; Religious Beliefs and Practices.

Further Reading

Gregory, James. *Of Victorians and Vegetarians: The Vegetarian Movement in Nineteenth-Century Britain*. London: Tauris, 2007.

Kingsford, Anna. *The Perfect Way in Diet: A Treatise Advocating a Return to the Natural and Ancient Food of Our Race*. London: Kegan Paul, Trench and Company, 1881.

Kingsford, Anna, and Edward Maitland. *Addresses and Essays on Vegetarianism*. London: John M. Watkins, 1912.

Pert, Alan. *Red Cactus: The Life of Anna Kingsford*. Watson's Bay, Australia: Books and Writers Network, 2006.

Williams, Howard. "Anna Kingsford, the First Prophetess of the Humaner Life." In *The Ethics of Diet*, 236–42. Manchester, UK: Albert Broadbent, 1907.

Gary K. Jarvis

LAPPÉ, FRANCES MOORE (1944~)

Frances Moore Lappé is a leading global food and hunger expert and democracy activist. Her 1971 seminal work *Diet for a Small Planet* set in motion a new way of thinking about food, economics, and democracy by positing that a vegetarian diet would make it possible to end starvation and that worldwide hunger is not the result of a scarcity of food but of a scarcity of democracy.

Lappé was born on February 10, 1944, in Pendleton, Oregon, and raised in Fort Worth, Texas. In 1966, she graduated from Earlham College in Indiana with a bachelor's degree in history and soon began working as a community organizer in a national nonprofit in Philadelphia that assisted welfare recipients in low-income communities to receive government benefits. After two years, she left her job for graduate studies at the University of California, Berkeley's School of Social Work to gain an understanding of the underlying causes of hunger and poverty, but she dropped out of the program a year later. Frustrated with traditional education, the 26-year-old Lappé began the independent research project in Berkeley's agricultural library that would eventually become the groundbreaking book *Diet for a Small Planet*.

A radical notion on its release in 1971, *Diet for a Small Planet* showed that a meat-laden diet was unnecessary for human nutrition and contributed to the global food shortage. It put forth an alternative diet whereby humans could meet nutritional requirements by consuming complementary proteins found in plant-based sources, an idea that placed the ability to end world hunger in the hands of ordinary citizens. The book became a best seller and launched Lappé's career.

At a World Food Day event in 1975, Lappé met Joseph Collins, a like-minded global hunger advocate who worked at the Institute for Policy Studies in Washington, D.C. That year, the two cofounded the Institute for Food and Development Policy (also called Food First) to conduct research on and educate Americans about the political and economic causes of global hunger. Lappé later expanded the organization's mission to include travel to developing nations to gain firsthand

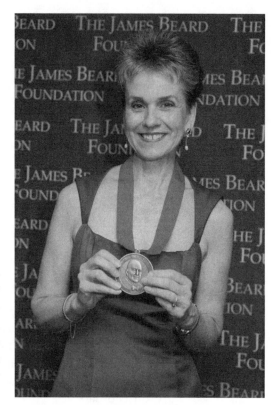

Author Frances Moore Lappé poses with her Humanitarian of the Year award at the 2008 James Beard Foundation Awards, 2008, at Avery Fisher Hall at Lincoln Center in New York. The awards recognize culinary professionals for excellence and achievement in their field. (AP Photo/Diane Bondareff)

knowledge of the issues facing local communities. The Institute for Food and Development Policy is now the nation's leading think tank on food policy and hunger issues.

Unsatisfied with her role as a social critic and desiring to get more people involved in global food activism, Lappé cofounded the Center for Living Democracy in 1990 with Paul Martin DuBois. The Center for Living Democracy was a 10-year initiative based in Brattleboro, Vermont, designed to encourage individuals to be accountable for their actions and resist market forces, such as advertising. Its mission was to increase the visibility of and accelerate the spread of democratic innovations by teaching ordinary citizens with a commitment to feeding the world how to use their skills and resources to solve world hunger. It did so through providing intensive skills-building workshops to teach successful problem solving and launching the American News Service to disseminate information about the successful use of innovative interventions whereby people are able to nourish themselves.

In 2001, Lappé shifted directions again, cofounding the Small Planet Institute and writing the 30th-anniversary sequel to *Diet for a Small Planet,* titled *Hope's Edge: The Next Diet for a Small Planet,* with her daughter, Anna. The Small Planet Institute channels resources to democratic social movements worldwide through the administration of funds to groundbreaking work such as Muhammad Yunus's Grameen Bank in Bangladesh and Wangari Maathai's Green Belt Movement in

Health Consequences of a Meat-Based Diet

Activist and author Frances Moore Lappé has described the standard high-sugar, high-fat diet of most Americans as "the greatest experiment ever attempted on human beings, and we, the guinea pigs, aren't faring very well!" Furthermore, she writes,

> The health consequences are staggering. This experimental diet puts the weight on at unprecedented rates. Across the planet, more than one billion people are now overweight—that's one in every six of us.
> . . . Extra weight itself heightens the risk of a great many diseases, including hypertension, heart disease, and certain cancers, such as late-life breast cancer. Therefore, obesity now ranks second only to smoking as a cause of mortality in America, resulting in 300,000 deaths each year. Think about it: In America our diet claims ten times more lives each year than does gun violence.

Source: Frances Moore Lappé and Anna Lappé. *Hope's Edge: The Next Diet for a Small Planet.* New York: Tarcher, 2002, p. 39.

Kenya and the creation and dissemination of solution-oriented media. Lappé has authored 17 books and has received numerous awards for the impact her lifelong work has had on the way people think about food, nutrition, and agriculture.

See also Activism and Protests; Agribusiness; Global Warming; Physiological Benefits; Policy; Reform; World Hunger.

Further Reading

Lappé, Frances Moore. *Diet for a Small Planet.* New York: Ballantine Books, 1971.
Lappé, Frances Moore, and Anna Blythe Lappé. *Hope's Edge: The Next Diet for a Small Planet.* New York: Tarcher, 2002.
Small Planet Institute. http://www.smallplanet.org/.

Mandy Van Deven

LYMAN, HOWARD F. (1938–)

One of America's leading spokespeople for vegetarian nutrition, Howard Lyman (aka the Mad Cowboy) is a fourth-generation cattle rancher from Montana. Lyman has dedicated his life to revealing falsehoods propagated by the meat and dairy industries by showing that a meat-based diet is the major cause of illness, such as certain types of cancer, heart disease, and obesity, in the United States.

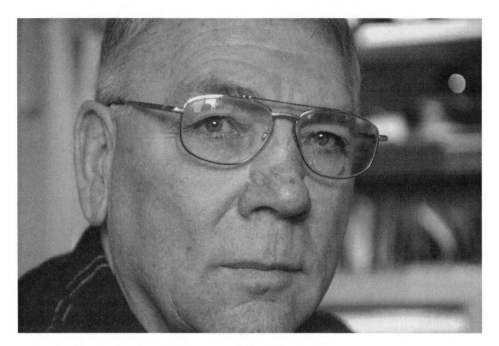

Howard Lyman, 2004. (AP Photo/Gerald Herbert)

Born on September 17, 1938, Lyman grew up on his family's organic dairy farm. Before joining the U.S. Army in 1961, Lyman earned a bachelor of science degree in agriculture from Montana State University. He returned to farming in 1963 when his brother's debilitating Hodgkin's disease and his father's declining health made it impossible for either of them to continue to manage the farm. Recognizing the organic method as not sufficiently profitable, Lyman made the changeover to chemically based techniques. Though the operation was running at nearly $5 million per year, the 40-acre farm remained unable to turn a profit.

In 1979, when the diagnosis of a spinal tumor threatened Lyman's life, he made a vow to himself: If he survived the operation to remove the tumor, he would return to organic farming. Lyman came through the surgery but was paralyzed from the waist down. Nevertheless, he was ecstatic, particularly when, after an arduous rehabilitation, he regained the ability to walk.

Fulfilling his promise, Lyman returned to organic farming and used integrated pest management (IPM) techniques. While learning about these methods, Lyman also learned about the harmful effects of unsustainable agriculture on food production worldwide. He learned about the connections between soil erosion, animal rights, and world hunger, which prompted first his conversion to vegetarianism and, a year later, veganism. Though this dietary change was only temporary, when Lyman lost over 100 pounds, lowered his cholesterol by over 150 points, and brought his blood pressure to a normal range, he began to think about the relationship between farming, diet, and health.

"Message for My Meat-Eating Friends"

In a chapter titled "Message for My Meat-Eating Friends" from the 2006 *No More Bull! The Mad Cowboy Targets America's Worst Enemy: Our Diet,* Howard Lyman rails at nonvegetarians:

> You shouldn't feel satisfied. Look at yourselves. You stand in the majority. You have government and industry on your side. Hell, your Department of Agriculture actually mandated, believe it or not, the "Got Milk?" and "Pork: The Other White Meat" advertising campaigns. Your steaks and hamburgers are effectively subsidized by national land and water policy. (If they were not, McDonald's hamburgers might well cost $5.00 each.) . . . Best-sellerdom is regularly achieved by diet book authors who, dripping with Orwellian logic, claim fatty animal foods will help you lose weight, as they strain to deny how the very eating habits they endorse have unleashed an obesity epidemic upon our nation. Burgers, pizza, hot dogs, and fried chicken all but reach out to your greasy fingertips on every highway and byway of the land. Your style of eating is brandished on billboards, and celebrated on television and in film as healthy, vital, and above all, normal—yet your existence could not be more precarious.
>
> First, by inducting yourself into the majority, you have compromised your own health. The scientific evidence of risk to your heart from eating the standard American diet rivals in depth, breadth, and uniformity the evidence that smoking causes cancer. Those who consume products derived from the carcasses and lactation of animals stand in markedly greater risk of developing heart disease, cancer, diabetes, obesity, osteoporosis, and a host of other illnesses than those who abstain from animal foods. By all accounts, vegetarians live seven to fourteen years longer on average than meat eaters, and enjoy better health while they're alive. And vegans live longer than vegetarians.
>
> . . . To state the obvious: vegetarians live longer than meat eaters simply and solely because we do not consume the filthy, fatty, disease-ridden, decaying flesh of animals.

Source: Howard F. Lyman, Glen Merzer, and Joanna Samorow-Merzer. *No More Bull! The Mad Cowboy Targets America's Worst Enemy: Our Diet.* New York: Scribner, 2005, pp. 60–61.

In 1982 Lyman ran for Congress and lost the election by only a small margin. He decided the following year to sell his farm in order to work with the Montana Farmers Union to help farmers in financial trouble. In 1987, Lyman moved to Washington, D.C., and became a professional lobbyist for the National Farmers Union. Over the next five years, Lyman worked toward the passage of the National Organic Standards Act, which was ultimately successful. In the process, he became convinced that the only way to enact more immediate change was to work directly with producers and consumers on a grassroots level.

In 1990, Lyman made a permanent switch to vegetarianism, followed again by becoming vegan. In 1995, he founded Voice for a Viable Future, a nonprofit organization whose mission is to encourage people to make choices that do not endanger the environment or their health. The following year, Lyman became a popular, and somewhat controversial, public figure after making an appearance on the *Oprah Winfrey Show*. Lyman explained the link between ruminant (cud-chewing hoofed animals) feeding and mad cow disease, which prompted Winfrey to declare that she would no longer eat hamburgers. As a result, both Lyman and Winfrey were sued by a group of cattle ranchers for violating a Texas law that forbids making false statements about agribusiness, but eventually they were found not liable.

From 1996 to 1999, Lyman served as the president of the International Vegetarian Union. He continues to advocate for a vegetarian lifestyle by writing books and speaking at events.

See also Activism and Protests; Agribusiness; Physiological Benefits; Policy; Reform; Veganism.

Further Reading

Lyman, Howard F. *Howard Lyman: Mad Cowboy.* http://www.madcowboy.com/.

Lyman, Howard F., and Glen Merzer. *Mad Cowboy: Plain Truth from the Cattle Rancher Who Won't Eat Meat.* New York: Scribner, 1998.

Mandy Van Deven

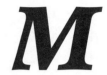

MACFADDEN, BERNARR (1868~1955)

Bernarr Macfadden was an American author who became famous as a health reformer with his unique and vital contribution to physical culture, which combined bodybuilding and nutritional and health theories. He was an inspiration for millions to live more healthfully and actively. In addition, he was received favorably in vegetarian circles because of his mistrust of growing urbanization and biological medicine as well as his tireless praise of the relationships between proper health and physical fitness, outdoor exercise, natural food, and natural medications.

Born in 1868 in Mill Spring, Missouri, to an alcoholic father and tubercular mother, Macfadden was orphaned before age 10. A skinny and sickly child who was frequently ill, he fought to recover by means of dumbbells and distance walking. He gradually became strong enough to teach gymnastics and win professional wrestling matches. By 1894 in New York City, Macfadden enjoyed a good clientele of people who paid him as their personal trainer and physical therapist. His self-image changed so much that he changed his first name to Bernarr because it sounded like a lion's roar—much stronger than Bernard—and also changed the spelling of his last name because Macfadden was more distinctive than McFadden.

Virtually self-taught, Macfadden spared no effort to achieve his greatest ambition, which was to educate people on the importance of physical culture in maintaining one's good health. Macfadden's books sold well, and his *Physical Culture* magazine enjoyed one of the highest circulations of any magazine in America for almost 50 years. Macfadden combined a genuine faith in the power of exercise with an obvious head for business that led him from rural poverty to the command of a vast publishing empire. Both his health and rise to outstanding financial success were a true-life rags-to-riches story.

By 1887, he opened his first studio under the title of "professor of kinesitherapy" and soon broadened his interests to incorporate the current themes of

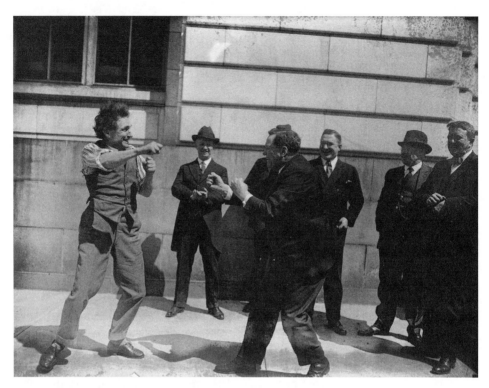

Bernarr Macfadden leads six senators in exercises in Washington, D.C., 1924. (Courtesy of the Library of Congress)

the preventive health gospel, which he called "physical culture." The magazine he launched in 1899 established the Physical Culture Publishing Company. The company expanded unceasingly, including by the 1920s newspapers and magazines such as *True Romances* and *True Detective,* and some on a gamut of health-related themes, making Macfadden a multimillionaire.

In 1911, he published the first edition of his five-volume opus, Macfadden's *Encyclopedia of Physical Culture,* revealing the system then practiced in his numerous physical culture "Healthatoriums," including one in his short-lived experiment in communal hygiene, Physical Culture City, in New Jersey and another in Battle Creek, Michigan, in front of the Kellogg's sanitarium. His Healthatoriums employed well-trained people, who contributed to the great success and helped to establish Macfadden as a leader in the field of alternative health care. Macfadden then created the Bernarr Macfadden Institute, a school that trained students in his physical culture methods, which he called "physcultopathy." The curriculum covered anatomy; physical training; hygiene, including diet, exercise, sunshine, fresh air, and cleanliness; and instruction in natural methods of treating illness.

Far from being limited to just the body, the physical culture scheme is conducive to self-perfection by way of its holistic reach; it is an intricate combination of physical, intellectual, and moral capacities, thereby reviving the timeless link established between a sound mind and a sound body. In particular, Macfadden was convinced that securing absolute purity of the blood, by means of a pure diet, was the best way to block any disease. In his 1915 *Vitality Supreme,* Macfadden worked out this principle: Blood is life, so people are what they are because of the blood that circulates in their body. To have enough pure blood in the body, proper digestion and absorption of nutrients are necessary. The diet is to be fortified with foods providing complete nutrition so that the blood will be pure and perfect. Though his gospel of physical regeneration—the reestablishment, as far as practicable, of the conditions to which human bodies became adapted during the ages before indoor life and prepared foods—included a great amount of healthy and natural diet, Macfadden's doctrine did not require vegetarianism. He acknowledged that meat was a vehicle for bringing impurities into the body and was more stimulating than vegetables, but he viewed sound physical culture practice as counterbalancing meat defects, by giving the eater enough potency to expel those impurities and live as happily and healthfully as any vegetarian. Because desire for food was an expression of natural instinct, Macfadden approved of fasting as a way to promote a healthy appetite. The success of physical culture is when the faithful follower pursues the cult of the body and actively seeks a physical wellness that results from natural hygiene and diet. The philosophy on which physical culture was founded continues to have adherents and will continue as long as the spirit of self-perfection pervades American society.

See also Alternative and Holistic Medicine; Colonies, Communal Societies, and Utopias; Physiological Benefits; Reform.

Further Reading

Ernst, Robert. *Weakness Is a Crime: The Life of Bernarr Macfadden.* Syracuse, NY: Syracuse University Press, 1991.

Whorton, James C. *Crusaders for Fitness: The History of American Health Reformers.* Princeton, NJ: Princeton University Press, 1982.

P. Arouna Ouédraogo

MEAT AND VIOLENCE

The status of animals in the human world has been debated for millennia by philosophers and jurists alike on a number of grounds, and vegetarianism has been linked to nonviolence in a number of religious and social milieus. Such concern has perhaps been most convincingly stated in recent times in the social science and feminist communities, which have studied parallels and correlations between violence toward animals and violence toward humans, especially women and children, and in studies of violence toward animals in connection with masculinity.

Many vegetarians cite violence against animals—ranging from the caging and tethering of companion animals to the well-documented abuses of zoo and circus animals to the corporatized factory farming industry—as reasons for their initial and continuing vegetarian lifestyles. People for the Ethical Treatment of Animals (PETA) has perhaps been the leading organization in introducing the general public to these forms of violence through its extensive ad campaigns featuring celebrities and through its activist tactics that range from boycotts to public-square activism involving nudity or the throwing of red paint on people wearing fur. PETA has been criticized in some quarters for using women's bodies and highly sexualized ad campaigns to achieve its ends.

Much concern about violence and vegetarianism focuses on humans' ability to separate animals into various categories or purposes. Feminist theorist Carol J. Adams has written broadly on the "absent referent" as the mechanism that allows humans to separate living and dead animals, one understood as a living being (for example, the calf), the other understood as food (for example, veal). Others have noticed a similar process at work in separating companion animals, such as dogs and cats, who are cherished and often considered to be members of the family, from noncompanion animals bred, raised, and slaughtered solely for consumption. Highlighting this incongruity has been central to the work of many vegetarians and animal rights advocates as well as academics working in fields ranging from social welfare to critical theory.

In recent years, a number of studies have connected violence toward animals with domestic violence toward women and children, documenting how childhood violence toward animals is often a precursor to adult violence. Studies have also indicated that companion animals are often used as pawns to intimidate human victims of domestic violence. As many as 85 percent of women who enter domestic violence shelters report instances of animal abuse in the home prior to or concurrent with the human abuse. Substantial work in this area focuses on intervention and prevention as well as tightening laws against animal cruelty.

Related work on advertising and on pornography has revealed similar connections between meat and violence. From the infamous June 1978 cover of *Hustler* magazine that featured a female being fed through a grinder and emerging as ground meat to seemingly less violent advertising that mixes references to animals and women, these images have been used to advertise everything from restaurants to clothing. Some researchers suggest that the conflation of animals and females has resulted in a desensitization with respect to violence toward both.

See also Advertising; Animal Rights and Animal Welfare; Ecofeminism; Ethical Vegetarianism.

Further Reading

Adams, Carol J. *The Sexual Politics of Meat: A Feminist-Vegetarian Critical Theory.* New York: Continuum, 1990.

Ascione, Frank, and Phil Arkow, eds. *Child Abuse, Domestic Violence, and Animal Abuse: Linking the Circles of Compassion for Prevention and Intervention.* West Lafayette, IN: Purdue University Press, 1999.

Luke, Brian. *Brutal: Manhood and the Exploitation of Animals.* Champaign: University of Illinois Press, 2007.

Nibert, David. *Animal Rights, Human Rights: Entanglements of Oppression and Liberation.* Lanham, MD: Rowman & Littlefield, 2002.

Milton W. Wendland

MEATLESS DIETS BEFORE VEGETARIANISM

The concept of vegetarianism as a choice of diet to match a humanitarian lifestyle became established in the mainstream of Western thinking only in the mid-19th century. Before this time, however, there were a number of manifestations of diets in which abstention from animal products was central. The term "vegetarian" was coined by the founding members of the Vegetarian Society in England in 1847.

Major Eastern religions, especially Hinduism, Jainism, and Buddhism, require devout adherents to abstain from animal products, although, in practice, the extremely loose organization of these creeds and their extreme diversity in terms of both geographic distribution and cultural contexts mean that the actual practice of a vegetarian diet in the societies in which these religions were predominant varied quite considerably, not only between individuals and groups but also over time. In the Western world, the Eastern Orthodox variety of Christianity—dominant in Greece and the Balkans, Russia, and large parts of eastern Europe—and Christianity in general before the Great Schism of 1057—have required the faithful to adopt a strict vegetarian diet, including abstention from alcohol and dairy products, not only on the Wednesday and Friday of every week but also during a number of fasts preceding the great feasts of the Dormition, the Nativity, the Apostles, and Pascha. In Orthodox monasteries, vegetarianism is also the norm, but among lay believers the practice varies sharply. In both East and West, then, religious observance has often required a vegetarian diet among a mass of believers—in some countries (such as Greece), the clear majority of citizens. There is also a strong affinity to vegetarianism in Judaism and in the ancient Persian religion of Zoroastrianism.

In the classical world a vegetarian diet is most commonly associated with the philosopher Pythagoras (580–500 BC) and his followers. For Pythagoras, abstention from meat seems to have been based on two things. The first of these was the concept of metempsychosis, by which souls might migrate from one being to another in a form of reincarnation; avoiding meat was obviously a good way of avoiding damage to the process of being in this scheme. Second, there was the belief that meat eating created an aggressive and savage temper in the human meat eater. Vegetarian beliefs, some influenced by Pythagoras and some not, can be found threaded throughout the Greco-Roman world. The late platonic philosopher Porphyry (233–304) produced a major work on vegetarianism, while Seneca (5 BC–AD 65), the Roman Stoic philosopher, was a convinced abstainer from meat. In spite of the many examples, however, in the classical period vegetarianism was not a mass phenomenon and was associated either with specific religious or philosophical cults or with isolated individuals.

In the Middle Ages and the Renaissance, vegetarianism remained a minority diet except in the monasteries, and not until the Enlightenment was there a growth of coherent secular philosophies of vegetarianism and the beginnings of the collective discussion that would lead to the formation of organized vegetarian movements in the 19th century. Perhaps the first figure of note is Thomas Tryon (1634–1703), who combined a Christian sensitivity toward the works of creation with a view that meat eating encouraged viciousness and immorality. In particular, Tryon associated the degradations of meat eating with the cruelty to animals and human beings that he saw among the slave-owning planters of the West Indies. In doing this he began a line of thought equating animal and human rights—and, especially, the rights of animals and the rights of slaves—that was to persist well into the 19th century. For example, Benjamin Franklin (1706–1790) was so influenced by what he read from Tryon that he became a vegetarian and according to some accounts remained one for 17 years. John Newton (1725–1807), a reformed slave trader and author of the famous hymn "Amazing Grace," was also a vegetarian.

In the 19th century, vegetarian practices became associated with radical politics spurred on by two major influences: the idea of the rights of man as a philosophical position that extended benevolence to the whole of creation and the European, especially the British, discovery and study of the cultures and beliefs of the Indian subcontinent—a theme picked up in the United States by the philosopher Ralph Waldo Emerson (1803–1882). English writers such as George Nicholson (1760–1825), Joseph Ritson (1761–1803), and John Oswald (1730–1803) were all producing major works advocating and explaining the vegetarian diet and blending their views about the duties of humanitarianism with radical politics of varying extremity. This blend of radicalism and vegetarianism became the hallmark of a certain kind of romanticism best exemplified by the important British poet Percy Bysshe Shelley (1792–1822), who wrote both poetry and prose tracts advocating a vegetarian diet and whose radical politics made him a highly influential figure for those who followed in the 19th century. Lewis Gompertz (1779–1865) was another influential vegetarian who combined advocacy for a vegetarian diet with a practical approach toward animal welfare and was the first president of the Society for the Prevention of Cruelty to Animals.

The beginnings of an organized vegetarian movement in Great Britain and the United States can probably be first seen in the work of the Reverend William Cowherd (1763–1816), who founded the Bible Christian Church in 1809. This was a breakaway group from a sect of Swedenborgians, a religious group that was popular at the time, and Cowherd's congregation was expected to adhere to a strict meatless diet. In 1817, one of Cowherd's disciples, the Reverend William Metcalfe (1788–1862), left Britain for the United States and set up a branch of the Bible Christian Church in Philadelphia. Here, also, members were expected to abstain from meat. This community contributed significantly to the growth of vegetarianism in the United States throughout the rest of the century and into the early 20th century. In particular, many of the period's most influential diet reformers, such as Sylvester Graham (1795–1851), attributed their interest in abstention from meat to the teachings of Metcalfe and other Bible Christians.

Together with William A. Alcott (1798–1859), Graham founded the American Physiological Society (APS) in 1837. This was, in essence, a vegetarian society, as its main aim was to promote the understanding and practice of a meatless diet based on both medical and moral principles. Bible Christians from Metcalfe's congregation represented a significant part of the society's membership. In 1850, a meeting between Metcalfe, Alcott, and Graham led to the organization of the American Vegetarian Society along the lines of the one that had been recently established in Great Britain. In the United States, as in Britain, this inspired the formation of many local branches and independent societies.

Out of the English Bible Christian Church but also showing clear connections to the radical romanticism of a slightly earlier time came Joseph Brotherton (1783–1857). Brotherton was a wealthy mill owner and also member of Parliament for the northern English industrial town of Salford. Brotherton combined philanthropy for his workers with the doctrine and practice of vegetarianism derived from the Bible Christian Church. Brotherton was involved in the prosecution of the free-trade agenda, in labor reform, and in pacifism and general humanitarian causes, but his vegetarian beliefs had a far-reaching consequence for all vegetarians even today, as in 1847 he founded the Vegetarian Society in Britain. This was the first of its kind in the world and a model for all to follow; among its other achievements, it popularized the term "vegetarian." This society continues to exist today as the Vegetarian Society of the United Kingdom.

While in ancient and medieval times abstention from meat was largely associated with communities bound together by common religious or philosophical beliefs, by the 17th century and up until the mid-19th century a more complex position was developing. The earliest vegetarian organizations were also associated with particular religious groups, notably the Bible Christians, but the social mission of these groups, and, in particular, their broader sense of the necessity of humanitarianism for world peace, meant that their ideas were bound up with other more secular notions and contextualized by the broader political movements of their time. Before vegetarianism became common usage meatless regimens thus had both a religious and a radical political character that, in many ways, might be said to persist into the present time.

See also Alcott, William A.; American Vegetarian Society; Animal Rights and Animal Welfare; Bible Christians, English; Bible Christians, Philadelphia; Eastern Religions, Influences of; Ethical Vegetarianism; Graham, Sylvester; Pythagoras; Reform; Religious Beliefs and Practices; Vegetarian Society of the United Kingdom.

Further Reading

Iacobbo, Karen, and Michael Iacobbo. *Vegetarian America: A History.* Westport, CT: Praeger, 2004.
Perkins, D. *Romanticism and Animal Rights.* New York: Cambridge University Press, 2003.

Spencer, Colin. *The Heretic's Feast: A History of Vegetarianism.* London: University Press of New England, 1995.

Stuart, Tristram. *The Bloodless Revolution: A Cultural History of Vegetarianism from 1600 to Modern Times.* New York: W.W. Norton, 2007.

John Simons

METCALFE, REV. WILLIAM (1788–1862)

A minister of the vegetarian Bible Christian Church, the Reverend William Metcalfe emigrated from England to Philadelphia to found a new congregation. Through links with leading dietary reformers, he spread a Christian vegetarian gospel into mainstream culture and commerce. Born on March 11, 1788, at Orton in Cumbria to Jonathan and Elizabeth Metcalfe, Metcalfe moved to Keighley, Yorkshire, at 19 years of age to work as a clerk. He joined the Swedenborgian congregation of the Reverend Joseph Wright, who arranged for him to study and teach at the academy of William Cowherd at Salford, an important working-class center of vegetarianism near Manchester. Cowherd, a former Anglican, had in 1809 founded the Bible Christian Church. In 1810, Metcalfe married Wright's daughter Susanna. Metcalfe was ordained the following year and returned to Yorkshire to minister at Addingham.

Metcalfe emigrated to Philadelphia in the spring of 1817 with 40 church members, opened a schoolroom, held services, and promoted vegetarianism and temperance through preaching, teaching, and tracts. In 1823, the church purchased premises and dedicated a new building in 1847. The congregation was never large or wealthy, comprising at most 100 people, yet it spread its vegetarian gospel by helping to inspire others who could spread the word. In 1830, the Presbyterian minister Sylvester Graham was introduced to Bible Christians while working as a temperance lecturer and health reformer. Metcalfe met him and also contacted another prominent reformer, William A. Alcott, beginning lifelong correspondences with both men.

Metcalfe taught that the Bible contains a spiritual sense that is progressively revealed to humankind. He argued that religious doctrines should conform to human reason, held a unitarian concept of God, and saw the world as harmoniously ordered by divine providence. He believed that Jesus was completely vegetarian, that accounts of him eating fish were mistranslations, and that God had dwelt fully in Jesus. He interpreted resurrection spiritually and thought that moral virtue could be cultivated by free will. Metcalfe also opposed war, capital punishment, and slavery.

After giving up teaching in 1832, Metcalfe worked in journalism, publishing, and medicine, in addition to his ministerial duties. In 1850, he was elected president of the American Vegetarian Convention, which founded the American Vegetarian Society, of which he was elected corresponding secretary later that year in Philadelphia. In 1851, he visited Great Britain to preach and teach. His wife died in 1853, and he then married congregation member Mary Caxiss, with whom he made a second visit to England from 1855 to 1857 for further his ministry. He was elected president of the American Vegetarian Society in 1859. On his death on October 16, 1862, he was succeeded as minister by his son Joseph. Other family members held positions in the Bible Christian Church into the 20th century, although the American Vegetarian Society disbanded following his death.

See also Alcott, William A.; Alternative and Holistic Medicine; American Vegetarian Society; Bible and Biblical Arguments; Bible Christians, English; Bible Christians, Philadelphia; Reform; Religious Beliefs and Practices.

Further Reading

Metcalfe, William. *Out of the Clouds: Into the Light. With a Memoir by His Son, Reverend Joseph Metcalfe*. Philadelphia: J.P. Lippincott, 1872.

The Philadelphia Bible Christian Church. *History of the Philadelphia Bible-Christian Church for the First Century of Its Existence from 1817 to 1917*. Philadelphia: J.B. Lippincott, 1922. www.ivu.org/history/usa19/history_of_bible_christian_church.pdf.

David Grumett

NETHERLANDS, THE

Throughout the West, the Netherlands has acquired a reputation for being a liberal country. Dutch contemporary culture is perceived to be permissive with regard to sexual mores, drug policies, and free speech. Nonconventional lifestyles, including vegetarian culture, are another part of Dutch society. These lifestyles began emerging at the end of the 19th century. Since then, Dutch vegetarians have voiced provocative ideas about politics and the self, culture and science, peace and violence. At three peak moments in the Netherlands' history, the practice of not eating meat prompted different sorts of anarchist-like revolutions.

The first vegetarian peak occurred at the beginning of the 20th century (1900–1940) and was driven by nonconventional intellectuals such as Ferdinand Domela Nieuwenhuis (1846–1919) and Felix Louis Ortt (1866–1959). Nieuwenhuis, a pioneer of Dutch socialism, was a former clergyman turned atheist. After the incorporation of most socialists into the Social-Democratic party (1894), Nieuwenhuis followed the minority in a more anarchistic direction. After reading the German Edward Baltzer (another German clergyman turned atheist and vegetarian), he advocated vegetarianism as a means to integrate social and personal reform. Ortt, a second proponent of early vegetarianism, was a civil engineer. Instead of leaving Protestantism altogether, Ortt adopted his beliefs to the teachings of the Russian novelist Leo Tolstoy. Inspired by this so-called Christian anarchism and by German vegetarianism, Ortt became vegetarian in 1892. In 1900, he animated the short-lived vegetarian colony International Brotherhood in the village of Blaricum. Together with Nieuwenhuis and others, he also fought the practice of animal vivisection.

Although Nieuwenhuis's and Ortt's beliefs had been perpetuated since 1894 by a long-standing vegetarian publication, the *Vegetarische Bode* (Vegetarian Courier) and an associated organization, the Nederlandse Vegetariërs Bond (Dutch Vegetarian League), the cultural aura of Dutch vegetarianism receded from the interwar years onward. In the eyes of many, the German occupation of Dutch territory during World War II permanently compromised the primary source from which Nieuwenhuis and Ortt had obtained their vegetarian beliefs. Not until the 1960s and 1970s could a new wave of Dutch vegetarianism gain from international youth activism. Roel van Duyn, the leader of the Amsterdam-based anarchist student group Provo, was the first to link vegetarianism to activist culture. In 1969, he launched the so-called dwarf movement. His "dwarfs" aimed to create a technical and scientific postwar order. They criticized the perceived environmental crisis of industrial society and reached for reliable (vegetable-based) good food.

In the 1980s and 1990s, an aversion to agribusiness was added to these environmental concerns. Whereas the new group Lekker Dier (Tasty Beast) manifested peacefully against the suffering of industrially produced animals, more radical animal activists gradually took recourse to illegal action. Militants of the Dierenbevrijdingsfront (Animal Liberation Front) liberated small farm animals but also set fire to butchers' shops. The murder of the right-wing politician Pim Fortuyn in 2002 by the radical animal rights activist Volkert van der Graaf may be seen as a late culminating point of these campaigns.

See also Activism and Protests; Agribusiness; Animal Liberation Front; Animal Rights and Animal Welfare; Antivivisection; Ethical Vegetarianism; Europe; Global Warming; Periodicals; Policy; Reform; Youth.

Further Reading

Verdonk, Dirk-Jan. *Het dierloze gerecht: Een vegetarische geschiedenis van Nederland.* Meppel, the Netherlands: Boom, 2009.

Evert Peeters

NEWKIRK, INGRID (1949–)

Animal rights activist Ingrid Newkirk is the president of People for the Ethical Treatment of Animals (PETA), a worldwide organization she cofounded in 1980. Newkirk is best known for instigating the use of sensational and theatrical tactics of civil disobedience to raise awareness about animal abuse through garnering media coverage. This has resulted in her being arrested over 20 times. Newkirk supports the work of more radical groups like the Animal Liberation Front. Her ultimate goal is to put an end to the suffering of animals around the globe.

Born June 11, 1949, in Surrey, England, Newkirk (whose family name is Ward) left Europe at seven years of age when her family relocated to Delhi, India. As a child, Newkirk was exposed to volunteer work through the benevolent actions of her mother, who worked at several charitable organizations. One such organization was Mother Teresa's Missionaries of Charity, which aided groups who were outcast from society, including people with leprosy, unwed mothers, and orphans. When she was not in the Himalayas attending a convent-run boarding school for

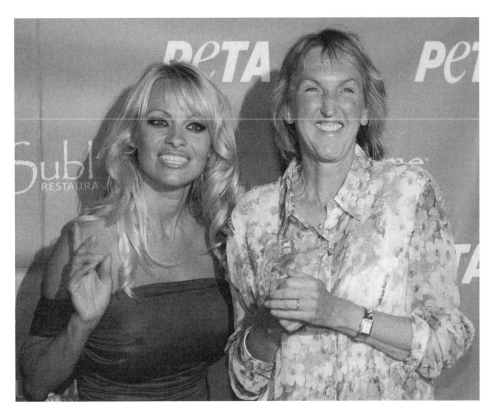

PETA president Ingrid Newkirk, right, with actress and animal rights activist Pamela Anderson, at Anderson's 40th birthday party at the Sublime Cafe in Fort Lauderdale, Florida, 2007. (AP Photo/J. Pat Carter)

children of affluent families, Newkirk would accompany her mother to the leper colony to lend assistance wrapping bandages, feeding stray animals, and other necessary tasks. She credits this formative experience with instilling the message that all creatures are valuable.

When she was 18 years old, Newkirk's engineer father got a job in Florida working for the U.S. Air Force and moved the family once again. In the Sunshine State Newkirk met her now ex-husband, race car driver Steve Newkirk. The couple married in 1968 and soon moved to Poolesville, Maryland, where Newkirk began her studies with the intention of becoming a stockbroker.

The seminal incident that changed Newkirk's life happened when she was 22 years old. She took a box of abandoned kittens she had found to a local animal shelter, where they were put down within the hour. Newkirk misunderstood the staff's intention, and the horror she felt after learning about the kittens' demise prompted her to change career paths the very next day. She convinced the manager of that same shelter to give her a job cleaning the kennel.

In a hint of what was to come a decade later, Newkirk's first act of direct action was to expose the abuse of the animals housed at the shelter in which she worked. This bold move helped to land her a job as a deputy sheriff of Montgomery County, where she vigorously investigated incidents of animal cruelty until 1976. Newkirk then became the first female poundmaster, managing animal disease control for the Commission on Public Health in Washington, D.C. During her time in this position, she successfully led campaigns that passed legislation to create the first spay and neuter clinics, animal adoption programs, and publicly funded veterinary services in the nation's capital. Newkirk's work was recognized in 1980 when she was named Washingtonian of the Year.

Inspired by Peter Singer's book *Animal Liberation,* Newkirk cofounded PETA with friend and colleague Alex Pacheco. PETA is now the largest animal rights organization in the world. Newkirk's media savvy, eccentric methods of activism, and ability to garner celebrity endorsements have made PETA a household name.

See also Activism and Protests; Animal Liberation Front; Animal Rights and Animal Welfare; Ethical Vegetarianism; Pacheco, Alex; People for the Ethical Treatment of Animals; Policy; Reform; Singer, Peter.

Further Reading

Galkin, Matthew. *I Am an Animal: The Story of Ingrid Newkirk and PETA.* New York: HBO Home Video, 2008.

Ingrid Newkirk. http://www.ingridnewkirk.com.

Newkirk, Ingrid, and Jane Ratcliffe, eds. *One Can Make a Difference: How Simple Actions Can Change the World.* Cincinnati, OH: Adams Media, 2008.

Mandy Van Deven

ORGANIC FOODS AND TECHNOLOGY

The rise of organic technology came to the forefront of agriculture after World War II. Chemical pesticides and fertilizers were developed from ammonium products used for weapons during the war. Those chemicals leave harmful residues on food and pollute the air and water supply. Traditional organic farming techniques are aimed not only at producing food free of pesticides but also at managing and maintaining the fertility of farmland for continued long-term productivity. Organic standards are legally defined and enforced by individual countries and states. Organic plants are grown without the use of synthetic fertilizers, sewage sludge, pesticides, or herbicides. Organic meat comes from livestock fed organic food and not routinely treated with antibiotics or hormones.

Additionally, certain technologies are excluded from the production of organic crops and livestock. These include genetic modification (also known as genetic engineering or biotechnology), cloning, and irradiation. In genetic engineering, the genome of a plant or animal is manipulated to produce new characteristics, such as resistance to pesticides, longer shelf life, or a leaner muscle mass. Cloning is the artificial, exact replication of a plant or animal. Ionizing radiation rids foods of harmful organisms and germs. The exclusion of conventional techniques has given rise to new technology specially designed for organic production, as well as continued use of traditional, natural methods for pest management and soil fertilization.

Crops draw nutrients from the soil. Nitrogen, phosphorus, and potassium (NPK) are three major nutrients important for plant growth. Without synthetic NPK mixtures, organic farmers find alternative sources of fertilizer using naturally occurring minerals. Rock phosphorus and greensand, which is high in potassium, are two such sources. Planting legumes is a common method for increasing soil nitrogen, because the plants take nitrogen from the air and fix it in the soil. Legumes can be planted in fields among crops or in fallow fields. Manure and compost are also important sources of nutrients. Manure can be sourced from farm

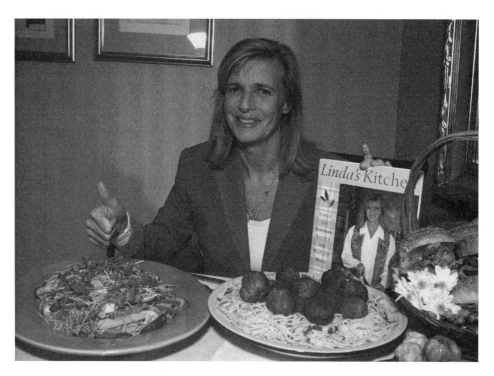

Linda McCartney poses with some of her favorite vegetarian dishes during an interview in New York, 1995. Before her death in 1998, McCartney, the wife of former Beatle Paul McCartney, built a food empire around her interrelated crusades for vegetarianism and organic food, including several cookbooks and an environmentally conscious line of meatless frozen dinners. (AP Photo/Marty Lederhandler)

animals, and manure from some livestock, such as chickens, is high in nitrogen. Compost is made by combining rotting food and plant waste and allowing bacteria and worms to break it down.

It is common for organic farmers to eschew the use of even natural pesticides as a regular practice, dealing with troublesome pests on an as-needed basis. Encouraging the growth of competing, nonpest species, including certain birds, is a strategy for avoiding the application of pesticides. Traps and coverings can also prevent crop damage from pests. Rather than spraying crops with herbicides to prevent weeds in their fields, organic farmers practice mechanical weeding, using their hands or automated machines to physically remove pest plants. Preventing weeds by using mulch or physical barriers is the first step. Planting cover crops that compete with weeds for space and nutrients is another effective strategy. Infrared weeders are machines that look like spray cans but can target weeds and kill them thermally.

Food produced by organic agriculture is considered healthier than conventional food because the products are free from harmful chemical residues. Eating organic food and maintaining a vegetarian diet are correlated because both offer health benefits to the consumer. Furthermore, eating organic and vegetarian foods preserves the health of the land.

See also Advertising; Agribusiness; Consumer Products; Policy; Reform.

Further Reading

Bond, W., and A.C. Grundy. "Non-Chemical Weed Management in Organic Farming Systems." *Weed Resistance* 41 (2001): 383–405.

Trewaras, Anthony. "Urban Myths of Organic Farming." *Nature* 410 (2001): 409–10.

Virbickaite, R., et al. "The Comparison of Thermal and Mechanical Systems of Weed Control." *Agronomy Research* 4 (2006): 451–55.

Wiswall, Richard. *The Organic Farmer's Business Handbook: A Complete Guide to Managing Finances, Crops, and Staff—and Making a Profit.* White River Junction, VT: Chelsea Green, 2009.

Ansley Watson

PACELLE, WAYNE (1965~)

Called "enemy number one" by the head of the U.S. Sportsmen's Alliance, Wayne Pacelle is the president and chief executive officer of the Humane Society of the United States, which, with 11 million members and constituents, is the largest and most affluent animal advocacy organization in the country.

A lifelong lover of animals, Pacelle grew up in New Haven, Connecticut. He had little exposure to careers connected with animals during his childhood. He developed a political consciousness about animal rights while attending Yale University, where he studied history and environmental science, the latter of which sensitized him to the ecological impact of animal cruelty. Seeing concern for animals and the environment as inextricably linked, Pacelle stopped eating and wearing all animal products and started the Student Animal Rights Coalition. He launched his career as an animal-protection activist by advocating for vegan food to be offered in his dormitory dining hall and protesting deer hunting on the university lands as well as cruel experimenting on animals in the medical school.

In 1987, Pacelle graduated from Yale University and became the associate editor of the *Animals' Agenda,* a national magazine of the animal rights movement. The following year Pacelle was hired by animal rights crusader and author Cleveland Amory to be the national director of the Fund for Animals, an antihunting group. (The fund merged with the Humane Society in 2005.) Pacelle engaged in direct action and civil disobedience to disrupt hunters' ability to kill animals. The politically savvy Pacelle also worked to pass ballot initiatives in several western states—including California, Oregon, Arizona, and Colorado—outlawing cruel hunting and trapping practices such as leghold traps, snares, and poisons on public lands.

Hired as the chief lobbyist and spokesperson for the Humane Society in 1994, Pacelle handled government affairs for the organization at the local, state, and federal levels as well as public relations until he became the president and chief

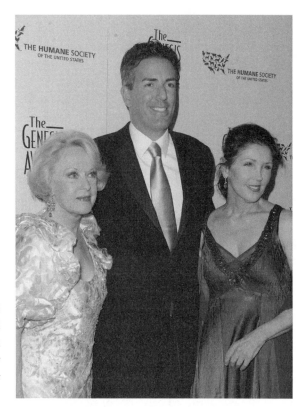

Wayne Pacelle, with actress Tippi Hendren on his left, and Beverly Kaskey, at the 24th Genesis Awards, 2010, in Beverly Hills, California. (AP Photo/Katy Winn)

executive officer of the nonprofit a decade later. Under his leadership, the Humane Society takes a "pragmatic not dogmatic" stance toward tangible reform to eliminate the unjust harm done to animals by humans. This harm includes puppy mills, rodeos, the fur trade, and dogfighting. Pacelle refashioned the Humane Society using the National Rifle Association's proactive, aggressive tactics as a model for gaining political strength. The organization doggedly works within the American legislative and judicial systems to implement legal barriers to animal abuses while also courting public opinion through mass media and awareness-raising campaigns aimed at a broad audience. The founding of the Humane USA, a nonpartisan political action committee, in 1999 and of the Humane Society Legislative Fund, a 501(c)(4) social welfare organization, in 2004 established a solid avenue for Pacelle to engage in both lobbying and electoral politics. These groups work to advance the careers of humane-minded political candidates who advocate animal protection through enacting animal welfare legislation and to challenge candidates with a poor animal rights record. In 2006, he helped to create the National Federation of Humane Societies, a trade association that works for the collective interest of local animal welfare organizations, animal shelters, rescue groups, and animal care and control agencies across the nation.

Pacelle blogs daily about current animal issues at *A Humane Nation,* the blog on the Human Society Web site, and he has contributed to several books, including

A Primer on Animal Rights (2002), *Making Burros Fly: Cleveland Amory, Animal Rescue Pioneer* (2006), and *The Inner World of Farm Animals* (2009).

See also Activism and Protests; Animal Rights and Welfare; Policy; Reform.

Further Reading

Hall, Carla. "Wayne Pacelle Works for Winged, Finned, and Furry." *Los Angeles Times,* July 19, 2008.
A Humane Nation. http://hsus.typepad.com/wayne/.
The Humane Society. http://www.hsus.org/.

Mandy Van Deven

PACHECO, ALEX (1958–)

Alexander Fernando Pacheco is a longtime animal rights activist, cofounder of People for the Ethical Treatment of Animals (PETA), and principal plaintiff in the Silver Spring Monkey case, which began in 1981 and lasted for more than 10 years, and is often credited with jumpstarting the animal rights movement in the United States.

Pacheco became interested in animal rights at the age of 20 after a visit to a slaughterhouse, and he quickly immersed himself in animal rights issues and activism, including a stint with the Sea Shepherd Conservation Society, policing ocean whale and fishing operations. Shortly thereafter, Pacheco cofounded PETA with Ingrid Newkirk as a grassroots organization designed to put animal rights issues in the public eye. Pacheco, PETA, and animal rights more generally received international media attention when, in the 1980s, Pacheco went undercover as a lab assistant at the Institute for Behavioral Research in Silver Spring, Maryland, near Pacheco's and PETA's home in Washington, D.C. Pacheco used his access to the lab to document mistreatment and abuse of the macaque monkeys being used in experiments testing sensory abilities. Based on Pacheco's photographs and notes, lead researcher Edward Taub was charged with over 100 counts of animal cruelty, most of which were eventually dismissed as courts wrangled over whether animal-cruelty statutes applied to researchers. The ensuing battle over custody of the monkeys, the criminal case against Taub, and public outcry (based in large part on a now-iconic photograph of one of the monkeys forcibly splayed out in a restraint chair) involved the media, the courts, and Congress, eventually leading to the 1985 Animal Welfare Act and significant changes in government regulations regarding the use of animals in experiments and research. Allegations that many of the photographs were staged remain unproven to this day, but police reports, court records, and congressional hearings acknowledged the presence of widespread abuse of various sorts.

Pacheco's media savvy in the Silver Spring case also propelled PETA into international prominence. Pacheco is credited with encouraging PETA's celebrity-heavy media campaigns against fur, factory farming, and other animal rights abuses but has also garnered criticism for using sexism and sensationalism to promote PETA's work. Many of Pacheco's public comments have been taken out of context and used to discredit him and the animal rights movement more generally. Among these is Pacheco's infamous comment that "arson, property destruction, burglary and theft are acceptable crimes when used for the animal cause." Statements like this have been used to cast Pacheco and PETA as animal rights terrorists, and Pacheco is alleged to be connected with the Animal Liberation Front, a group known for its incendiary and criminal tactics. Pacheco ended his involvement with PETA in 2000, but he continues to be a leader in the animal rights movement. More recently, he has founded or been affiliated with groups such as All American Animals and 600 Million Stray Dogs Need You.

See also Activism and Protests; Animal Rights and Animal Welfare; Antivivisection; Newkirk, Ingrid; People for the Ethical Treatment of Animals; Policy; Reform.

Further Reading

Guillermo, Cathy Snow. *Monkey Business: The Disturbing Case That Launched the Animal Rights Movement.* Washington, DC: National Press Books, 1993.
Pacheco, Alex, and Anna Francione. "The Silver Spring Monkeys." In *In Defense of Animals*, edited by Peter Singer, 135–47. New York: Blackwell, 1985.

Milton W. Wendland

PEOPLE FOR THE ETHICAL TREATMENT OF ANIMALS

People for the Ethical Treatment of Animals (PETA) is the largest and best-known animal rights organization in the world. Founded in 1980 by Ingrid Newkirk and Alex Pacheco, PETA is based in Norfolk, Virginia, and has approximately two million members, with affiliates in the United Kingdom, Germany, Spain, France, the Netherlands, India, and the Asia-Pacific region. It is registered as an international nonprofit charitable and tax-exempt organization. With its motto, "Animals are not ours to eat, wear, experiment on, or use for entertainment," PETA is an abolitionist organization that seeks the eradication of all forms of animal exploitation.

Born in Britain and raised in India, Newkirk had acted as director of cruelty investigations for the Washington Humane Society and as chief of animal disease control for the Commission on Public Health in Washington, DC, where she met Pacheco and cofounded PETA with him. At the time, Pacheco was an American college student at George Washington University. PETA began as a national grassroots organization with several local chapters but eventually closed its local offices in the mid-1980s and centralized its operations. PETA rapidly rose to national prominence as early as 1981 as a result of its undercover investigation and exposé of the violent deafferentation experiments conducted on macaque monkeys in Edward Taub's laboratory at the Institute for Behavioral Research in Silver

Spring, Maryland. Posing as an aspiring medical researcher, Pacheco was hired by Taub to assist in his experiments, which involved cutting the roots of dorsal nerves attached to the limbs of the monkeys. PETA's release of videotape footage of the deplorable conditions in the laboratory resulted initially in Taub's arrest and criminal conviction for cruelty but led eventually to an eight-year legal battle in a case that was brought twice before the U.S. Supreme Court. Although Taub's conviction was ultimately reversed, the conviction of an animal experimenter for cruelty was the first of its kind in the United States and is largely considered a watershed case in the contemporary animal rights movement.

Other historic achievements resulting from PETA's undercover investigations in laboratories, factory farms (intensive industrialized farming facilities), slaughterhouses, and fur farms include the termination of crash-test experiments on animals by General Motors; commitments by several fast food chains such as McDonald's, Burger King, and Wendy's to insist on improved welfare standards for animals from their suppliers; the first felony indictments of farmworkers for cruelty at pig-breeding factory farms in North Carolina and Oklahoma; and decisions by several retailers such as J. Crew and Ann Taylor to terminate the sale of fur products and by top designer Ralph Lauren to abandon the use of fur in his designs.

In addition to exposing cruelty and seeking legislative reform through undercover investigations, PETA conducts boycotts, stages demonstrations, and disseminates other educational materials promoting a vegan lifestyle. PETA has also won endorsements from celebrities such as Sir Paul McCartney, Alec Baldwin, Pamela Anderson, Alicia Silverstone, Chrissie Hynde, and others, many of whom are also actively involved in its campaigns.

Despite its notable successes, PETA has been the center of controversy for its use of what are deemed sensationalist tactics and its tendency to rely on shock value and explicit imagery to draw attention to animal exploitation. PETA has been especially criticized by feminists within the animal rights movement for reinforcing sexism and the objectification of women by, for example, exhibiting antifur billboards with nude female models as part of its ongoing "Fur Is Dead" campaign or using young women, dubbed "lettuce ladies" and wearing only "lettuce-leaf bikinis," to hand out soy sandwiches in front of 7-Eleven stores in its 2008 "Turn Over a New Leaf" campaign. Such images, critics argue, indicate PETA's failure to recognize the inextricable link between the subjugation of women and other animals in patriarchal, capitalist society—a myopia that does a disservice not only to women but also to other animals. PETA's supporters have defended the use of such tactics as an attempt to appeal to the more mainstream element in mass culture and to present a cruelty-free lifestyle in an ostensibly appealing light.

PETA has also been accused of anti-Semitism by groups like the Jewish Anti-Defamation League for its comparison of factory farms to concentration camps, as in its 2004 "Holocaust on Your Plate" campaign. The charge of racism has also been leveled against PETA for its 2005 campaign, "Are Animals the New Slaves?" in which PETA argued that institutional violence against animals is the contemporary equivalent to the historical enslavement and abuse of African Americans and Native Americans in the United States. Although PETA eventually suspended the "New Slaves" campaign, PETA spokespeople continue to defend these analogies between human and nonhuman exploitation. Its failure to recognize the relationship between the exploitation of women and animals notwithstanding, PETA argues that these comparisons are not intended to degrade humans but, to the contrary, are meant to highlight the common roots of all systemic violence and of all discriminatory ideologies that designate one group as inferior to another in order to justify atrocities against the maligned group.

Perhaps most controversial is PETA's involvement with and vocal public support of the Animal Liberation Front (ALF), an organization that uses direct-action tactics such as economic sabotage, effected through the destruction of property in laboratories, factory farms, and so on, and the rescue and rehabilitation of animals held in these places. Though PETA is not officially affiliated with the ALF, Newkirk openly endorses the ALF's illegal direct-action methods and acknowledges that PETA assists the ALF in the release of video footage documenting their acts of sabotage and liberation. The ALF, during a 1984 raid of Thomas Gennarelli's laboratory at the University of Pennsylvania, obtained 60 hours of footage of head-injury experiments on baboons, taken by the experimenters themselves, in which the latter are seen laughing at and tormenting the unanesthetized animals. PETA edited the footage into a 20-minute film that they released later that year, ironically entitled *Unnecessary Fuss,* taken from Gennarelli's contention, in a newspaper interview, that he ought not to discuss his experiments because in doing so he would cause an "unnecessary fuss." Subsequent to the release of the footage, the experiments were terminated, the chief veterinarian was fired, and the University of Pennsylvania was put on probation.

While Pacheco left the organization in 1999, Newkirk continues to be the driving force behind PETA's campaigns. As a result of both its significant achievements, its controversial tactics, and its celebrity endorsements, PETA remains one of the most, if not the most, high-profile animal rights organizations in the world.

See also Activism and Protests; Agribusiness; Animal Liberation Front; Animal Rights and Animal Welfare; Antivivisection; Newkirk, Ingrid; Pacheco, Alex; Reform; Social Acceptance; Veganism; Vegetarians and Vegans, Celebrity.

Further Reading

Finsen, Lawrence, and Susan Finsen. *The Animal Rights Movement in America: From Compassion to Respect.* New York: Twayne, 1994.

Francione, Gary L. *Rain without Thunder: The Ideology of the Animal Rights Movement.* Philadelphia: Temple University Press, 1996.

Galkin, Matthew. *I Am an Animal: The Story of Ingrid Newkirk.* New York: HBO Home Video, 2008.

Guillermo, Kathy Snow. *Monkey Business: The Disturbing Case That Launched the Animal Rights Movement.* Washington, DC: National Press Books, 1993.
"PETA's History: Compassion in Action." http://www.peta.org/mc/factsheet_display. asp?ID=107.

Zipporah Weisberg

PERIODICALS

Historians generally look to early 19th-century England when identifying the start of the modern vegetarian movement in the Western world. At this time the movement's first attempts to express—and develop—its philosophies, practices, and prescriptions in serial print took place. Since that time and place, the story of vegetarian periodicals has been neither linear nor neat: Filled with changing names and leadership; starts, stops, and pauses; mergers and diversification, it is a tale of ongoing evolution. What has remained consistent about these periodicals is their espousal of the core vegetarian tenet: principled abstinence from the flesh of nonhuman animals.

The intellectual energies that gave birth to the first vegetarian periodical can be traced to an offshoot of the Church of England called the Bible Christians, the leader of which, William Cowherd (1763–1816), cited impassioned readings of Scripture as support for vegetarianism. Decades after his death, Cowherd's teachings inspired a small group of activists in Kent to form the Vegetarian Society (1847), the first formal organization devoted to the cause. By the end of its second year the society, by then 500 members strong, had begun producing monthly issues of a penny magazine called the *Truth Tester.* That title changed to the *Vegetarian Advocate* in 1850; in 1851 it assumed the name it would keep for nearly a century, the *Vegetarian Messenger.* All the while, the magazine kept growing in popularity, selling more than 5,000 copies the year it debuted and 20,000 copies a year by the mid-1850s.

Like most serial publications, the *Messenger* was shaped by, and helped to shape, the historical moment in which it found itself. For much of the 19th century this meant an ongoing dialog with the temperance movement, which endorsed vegetarianism as a means to better health. The salutary aspects of vegetarianism would remain the *Messenger*'s focus into the early 20th century, when rising political concerns started coming to the fore. During each World War, the magazine promoted a vegetarian diet as more patriotic (because less costly) than meat eating and advocated on behalf of vegetarian soldiers.

It is hard to overstate the extent to which the Bible Christians influenced the early vegetarian movement—and thus its print material like the *Messenger*—not only in the United Kingdom but also in the United States. Although Cowherd died before he was able to travel to America with his vegetarian message, one of Cowherd's followers did so in his place. Joined by 41 Bible Christians, William Metcalfe (1788–1862), an ordained minister, arrived in Philadelphia in 1817 and proceeded to throw himself into writing about vegetarianism and establishing his church. In 1850, together with some of vegetarianism's leading U.S. advocates, including William A. Alcott and Sylvester Graham, Metcalfe would launch the American Vegetarian Society (AVS).

The AVS's periodical, the *American Vegetarian and Health Journal,* started circulating in 1851. The *Journal* profiled famous as well as everyday vegetarians, printed letters between Metcalfe and his contemporaries, and enumerated the overlapping physical, moral, spiritual, and financial benefits of a vegetarian life. Yet despite its broad appeal, the periodical was forced to fold just four years after its start, in 1854, when the AVS could no longer pay the printing bills.

It would take several decades for Americans to see their next vegetarian periodical; when it appeared, a Bible Christian once again would be to thank. Henry S. Clubb (1827–1921) was a charismatic Bible Christian and journalist who reinvigorated the U.S. vegetarian movement after the Civil War. In 1886, Clubb organized the Vegetarian Society of America (VSA); from 1889 on, he edited the VSA's publication *Food, Home and Garden.* Like its predecessors, *Food, Home and Garden* underwent several name changes, becoming the *Vegetarian Magazine* when the VSA merged with the Chicago Vegetarian Society (1899–1900). The periodical subsequently was called *The Vegetarian and Our Fellow Creatures* (1901–1903), the *Vegetarian Magazine* (1903–1925), the *Vegetarian Magazine and Fruitarian* (1925–1926), and *The Vegetarian and Fruitarian* (1926–1934). Throughout these name changes, the content and purpose of the VSA's signature periodical largely remained consistent. Throughout the early 20th century it would attract a steady readership.

These publications played a key unifying role. Until the mid-19th century, vegetarianism had found enthusiastic support among many Americans, from laypeople to medical and religious leaders; in a vast and expanding country, however, these constituents remained isolated from each other. In the words of Alcott, one of the founders of the AVS, "They have no bond to hold them together; no standard to rally round; no written constitution or creed; no associations and no periodical." It was the hope of Alcott and his peers that a serial publication would confederate the movement's "scattered friends."

That is exactly what vegetarian periodicals long have done. To offer one prominent example, members of the Chicago Vegetarian Society (1889) credited *Food, Home and Garden* with introducing them to the VSA; the two groups merged not long after, resulting in one of the largest vegetarian organizations to date. Similarly, letters to the editor in vegetarian periodicals dating from the early 19th century suggest that these publications helped like-minded people find each other—an essential function for any community but especially one whose members often find themselves on society's fringe.

Throughout the 20th century and into the 21st, vegetarians have been able to choose from an increasingly wide array of periodicals. Some, like *Good Medicine* (published by the Physicians Committee for Responsible Medicine), *Ahimsa* (published by the American Vegan Society), or *Vegetarian Voice* (published by the North American Vegetarian Society), frame vegetarianism as part of a comprehensive lifestyle motivated by a desire to do the least harm. These publications tend to include profiles of animal rights and environmental activists, evidence for a plant-based diet as part of a "green" strategy, and advertisements from food, clothing, and housewares companies that do not use animals or animal ingredients to make their products.

Other types of vegetarian periodicals focus more narrowly on vegetarianism as a dietary choice, offering their readers culinary techniques, recipes, and health suggestions. Popular examples here include the *Vegetarian Times* and *Vegetarian Gourmet,* and the BBC's *Vegetarian Good Food Guide.* Although accused by some of being too accepting of meat eaters and of failing to point out vegetarianism's wider exigencies, such periodicals have been applauded for presenting vegetarianism as easy, appealing, and even fun. After all, this is a goal shared by nearly all vegetarian periodicals, from the mid-19th-century penny magazine to the glossy magazines and online journals of today: shifting the movement to the mainstream.

See also Alcott, William A.; Alternative and Holistic Medicine; American Vegetarian Society; Clubb, Henry S.; Graham, Sylvester; Metcalfe, Rev. William; Reform; Religious Beliefs and Practices; Social Acceptance; United Kingdom; Vegetarian Society of America; Vegetarian Society of the United Kingdom; World Wars in England.

Further Reading

Alcott, William A. "Vegetarianism in the United States." *The Vegetarian Advocate* (April 1850). http://www.ivu.org/congress/1850/history.html.

Gregory, James. *Of Victorians and Vegetarians: The Vegetarian Movement in Nineteenth-Century Britain.* New York: I. B. Tauris, 2007.

Iacobbo, Karen, and Michael Iacobbo. *Vegetarians and Vegans in America Today.* Westport, CT: Praeger, 2006.

International Vegetarian Union. http://www.ivu.org/.

Spencer, Colin. *Vegetarianism: A History.* London: Grub Street, 2000.

Stuart, Tristram. *The Bloodless Revolution: A Cultural History of Vegetarianism from 1600 to Modern Times.* New York: W. W. Norton, 2007.

Unti, Bernard. "Vegetarian Roots." *Vegetarian Times* 152 (1990): 52–58, 82.

Melissa Tedrowe

PHYSICAL FITNESS AND ATHLETICISM

Throughout history, people have adopted meatless diets for a variety of religious, economic, ethical, or health-related reasons. For much of this time, however, vegetarians have had to deal with assumptions that they were weaker, were less healthy, or had less energy than individuals who ate meat. This became an increasingly vexing problem as the organized vegetarian movements of the 1840s in the United States and Europe continued to grow during the second half of the 19th century. Many within these modern vegetarian movements believed that the stereotype of the weak, enervated vegetarian was not only contrary to their own experiences but also a hindrance to the expansion of vegetarianism itself, and some actively sought to counter the negative connections by highlighting any evidence suggesting that vegetarians were just as healthy and strong—if not more so—than individuals who adhered to a traditional meat-based diet.

Some of the associations linking meat to virility or strength and vegetarianism to weakness and debility date back to the ancient Greeks and Romans, who valued physical fitness and enjoyed competitive athletics including wrestling, footraces, and swimming. Many Olympic runners allegedly competed on a nearly all-meat diet, and the athletic prowess of some of the most revered ancient athletes was often attributed to their prodigious intake of animal flesh. While reports that champion wrestler Milo of Croton ate some 20 pounds of meat a day were almost certainly exaggerated, they nonetheless suggest that athleticism and the consumption of meat were closely linked in the ancient world.

From the fall of the Roman Empire through the end of the Renaissance, there is little evidence about the connections between physical fitness and diet, primarily because few individuals outside ruling aristocracies possessed the luxury of either choosing their own diet or having time to engage in athletics. Starting around the 18th century, however, a handful of medical specialists began investigating the relationship between food and health, and the differences between plant-based and animal-based diets. In works like his 1724 *An Essay of Health and Long Life,* for example, English physician George Cheyne argued that many physical ailments could be remedied by forgoing meat in favor of bread, fruit, milk, vegetables, and seeds. By 1809, physician William Lambe went even further and declared that eating animal flesh was the cause of nearly all human disease and premature death.

Interest in the connections between diet, health, fitness, and disease soon increased dramatically. During the 1830s, American vegetarian pioneer Sylvester Graham lectured extensively on what he called "the science of human life," explaining that most disease and debility was caused by the overstimulating effects of meat consumption on the human body. Graham prescribed a vegetarian diet that included fruits, vegetables, whole grains, and plenty of water and noted that physical exercise and fresh air were also essential for good health. As the modern vegetarian movement in Europe and the United States gained momentum during the second half of the 19th century, Graham and other diet reformers' efforts were bolstered by rapid advances in organic chemistry, human physiology, and nutritional science. Protein became a central issue in the debate over vegetarian nutrition, especially once researchers discovered that the protein found in plants was virtually indistinguishable from that in animals, offering apparent scientific proof that vegetarians could be just as athletic and strong as meat eaters.

Still, the old stereotypes persisted, and for every discovery that supported the vegetarian cause it seemed that another undermined it. While most scientists came to agree that plant and animal proteins were nearly identical chemically, for instance, some insisted that meat was still nutritionally superior since animal tissue was more biologically similar to human tissue and thus more readily assimilated. Other critics of vegetarianism claimed a meatless diet was simply impractical, because the lower concentrations of protein found in most plant foods would require eating enormous quantities of vegetable matter to ingest the amount of protein found in an average serving of meat. As vegetarians learned that foods like legumes and nuts were dense in protein (and since they typically consumed at least some animal protein anyway, in the form of eggs or dairy products), the warning from one physician that they would need to "eat straw like an ox" to meet their need for protein was probably not a source of concern.

Meanwhile, some vegetarian advocates noted that while they embraced the intellectual evidence supporting their diet, most did little to counter physically the widely held assumptions linking strength and stamina to meat consumption. That started to change during the 1880s, as vegetarians began competing in various races and athletic contests and also organized clubs devoted to swimming, cycling, running, and walking. Within years of its founding in 1888, members of London's Vegetarian Cycling Club were not only competing—and winning—against non-vegetarians but also setting various endurance records. By the early 1900s, vegetarian Eustace Miles had won four major amateur tennis championships, and George Antony Olley, another vegetarian athlete, was named the "best all-round amateur cyclist in Britain." In the United States, vegetarian boxer William "Kid" Parker amassed an 18-match undefeated streak, while a 1907 study in the *Yale Medical Journal* concluded that the physical endurance of vegetarian athletes far surpassed that of nonvegetarians. That fall, the coach of the University of Chicago football team—himself a vegetarian—encouraged his entire squad to give up meat.

Interest in vegetarian athleticism declined along with the wider diminution of the vegetarian movement following World War I, though a number of prominent vegetarian athletes continued to undermine the old stereotypes. Distance runner Paavo Nurmi, for example, set 20 world records and took home nine gold medals in the 1920, 1924, and 1928 Olympic Games, and weightlifter Roy Hilligenn won the 1951 Mr. America title. More recently, vegan sprinter Carl Lewis set the 100-meter world record at the 1991 Tokyo World Championship meet, and ultramarathoner Scott Jurek, who adopted a vegan diet in 1999, won the Western States 100-mile endurance run seven consecutive times. Even some within the masculine culture of team sports—like National Basketball Association players Salim Stoudamire and Raja Bell and Milwaukee Brewers' first baseman Prince Fielder—have publicly discussed their vegetarian diets.

Perhaps most important, the medical establishment that as recently as the 1970s called vegetarianism a thoroughly unscientific example of food faddism now agrees that a meatless diet can be safe, nutritious, and healthy, even for athletes. The American Dietary Association acknowledged as much in 1980, and the official U.S. Government Dietary Recommendations finally included vegetarianism as an "acceptable option" in 1995. Moreover, multiple studies continue to demonstrate that, on the whole, modern vegetarians have a lower risk of obesity, heart disease, and certain cancers than those consuming a typical meat-based diet. It may have taken a while, but the image of a robust and healthy vegetarian seems to have finally displaced the old stereotypes.

See also Alternative and Holistic Medicine; Backlash; Physiological Benefits; Reform; Social Acceptance; Vegetarians and Vegans, Celebrity.

Further Reading

Carlson, Peggy. *The Complete Vegetarian: The Essential Guide to Good Health.* Urbana: University of Illinois Press, 2006.

Dorfman, Lisa. *The Vegetarian Sports Nutrition Guide: Peak Performance for Everyone from Beginners to Gold Medalists.* New York: John Wiley & Sons, 1999.

Forward, Charles W. *The Food of the Future: A Summary of Arguments in Favor of a Non-Flesh Diet.* London: George Bell & Sons, 1904, 89.

Gregory, James. *Of Victorians and Vegetarians: The Vegetarian Movement in Nineteenth-Century Britain.* New York: Tauris, 2007.

Iacobbo, Karen, and Michael Iacobbo. *Vegetarian America: A History.* Westport, CT: Praeger, 2004.

Light, H. "Some Results of Vegetarian Athleticism." *Humane Review* 1 (April 1900): 92.

Younkin, Edwin. "Dr. Younkin's Reply." *Chicago Vegetarian* 3 (April 1899): 7.

Gary K. Jarvis

PHYSIOLOGICAL BENEFITS

Diet is a key factor in determining wellness and vitality and can be critical in mitigating the effects of certain illnesses. From heart disease to cancer to diabetes, one of the simplest ways to prevent or control disease is through the development of a healthy lifestyle, including a well-balanced diet. Recent medical studies confirm that a vegetarian or vegan diet has certain physiological advantages when compared with the diet of omnivores. A diet rich in green, leafy vegetables, whole grains, fruit, and soy, coupled with a reduction of animal fats, can help to mitigate many disease processes and help individuals enjoy longer, healthier lives. The benefits suffuse every segment of human health.

Cardiovascular Health When coupled with healthy lifestyle choices, the vegetarian diet can result in lower overall blood pressure and better cardiac health. This is due, in part, to the overall leanness and active lifestyle of vegetarians, but these benefits may also be attributed to a diet rich in green vegetables, fresh fruit, whole grains and legumes, which is a decisive factor in determining cardiac health. The well-balanced vegan or vegetarian diet provides better nutrition with fewer calories and additives. It also increases levels of dietary fiber and whole grains and helps to lower levels of cholesterol and saturated fat in the blood and reduce serum lipids. As a result, vegetarians tend to have lower levels of saturated fat, low-density lipoprotein (LDL) and total cholesterol, and generally experience a lower body mass index (BMI, or body fat). The lower cholesterol also helps reduce the risk of coronary artery disease.

Improved cardiac health can also depend on those elements that are absent from the diet. Vegetarians typically eat fewer highly processed fast foods that contain high levels of fat and calories and increased amounts of sodium and sugar. A diet rich in fresh fruits and vegetables is generally lower in sodium; the increased level of raw or minimally cooked foods also helps to replace processed foods that have more salt. Less sodium in the diet can mean less water retention, less stress on the cardiovascular system, and often lower blood pressure.

Gastrointestinal Health Diets that are high in dietary fiber and low in fat and cholesterol are associated with lower incidences of gastrointestinal disease

Benefits of a Vegetarian Diet

These excerpts from an American Dietetic Association article tout the benefits of a vegetarian diet:

> A considerable body of scientific data suggests positive relationships between vegetarian diets and risk reduction for several chronic degenerative diseases and conditions, including obesity, coronary artery disease, hypertension, diabetes mellitus, and some types of cancer. . . . Although most vegetarian diets meet or exceed the Recommended Dietary Allowance for protein, they often provide less protein than nonvegetarian diets. This lower protein intake may be associated with better calcium retention in vegetarians and improved kidney function. . . . Further, lower protein intakes may result in a lower fat intake with its inherent advantages, because foods high in protein are frequently high in fat also.
>
> . . . Infants, children, and adolescents who consume well-planned vegetarian diets can generally meet all of their nutritional requirements for growth. . . . Well-planned vegetarian diets can (also) be adequate for pregnant and lactating women.

Source: American Dietetic Association. "Position of the American Dietetic Association: Vegetarian." *Journal of the American Dietetic Association* 93, no. 11 (November 1993): 1317, 1319.

such as colon cancer, diverticulitis, and gallstones. Colon cancer rates increase as more animal fat and red meat are added to the diet and as fat and cholesterol levels increase. Possible causes include increased secretion of bile acids, increased serum cholesterol, and enhanced development of adenomas, which are a form of precancerous growth. Differences in dietary fiber between vegetarian and semi-vegetarian populations also correlate to mortality rates from colon cancer. There is evidence that the type of colon cancer also depends on diet. Rates of left-sided colon and rectal cancers are higher in nonvegetarians; right-sided colon cancer is more prevalent in vegetarians. Incidence of diverticulitis is decreased in populations that have diets higher in cereal fiber, fruits, and vegetables. Dietary fiber increases fecal bulk, which may lessen the pressure required to clear the bowel of contents. Adding fiber to the diet may reduce symptoms.

Obesity and high-calorie diets are implicated as strong risk factors for cholesterol gallstones, which occur at a higher rate in nonvegetarian populations. Vegetarians are leaner and have a higher intake of dietary fiber, which leads to a reduction in the incidence of gallstones. Other issues, including the use of oral contraceptives and postmenopausal estrogen therapy, may contribute to gallstones. Rates of estrogen therapy usage in vegetarians also tend to be lower, further reducing the risk.

Diabetes   A diet rich in complex carbohydrates and fiber from beans, whole grains, and fruit helps to maintain control of blood glucose levels and lower insulin requirements. Because vegetarians have lower body fat and greater dietary diversity, they appear to be at lower risk for non-insulin-dependent diabetes. Research also suggests that plant-based diets may reduce the risk of type II, or adult-onset, diabetes. Complex carbohydrates slow carbohydrate metabolism, and the presence of legumes slows digestion, reducing the postprandial rise in blood glucose levels. There is also evidence that a lower body mass index and increased intake of dietary fiber may increase tissue sensitivity to insulin, lowering blood glucose levels as well.

Cancer   Medical studies have long promoted a diet rich in fresh fruits and vegetables as one of the key ingredients in preventing cancer. Although cancer can result from both genetic and environmental elements, studies have linked certain cancers with increased levels of fat consumption, and roughly 70 percent of all fats come from animal products. Higher levels of fruits and vegetables can reduce the risk of cancer by one-half, especially the endothelial cancers.

Breast cancer has a number of risks related to diet and lifestyle. These include obesity, dietary fat, alcohol, dietary fiber, energy balance, and a history of weight gain and loss. Changes in leanness and physical-activity level may change risk status by altering the sex-hormone metabolism. There are dramatic differences between vegetarian and nonvegetarian women that relate to breast cancer risk and are not simply a question of diet. A balance of physical activity, diet, reduced alcohol consumption, and other factors can diminish the risks, but other factors must be considered. While advocating a balanced diet as a primary defense against cancer, the World Cancer Research Fund has identified specific foods as having protective properties against cancer, including cruciferous vegetables (broccoli, cauliflower, cabbage), whole grains, flaxseed and nuts, and a variety of other vegetables: carrots, celery, tomatoes, grapes, and berries.

Beneficial Vitamins and Minerals   A balanced vegetarian diet, consisting of fresh fruits and vegetables, nuts, legumes, and whole grains, is rich in vegetable fiber, folates, phytosterols, and antioxidants like vitamins A, C, and E and selenium. Each of these components provide specific benefits. Soluble fiber, which readily dissolves in water, is obtained from grains, legumes, and root vegetables and has been shown to protect against the development of heart disease by reducing cholesterol levels. Insoluble fiber, which does not dissolve in water, helps to reduce the risk of developing constipation, colitis, colon cancer, and hemorrhoids.

Folates are water-soluble B vitamins that provide protection against coronary artery disease. They can be found in cereals, leafy vegetables, okra, asparagus, fruits, legumes, mushrooms, orange juice, and tomato juice. Phytosterols (or plant sterols) are the plant equivalents of cholesterol, which is derived from animal products and manufactured through routine processes such as liver synthesis and intestinal absorption. Phytosterols help to reduce serum cholesterol levels and maximize cardiac function.

Antioxidants work to reduce oxidative stress and improve endothelial function. Beta carotene and vitamin A are associated with the prevention of epithelial cancers: skin, uterine, cervix, larynx, lung, gastrointestinal system, and breast. Vitamin A and carotenoids are found in brightly colored fruits and vegetables such as carrots, squash, broccoli, sweet potatoes, collards, peaches, tomatoes, cantaloupes, and apricots. Vitamin C helps to reduce cancer of the esophagus and stomach and is found most often in green leafy vegetables such as broccoli and green peppers as well as citrus, tomatoes, and strawberries. Vitamin E is found in nuts and seeds, whole grains, green leafy vegetables, and vegetable oils. Another antioxidant, selenium, is found primarily in animal products such as fish and eggs, but it can also be obtained from some grains and garlic.

A number of other beneficial compounds in the vegetarian diet act as antioxidants, including lycopene, lutein, and flavonoids. Flavonoids and polyphenols are found in soy, red and white wine, grapes, pomegranates, cranberries, and tea. Flavonoids are the most potent antioxidants. They protect LDL cholesterol from oxidation and inhibit clot formation. Increases in flavonoids are associated with a 60 percent lower mortality from heart disease and a 70 percent lower chance of stroke compared to those with a lower intake of flavonoids. Lycopene, a pigment that gives tomatoes, pink grapefruit, and watermelon their red color, has been linked to lower risk of prostate cancer and cardiovascular disease, and men who consume higher levels of lycopene have a reduced risk of myocardial infarction. Lutein, in addition to its antioxidant benefits, may also be linked to eye and skin health and is available in dark green vegetables. Lignans are phytoestrogens, or plant-based estrogens, which also act as antioxidants. The best sources for lignans are flax and sesame seeds, but they can also be found in broccoli and kale, oatmeal, barley, and rye.

One of the less obvious benefits of a vegetarian diet is the minimization of toxins in the body. Organic foods help to avoid the addition of toxic chemicals to the body, and the use of raw or minimally processed foods provides protection against the increasing use of preservatives in one's diet. Fresh produce also helps to eliminate toxins from the body by increasing the amount of vegetable fiber available to the system. Vegetarians also tend to avoid those food-borne illnesses created by undercooked meats or animal products.

Vitamin Deficiencies Vegetarians can be prone to certain vitamin and mineral deficiencies, including vitamin B_{12}, iron, calcium, and vitamin D. Precautions can be taken to avoid problems, either through carefully managed diet or via supplements. The only reliable sources of vitamin B_{12} (outside of supplements) are meat, dairy products, and eggs, although fermented soy products, seaweed, and certain algaes are being investigated as possible sources. Supplements of B_{12} are recommended for adults, especially vegans, and are considered critical for children who do not consume any animal or dairy products.

In addition to B_{12}, vegetarians may need to monitor iron levels. Iron from vegetable sources has lower bioavailability, so absorption can be compromised. Although iron-deficiency anemia can be found worldwide, it is most prevalent in developing countries where diets are mostly vegetarian. In contrast, Western countries do not experience iron-deficiency anemia due to the availability of fortified cereals and green leafy vegetables in the diet. Females between the ages of 18 and 45 should be particularly aware of their iron intake.

Calcium deficiency exists in vegetarians for two reasons: low calcium intake and an abundance of calcium-intake inhibitors such as dietary fiber and phytic and oxalic acid. Calcium levels in lacto-vegetarians are usually satisfactory as long as vitamin D levels are sufficient. Fortified soy and rice milk products, as well as vitamin-enriched fruit drinks, are available for vegetarians who do not consume milk products.

Infants and younger children of vegans who breast-feed are at higher risk for vitamin D deficiency than their lacto-vegetarian or nonvegetarian counterparts. Sunshine alone is insufficient to protect children from vitamin D-deficiency rickets. Supplements in the form of cod liver oil, vitamin D supplements, or fortified milk substitutes are available.

Other Considerations   High levels of fiber in the diet will cause an increase in internal gas production that may be problematic for some. These symptoms may be minimized by tracking which foods cause the most problems and avoiding or reducing them. The addition of supplemental enzymes may also be of some help while the body adjusts to the increases in dietary fiber.

Hormone levels will be affected by switching to a diet rich in soy and other phytoestrogens. Many vegetarian women have reported reduced menopausal symptoms, but amenorrhea (or absence of menstruation) has been reported in some vegetarian women prior to menopause. Dietary estrogen may also be linked to developmental issues. While the adoption of a vegetarian diet is generally considered a valid lifestyle choice, there are other considerations when preparing to choose a vegetarian diet. An individual's kidney and liver chemistry may determine what benefit she may gain from plant-based diets. As with omnivorous diets, the vegetarian diet is not one size fits all. The choice to adopt a vegetarian diet and lifestyle may be made for a number of excellent reasons, but the results are essentially the same. Increased consumption of fruits and vegetables may reduce incidence of cardiovascular diseases including heart attack and stroke (the leading causes of death for both men and women in the United States), diabetes, and certain cancers. If a balanced vegetarian diet is followed and precautions are taken to ensure adequate levels of proteins and vitamins, then the results can lead to greater longevity and increased productivity over time.

See also Alternative and Holistic Medicine; Childbearing and Infant Feeding; Childrearing; Organic Foods and Technology; Physical Fitness and Athleticism; Policy; Reform.

Further Reading

American Dietetic Association. "Position of the American Dietetic Association: Vegetarian Diets." *Journal of the American Dietetic Association* 93, no. 11 (November 1993): 1317–19.

Dwyer, Johanna T. "Health Aspects of Vegetarian Diets." *American Journal of Clinical Nutrition* 48, no. 3 (1988): 712–38.

Melina, Vesanto, and Brenda Davis. *The New Becoming Vegetarian: The Essential Guide to a Healthy Vegetarian Diet.* 2nd ed. Summertown, TN: Book Publishing Company, 2003.

Saunders, Kerrie K. *The Vegan Diet as Chronic Disease Prevention: Evidence Supporting the New Four Food Groups.* New York: Lantern Books, 2003.

Lisa Hudgins

POLICY

Nutrition-related policies of the U.S. government are developed to improve the health and quality of life of Americans. Policies and programs often address specific conditions such as under- or overnutrition, food allergies, heart disease, diabetes, and cancer. Many nutrition-related policies are administered by the U.S. Department of Agriculture (USDA) and the Food and Drug Administration (FDA). Nutrition policies and programs include *Dietary Guidelines for Americans*; food labeling acts; child nutrition programs such as the National School Lunch Program; and the Special Supplemental Nutrition Program for Women, Infants, and Children (WIC).

Policies vary in their impact on vegetarian culture. For example, no federal standards exist for the use of "vegetarian" or "vegan" on food labels, which can lead to inconsistencies and consumer confusion. Policies can affect the ease with which vegetarians are able to participate in specific programs.

The *Dietary Guidelines for Americans* are the cornerstone of federal nutrition policy. These guidelines are published every five years by the Department of Health and Human Services and the USDA. They provide advice about the role of dietary habits and exercise in health promotion as well as forming the basis for food programs like the child nutrition programs and nutrition education programs. Vegetarian diets were first mentioned in the *Dietary Guidelines* in 1995; they stated that vegetarian diets are consistent with the guidelines and can meet recommendations for nutrients. The 2000 *Dietary Guidelines* were the first to identify what had been previously titled the "Meat, Poultry, Fish, Dry Beans, Eggs, and Nuts Food Group" as the "Meat and Beans Group." This edition also recommended making plant foods the center of one's diet. The most recent edition (2005) of the *Dietary Guidelines* recommends that food preferences of vegetarians be incorporated into diet plans and educational materials. Vegans, and others who avoid milk products, are given a list of nondairy sources of calcium that includes soy-based beverages with added calcium, tofu made with calcium sulfate, and dark green leafy vegetables.

Earlier food guides provided little guidance for vegetarians and none for vegans. The USDA published their first food guide in 1916. Food groups included "meat, fish, and milk" and "butter and wholesome fats." The Basic Four Food Guide, developed in the 1950s, implied that one-fourth of the daily diet should come from the milk group and one-fourth from the meat group. This food guide could be used by vegetarians in a limited fashion by choosing eggs, beans, and peanut butter from the so-called meat group. Serving sizes of vegetarian foods were large, with 1½ cups of beans specified as a replacement for three ounces of meat. No alternatives to the milk group were listed.

The Food Guide Pyramid was issued in 1992 and modified in 2005. Food groups, which are displayed in proportion to the relative amount to be included in the diet, include grains, vegetables, fruits, meat and beans, and milk. A Web site, mypyramid.gov, allows consumers to develop a customized eating plan, which can be vegetarian or vegan. The meat and beans group includes eggs, beans, nuts, nut butters, peas, and soy products as choices for vegetarians. One-quarter cup of cooked beans or one tablespoon of nut butter is considered to be equivalent to one ounce of meat. The milk group does not include options for vegans, although calcium sources for those who do not consume milk products are listed in educational materials.

Although the federal government does not regulate the use of the words "vegetarian" or "vegan" on food labels, some labeling requirements are helpful for vegetarians. Foods containing the major allergens, which include milk, eggs, fish, and shellfish, must be clearly labeled with either the name of the ingredient source or a statement that the product contains specific allergens. For example, the ingredient list could either include whey (milk) or state after the list of ingredients "contains milk." While vegetarians still may not be able to identify meat and some shellfish derivatives from the ingredient listing, eggs, milk, fish, and crustacean shellfish-derived ingredients can be easily determined.

Child nutrition programs administered by the USDA include the National School Lunch Program and the School Breakfast Program. Schools are not required to serve vegetarian meals under these programs, although some nonmeat protein products are allowed. Cheese, eggs, dried beans and peas, yogurt, peanut butter, other nut or seed butters, peanuts, tree nuts, seeds, and some soy products can be served as partial or complete replacements for meat, fish, or poultry. School districts may, but are not required to, serve soy milk to students with a special need identified by parents or guardians. The school district must pay for any costs that exceed the reimbursement for dairy milk.

The WIC program provides vouchers for the purchase of specific foods for pregnant, postpartum, and breast-feeding low-income women, infants, and children up to the age of five years who are at nutritional risk. In some states, following a vegan diet is considered to be a nutritional risk factor. This would seem to be an arbitrary designation. The fact that this classification varies from state to state also seems confusing.

WIC vouchers cover some foods acceptable to vegetarians, including dried beans and peas, peanut butter, dairy milk, cheese, eggs, fruits, vegetables, and approved juices. Vegan participants and others who avoid dairy products can get vouchers for soy milk and tofu made with calcium sulfate in place of dairy milk, provided the participants provide medical documentation of need. This adds a level of complexity that may reduce participation in the program. In addition, health-care practitioners may not be willing to certify an individual's choice to avoid dairy products as a medical condition. Soy milk must meet specified criteria for nutrient content; only a limited number of brands meet the requirements.

See also Childbearing and Infant Feeding; Childrearing; Consumer Products; Physiological Benefits; Veganism.

Further Reading

History of Dietary Guidelines for Americans. U.S. Department of Health and Human Services Web Site. http://www.health.gov/DietaryGuidelines/history.htm.

Jacobson, Michael F. *Six Arguments for a Greener Diet.* Washington, DC: Center for Science in the Public Interest, 2006.

My Pyramid.gov. U.S. Department of Agriculture Web Site. http://www.mypyramid.gov/.

Nestle, Marion. *Food Politics: How the Food Industry Influences Nutrition and Health.* Berkeley: University of California Press, 2002.

Reed Mangels

PUNK ROCK

Punk rock emerged as a music genre in London and New York City in the mid-1970s. The cacophonous and edgy music provided an outlet for radical antiauthoritarian politics to be screamed into public consciousness by disaffected youth. As is the case with most subcultures, punk rock defined itself through lifestyle choices, methods of self-expression, and ethical principles that were distinctive from the culture at large. One way punk rock was set apart from the mainstream was through its members' belief in liberation. The concept of liberation in punk rock quickly came to include compassion for animals.

Punk rock is about living unconventionally. Poly Styrene (X-ray Spex) and the late Joey Ramone (The Ramones) were among the first punk rock musicians to claim to be vegetarians, and animal liberation was further made popular by anarchist punks, such as the radical, pacifist, feminist, vegetarian band Crass.

The punk rock scene most popularly associated with vegetarianism, particularly veganism, is straightedge. In the mid-1980s straightedge adopted veganism as an important part of its creed, and by the 1990s living a cruelty-free lifestyle was as important as abstaining from using drugs and alcohol. Straightedge frames veganism as the logical extension of living a positive, nonexploitative lifestyle, and bands like Earth Crisis and Minor Threat served to reinforce this belief in song lyrics.

While most punks focus on individual actions, some participate in animal rights organizations, such as the Animal Defense League. Food Not Bombs is also popular in punk rock communities because it combines elements of pacifism, vegetarianism, waste reduction, and feeding the hungry. Punk rock collectives, such as ABC No Rio, adopted the practice of providing vegetarian meals to the public. Some punks noticed a lack of restaurants catering to their community, and now—from Foodswings in New York to Ria's Bluebird in Atlanta—restaurants across the United States are owned and operated by punk rock vegetarians.

Despite anticorporate sentiment being a founding principle of punk rock, the scene has become quite commercial. Corporate-sponsored Vans Warped Tour hosts many mainstream punk rock bands as they tour around the United States and provides vegetarian food vendors that distribute information from People for the Ethical Treatment of Animals to the attendees. In recent years, there has been an influx of punk rock-themed cookbooks published by large publishing houses, such as *Vegan with a Vengeance* by Isa Chandra Moskowitz and *How It All Vegan* by Sarah Kramer and Tanya Barnard. Several cosmetic and clothing companies also exist to serve a punk rock vegetarian clientele. As both punk rock and vegetarianism became more popular, businesses began to take advantage of a newly emerging niche market, undermining the antiestablishment message of the founders of punk rock and pushing the scene in a new direction.

See also Activism and Protests; Animal Rights and Animal Welfare; People for the Ethical Treatment of Animals; Reform; Veganism.

Further Reading

Haenfler, Ross. *Straight Edge: Clean-Living Youth, Hardcore Punk, and Social Change.* New Brunswick, NJ: Rutgers University Press, 2004.
Maurer, Donna. *Vegetarianism: Movement or Moment.* Philadelphia: Temple University Press, 2002.

Mandy Van Deven

PYTHAGORAS

One of the earliest proponents of abstention from animal food in the Western tradition was Pythagoras (ca. 570–490 BC), who provided an ethical argument against eating meat. His argument was based on his religious conviction that human souls transmigrate from one life to another. Thus, death is not the end of existence for the soul; instead, it simply defines a step in the cycle of birth and death. This theory unites one generation to another, one culture to another, and one life-form to another. Various life-forms are just different evolutionary stages: Monkeys, cows, dogs, or humans find a common connection between themselves. Therefore, most philosophers who propagated the idea of the transmigration of soul also propagated vegetarianism.

This process of soul migration is popularly known as metempsychosis, transmigration of the soul, or reincarnation of the soul. The concept of metempsychosis states that the soul is immortal and transmigrates or reincarnates from one life-form to another. There is nothing comparable to the soul in modern science. Science does not deal with the existence of the soul. In most religions and cultures, however, the existence of the soul is central to their defining philosophies.

Pythagoras advocated vegetarianism on the basis of his belief in metempsychosis—his view of transmigration of the soul—but he also encouraged fasting as a way of purification and of acknowledging the sanctity of animal life. Pythagoras established a school of thought that, although religious in nature, influenced the ideas of Empedocles, Socrates, Plato, Porphyry, Plotinus, Apollonius, Plutarch,

Clement of Alexandria, and many other Greek philosophers. These philosophers also advocated vegetarianism and believed in the transmigration of soul.

For example, in Plato's *The Republic* (369d–373e), a model city is defined where all food needs are fulfilled by a vegetarian diet. Plato suggested barley and wheat loaves, roots and herbs, salt, olives, cheese, onion, greens, desserts made from figs, chickpeas, beans, berries, and acorns as ideal foods for human beings. Plato considered vegetarian foods as the foods of "health and peace," where peace indicates peace with animals.

In a popular story, Pythagoras saw a man beating a young dog. He recognized the voice of a recently demised friend in the dog's yelping and asked the man to stop the beating. The transmigration of soul theory is not unique to Pythagoras; it is also central in the Hindu religion. On the possible contact of Pythagoras with Indian philosophy, Apollonius of Tyana (AD 15–100), a Pythagorean who traveled widely within and outside the Roman Empire as a teacher of asceticism, wrote that Pythagoras was taught by Egyptian philosophers who were trained in Indian philosophy.

See also Ethical Vegetarianism; India; Meatless Diets before Vegetarianism; Vegetarians and Vegans, Noted.

Further Reading

Dombrowski, Daniel A. *The Philosophy of Vegetarianism.* Amherst: University of Massachusetts Press, 1984.

Dombrowski, Daniel A. "Was Plato a Vegetarian?" *Apeiron* 18 (1984): 1–9.

Guthrie, Kenneth Sylvan. *The Pythagorean Sourcebook and Library.* Grand Rapids, MI: Phanes, 1987.

Jones, Christopher P. *Philostratus: The Life of Apollonius of Tyana.* Cambridge, MA: Harvard University Press, 2005.

Walters, Kerry, and Lisa Portmess, eds. *Ethical Vegetarianism: From Pythagoras to Peter Singer.* Albany: State University of New York Press, 1999.

Alok Kumar

REFORM

Since antiquity, abstinence from meat has constituted a form of statement, and the act of rejecting animal flesh—up to the point of contesting its use as food—both describes and prescribes a specific worldview. In the Western tradition, vegetarianism has represented a minority trend in prevalently meat-eating societies, and therefore it has posed itself as an alternative relationship between humans and animals, the body and the soul, relations of humans among themselves, and the very idea of what food is, including how it influences the construction of one's body and identity and how dietary choices shape society. Due to all of these factors, the vegetarian choice, once promoted at a collective level, represents a form of social reform with far-reaching consequences.

In fact, the individual choice to abstain from meat, far from being a mere dietary preference, is to be included in a wider frame of references, where the individual food choice is accompanied by the concern to promote vegetarianism. The reasons for this proselytism are as varied as the rationales that can sustain the vegetarian choice. It can stem from ethical, religious, spiritual, hygienic, and/or political ideas and ideals. In Western societies, vegetarianism has developed into different strands over the last three centuries, as a result of the influence exerted by these different components and rationales, with one or some of them prevailing over the others during specific historical moments according to the mainstream cultural tenets of the time.

Vegetarianism as a Moral Physiology   Central tenets of vegetarianism during the 18th and 19th centuries might seem strange to vegetarians of today. While in the 20th and 21st centuries the rejection of the killing of animals plays a central and explicit role, previously, animal welfare concerns were secondary to other interests and rarely made explicit. Other concerns, somewhere in-between morality (religion) and physiology, were the main focus of the early vegetarian social movement in the West.

During the 18th and 19th centuries, a medical vegetarian movement gained popularity in Europe and eventually the United States. The promotion of vegetarianism as a form of preventive and therapeutic dietary medicine by physicians was so widespread in England that it became a mass movement. A meatless diet was advocated by orthodox physicians like George Cheyne (1671–1743), the most authoritative figure in this respect of his time, and William Lambe (1765–1847), who, on the basis of anatomical similarities between humans and herbivores, declared that eating meat was unnatural.

Although charismatic and authoritative figures such as these played an important role in the spread of vegetarianism, the work of middle-class social reformers was key as well. The physical improvement brought about by temperance (mainly associated with abstention from alcohol but also including for a time a restriction on tobacco, sweets, and other spicy or "stimulating" foods) and the adoption of a meatless diet both prompted and resulted in these social reformers' collective action against the appalling conditions of working people's diet. The emphasis on temperance, including moderation in both food and drink, also promoted the spiritual salvation of their fellows from the perceived moral decay of society. It was not only a question of health and hygiene; vegetarianism was a matter of physical as well as spiritual health, morality, religion, personal salvation, and social transformation. At a time when discourses on humans were imbued with religious statements, people's diet had to be consistent with Christian doctrine. Interpretations of the Bible suggested that eating meat was unnatural and that meat polluted the body and aroused evil instincts. Parallel to this, the idea of animal abuse paving the way to violent behavior against other human beings sprang from the current of humanitarianism. Overindulgence in meat was signaled by many advocates of a "natural" (vegetarian) diet as a habit leading to vicious and aggressive behaviors dominated by sexual urges. In many pamphlets and articles published in vegetarian magazines, even war and militarism were described as consequences of a meat-based lifestyle. In a more theoretically structured way, a strong link between the subjugation of animals and violence against women was—and still is—denounced by the vegetarian current within the feminist movement, just as vegetarian pacifists underlined the connection between the killing of animals and the killing of other human beings.

Vegetarian Societies   Both health concerns and humanitarian sentiments prompted vegetarianism among the Bible Christian churches. The Bible Christian Church was founded in Salford, England, at the beginning of the 19th century by the efforts of William Cowherd; then, in 1817, Rev. James Clark and Rev. William Metcalfe, envoys of the Salford dissenting churches, exported the doctrine to the United States, giving impetus to the American vegetarian movement, along with temperance and humanitarian campaigns—pacifism, abolition of the slave trade, temperance, and abolition of capital punishment.

Thanks to the spread and development of the ideas of these vegetarian pioneers in the United States, social reformers started considering vegetarianism as one of the fundamental principles of their programs. These reformers included the clergyman Sylvester Graham (1794–1851), advocate of a vegetarian lifestyle (which also prescribed abstinence from alcoholic beverages and sexual activity) to promote health and personal salvation; William Andrus Alcott (1798–1859), physician and first president of the American Vegetarian Society; and John Harvey Kellogg (1852–1943), medical doctor, Grahamite, member of the Seventh-day Adventists (a church founded in 1863 that recommends vegetarianism), and inventor of the popular corn flakes breakfast cereal.

In the meantime, with the same arguments, other popular figures livened up the debate around diet, health, and morality in Europe. The resulting mobilization of evangelical and humanitarian reformers, intellectuals, physicians, clergymen, and politicians saw the foundation of the first Vegetarian Society in Manchester in 1847. Joseph Brotherton (1783–1837) and other members from the Salford Bible Christian Church contributed significantly to the group's establishment. The Vegetarian Society in England was shortly followed by the launch of the American Vegetarian Society in 1850 and, two decades later, by the creation of the first German organization by the clergyman Edward Baltzer. The Vegetarian Federal Union—created in 1889—was the result of the spreading of vegetarian societies across Europe, in Austria, France, Switzerland, and Hungary, in the 1880s. The Vegetarian Federal Union was subsequently replaced by the International Vegetarian Union in 1908.

Animal Welfare   During the second half of the 19th century, this trend of social reforms, vegetarianism included, underwent a process of secularization and inner transformation. As a result, the rhetoric and even the hierarchical order of values expressed by the vegetarian movement changed. These reformers—who were concerned with vegetarianism, education, blood sports, temperance, and the plight of the working classes—also reflected on women's role in society, creating a strong link between animal advocacy and the women's rights movement. Parallel to this, humanitarian reformers interested in animal issues were fighting the battle for the abolition of the slave trade. Thus, vegetarianism was at the root of a series of reforms in different causes that vegetarians considered to be united in essence.

Gradually, the question of animal welfare grew in importance within the movement. Thanks to an effective humanitarian animal-protection campaign that denounced the dreadful conditions of animals in markets and slaughterhouses, a law for the protection of work animals was passed in 1822 in the United Kingdom (known as the Martin's Act). In the United States, a series of anticruelty laws were approved in the second half of the 19th century, following New York State's example in 1867. The passage of this legislation in New York can be largely attributed to the work of Henry Bergh, a prominent activist and founder of the American Society for the Prevention of Cruelty to Animals, and members across the country.

Animal Rights in the 20th Century   The development of vegetarianism continued from the 19th into the 20th century. The evolution of the vegetarian trend was characterized by a turning point in the 1960s and 1970s, both quantitatively and qualitatively. In the 1960s, meat avoidance gained in popularity in mainstream American society. Also, the ethical framework that gives meat avoidance its meaning was changing. The 1960s and 1970s counterculture movement challenged the established thinking about power, dominion, interhuman relationships, and also humans' relationships with animals and the environment. Dietary choices like vegetarianism became a very powerful form of protest and an effective political statement.

Currently, varied kinds of vegetarianism exist: ethical, spiritual, environmental, and health-related, with the ethical treatment of animals being at the core of today's mainstream vegetarianism. The vegetarian choice springs from the rejection of the killing of animals for food and, at a more general level, from a rethinking of human obligations toward nature and other sentient beings. The debate on speciesism, animal rights, and animal welfare characterizes modern ethical vegetarianism.

This ethical debate on animal issues—developed in Western countries in the 1970s and 1980s—was supported by the theoretical work of scholars like Richard Ryder, Peter Singer, and Tom Regan, in whose perspective vegetarianism and veganism are to be included in the framework of the animal advocacy theory. The term "speciesism," which was coined by Ryder and appeared in 1975 in his *Victims of Science,* indicates discrimination on the basis of the species difference. The book explicitly draws a parallel between speciesism, sexism, and racism.

This form of discrimination is challenged by the antispeciesist ethical attitude proposed first by Ryder and then by Singer. Singer introduced the concept of speciesism within a utilitarian philosophical frame. In *Animal Liberation* (1975), he argued for an "equal consideration of interests" not biased by species differences and therefore not excluding animals from the sphere of moral consideration. The expression "animal rights," which has recently become eponymous for the entire social movement, appeared in 1983 in Regan's *The Case for Animal Rights,* a philosophical dissertation on the rights of nonhuman beings as individuals that have an inherent value as subjects of a life.

Prior to this theoretical structuring of animal rights philosophy, vegetarianism as a social movement had already spread across social classes in the mid-20th century, parallel to the development of factory farming. Its aim has been to promote compassionate living, a lifestyle that abhors animal killing for food and the transformation of animals into machines. An important point of reference for the spread of these ideas was the book *Animal Machines* (1964) by Ruth Harrison, which called public attention to the shocking conditions of animals in factory farming, and *Diet for a Small Planet* by Frances Moore Lappé (1971), which, adopting a scientific approach to nutrition, hunger, and natural resources, demonstrated how vegetable proteins satisfactorily meet human nutritional requirements, guaranteeing not only a healthy diet to us but also a healthier planet.

Today, vegetarianism is a new social movement that calls for a radical change in society framed by a radically different cultural and ethical paradigm. The individual and daily act of avoiding meat means a lot more than refusing one food for another. Against the background of the antispeciesist perspective, this simple gesture symbolically subsumes the rejection of the humanistic view that describes the human being as the "measure of all things," along with the anthropocentric perspective that has framed every discourse on humanity and animality since Aristotle's times. Rethinking human-animal relationships constitutes a model to rethink other kinds of relations that have to do with gender, race, social classes, power, and hegemonic status and prompts the exploration of new ways of understanding the place of humans in the world. Given these premises, ethical vegetarianism, despite having become part of mainstream culture in the United States, questions and challenges some of America's core values and attempts to overthrow the established cultural paradigm.

See also Activism and Protests; Agribusiness; Alcott, William A.; Alternative and Holistic Medicine; American Vegetarian Society; Animal Rights and Animal Welfare; Bible Christians, English; Bible Christians, Philadelphia; Ethical Vegetarianism; Global Warming; Graham; Sylvester; International Vegetarian Union; Kellogg, John Harvey; Lappé, Frances Moore; Meatless Diets before Vegetarianism; Metcalfe, Rev. William; Physiological Benefits; Policy; Religious Beliefs and Practices; Seventh-day Adventists; Singer, Peter; United Kingdom; Vegetarian Society of the United Kingdom.

Further Reading

Iacobbo, Karen, and Michael Iacobbo. *Vegetarian America: A History.* Westport, CT: Praeger, 2004.
International Vegetarian Union. http://www.ivu.org.
Spencer, Colin. *Vegetarianism: A History.* London: Grub Street, 2000. (Originally published in 1993)
Stuart, Tristram. *The Bloodless Revolution: A Cultural History of Vegetarianism from 1600 to Modern Times.* New York: W.W. Norton, 2007.
Twigg, Julia. "Food for Thought: Purity and Vegetarianism." *Religion* 9 (1979): 13–35.

Sabrina Tonutti

RELIGIOUS BELIEFS AND PRACTICES

Food is central to the practice, ritual life, and belief systems of most religious traditions. Within their range of practices, many religions also include either brief periods of vegetarianism, as part of ascetic discipline, or extended periods of vegetarian eating, including one's entire life, as an ideal goal. While food practices change over time and place, and are sometimes dictated by climate and food availability, some practices of vegetarianism are also inherent to particular traditions. For organizational ease, the major world traditions are grouped here into those historically based in South Asia or in the Mediterranean.

The religions of South Asia—Hinduism, Buddhism, and Jainism—all include vegetarian ideals because of the centrality of the concepts of karma, *ahimsa,* and the transmigration of souls. While these religious ideas are extremely complicated and not necessarily monolithic in each of the traditions, their basic components are central to understanding the related vegetarian practices. Ahimsa is the principal doctrine of noninjury or nonharming and is considered one of the highest duties in the traditions of South Asia. Scholars trace the doctrine back to the pre-Aryan inhabitants of the subcontinent.

In Jainism, possibly the oldest of the three traditions (though dating their emergence and development is problematic), animal souls and human souls are equally important. Because of this belief, a central precept for Jains is never to harm another form of life. The most rigorous practitioners will not even eat root vegetables, as pulling them from the ground could harm the organisms attached to the root. While not all Jains are this strict, almost all are vegetarians. Some Jain holy people will even wear face masks to keep from accidentally breathing in, and thus killing, small flying creatures and will walk slowly while gently sweeping the ground in front of them to avoid stepping on insects.

Hinduism also focuses on ahimsa and the role of other animals, as evidenced in the great Hindu epic the *Mahabharata,* which proclaims that eating animals is like eating the flesh of one's own son. But with the exception of ascetics and other humans at certain stages of life, strict vegetarianism is not a necessary practice. As a matter of fact, some early forms of Vedic Hinduism included animal sacrifice. By 500 BC, however, evidence of the increasing significance of the sacred cow and *samsara,* which is the process of rebirth, means vegetarian practices were more widespread. The soul, or *atman,* which is identical in all living beings, transmigrates through endless incarnations. Killing or even harming another being increases the weight of karma that the soul carries and extends the process of transmigration, a process that one seeks to escape. In order to escape, attachments to worldly desires must be overcome. Therefore practicing vegetarianism and the nonharming of all living beings is integral to achieving *moksha,* the release from rebirth.

Buddhism, the third of the Indian-based traditions, is grounded in the life and teachings of Gautama Buddha, who lived in the sixth century BC. Central to his teachings is the end to killing of living beings. The Jataka tales, part of the body of sacred texts of Buddhism, often include interactions between humans and other animals. The Buddha's previous incarnations are sometimes in the form of other animals in these tales. Practices of renunciation are therefore central to Buddhism, and, for most monks and nuns, vegetarianism is part of their overall focus on a life of ahimsa and of release from the cycle of rebirth.

While an ideal in Buddhism, vegetarianism is not universally practiced. In part, this is due to the concept of intentionality. One might eat a dead animal without incurring the same karma as the one who actually killed the animal. If monks and nuns who beg for their food are given food containing meat, they will sometimes eat it since they did not intend the animal to be killed. Also, there are certain geographic areas where Buddhism flourished, such as Tibet, where vegetarianism would be almost impossible because of the climate and terrain.

Compassion toward other animals is certainly an element in all three of these traditions, but karma also plays a major role in dietary practices. In Buddhism, for instance, it is more harmful to kill an elephant than a dog because of the sustained intention required to kill the larger animal. This sustained intention leads to a more weighty accumulation of bad karma, and therefore an increased likelihood of rebirth into a lower form. This concept of karmic impact is key when considering the reasons for practicing vegetarianism in Buddhism, Jainism, and Hinduism.

The three world religions that emerged in the Mediterranean world—Judaism, Christianity, and Islam—all have quite varied eating practices as well. Judaism is the oldest and is, in some ways, the foundational religion for Christianity and Islam. Similar stories and texts are shared in the Jewish Scriptures, the Christian Bible, and the Muslim Qur'an.

In Judaism, the creation stories suggest that a vegetarian diet in a nonviolent paradise is the original plan God had for humans. After the fall of humanity into sin, sacrifices in the form of burnt animal offerings appear as a way to appease an angry God. This shift in the human condition is quickly followed by the story of the Great Flood, a punishment for sin. At this post-Flood juncture the Hebrew Scriptures state that humans are given permission by God, or more accurately are cursed by God, to eat animal flesh. While animal sacrifices have not taken place in Judaism for 2,000 years, the concept is central to the history of Judaism.

In addition, the Jewish law code includes a significant number of rules regarding what one eats and how one prepares food. This is particularly evident when one considers the animals marked clean, thus edible, or unclean, prohibited for consumption. For those animals that the kosher laws recognize as clean or edible, certain guidelines define how those animals can be slaughtered and prepared for consumption, with particular attention paid to the significance of blood. Thus, while some contemporary forms of Judaism include vegetarian practices, there is a complicated history of eating and sacrificing animals in the tradition.

Christianity is rooted in Judaism, Greek philosophical schools, and the mystery religions of the Mediterranean world, to mention just a few of the historical influences that lead to a variety of ideas regarding meat consumption. Though Orthodox Christianity does not follow the kosher eating laws of Judaism, most Christians, particularly in the Pauline and eventually Orthodox tradition, do focus on the scriptural texts that permit the killing of animals for food. Thus, dominant forms of Christianity rarely follow vegetarian practices; rather they insist that God gave humans dominion over all other animals, and therefore meat eating is not only allowed but assumed or even mandated.

Still, throughout Christianity's 2,000-year history, many individuals and groups—usually those considered radical, along with ascetics in the Orthodox traditions—ate a vegetarian diet. For example, the early desert ascetics abstained from the eating of flesh in order to purify their bodies from evil. Throughout medieval Christianity, food practices were particularly important for women who chose life in religious orders and for some influential heretical groups. Many prominent female ascetics, such as Catherine of Siena, likely died as a result of an extremely limited diet. Francis of Assisi, while not a pure vegetarian himself, still emphasized the spiritual nature of animals and the efficacy of vegetarian eating practices. There are still remnants of such vegetarian practices in the recognition of certain seasons such as Lent, the 40-day period of preparation prior to the Feast of the Resurrection, or Easter. Throughout this period certain renunciations are obligatory for some Christians, including abstaining from meat on Fridays. While this has a minimal impact in terms of overall consumption of meat, it is a reminder of the history and efficacy of vegetarian practices in the religion. Several movements, such as Catharism, a widespread and influential medieval heresy, focused on a lifestyle reflecting "perfection." For them the "Perfect," those who reached the highest levels of spiritual life, ate no meat as one of many signs of their perfection.

As a response to the Reformation, humanism, and the Enlightenment, some small groups within Christianity began to practice vegetarianism as part of their overall religious discipline. Sir Thomas More's influential work *Utopia* describes a world free of animal slaughter based on his Christian ideals. Leonardo da Vinci, among other prominent thinkers and theologians, was also a famous vegetarian. In addition to these individuals, various critics of new scientific methods, particularly those responding to the philosophy of Descartes, questioned the Christian-based precept of human dominion over the world. Eventually, movements to protect animals from vivisection and cruel agricultural practices grew both within and parallel to Christianity in Europe and the United States. The Swedenborgians and Seventh-day Adventists are among those groups who, by the 19th century, adopted a vegetarian diet both for personal health reasons and with an underlying critique of the treatment of other animals as well.

Islamic practices of vegetarianism are relatively rare, and the Qur'an is most often interpreted as advocating the eating of meat based on human dominion. In addition, Islam emerged in a desert environment; thus a vegetarian diet would have been almost impossible for humans in that area. Still, there are examples of Islamic ascetics, particularly some Sufis (mystics), who have abstained from meat eating for spiritual reasons, even though they were sometimes ridiculed for doing so.

In contemporary Judaism, Christianity, and Islam, vegetarianism does appear to be increasingly popular, though still on a relatively minor scale and for different reasons. In many cases, the choice of a vegetarian diet is primarily for either health- or environment-related reasons rather than out of a sense of compassion for other animals. But the centrality of compassion and its connection to animals in all three Mediterranean religions is growing in the 21st century. For many reasons, public awareness of confined animal feeding operations, or factory farming, is growing. Different campaigns, such as one launched by the Humane Society of the United States, are focusing on animals and religion with a particular emphasis on food animals and their plight in the midst of contemporary mass agricultural production. Increasingly, scholars and practitioners of Judaism, Christianity, and Islam are reexamining the place of vegetarianism in these traditions and providing resources for practitioners.

Vegetarianism in the myriad indigenous traditions is difficult to address, as the groups vary so widely across time and location. Usually, whatever native plants and animals are available for food are found in the diets of indigenous people. Taboo and totem practices, both of which designate certain animals that cannot be eaten, do limit the consumption of some animals by certain groups or individuals, though. This could be an important factor in population maintenance for a variety of animals.

While Christianity and Islam are growing rapidly in Africa, South America, and Southeast Asia, there are also a number of newly formed religions, often called new religious movements, growing in North America and Europe in particular. These often combine ancient pagan practices with Christianity and, at times, with other contemporary ideas such as environmentalism to create new religious or spiritual sensibilities that dictate vegetarianism.

See also African Hebrew Israelites; Ahimsa; Bible and Biblical Arguments; Bible Christians, English; Bible Christians, Philadelphia; Colonies, Communal Societies, and Utopias; Eastern Religions, Influences of; Ethical Vegetarianism; Ethnic and Racial Groups, U.S.; Gandhi, Mohandas; India; Jainism; Meatless Diets before Vegetarianism; Reform; Seventh-day Adventists; Shakers, The.

Further Reading

Bynum, Caroline Walker. *Holy Feast and Holy Fast: The Religious Significance of Food to Medieval Women.* Berkeley: University of California Press, 1987.

Foltz, Richard. *Animals in Islamic Tradition and Muslim Cultures.* Oxford: Oneworld, 2006.

Hamilton, Malcolm. "Eating Ethically: 'Spiritual' and "Quasi-Religious' Aspects of Vegetarianism." *Journal of Contemporary Religion* 15, no. 1 (2000): 65–83.

Hobgood-Oster, Laura. *Holy Dogs and Asses: Animals in the Christian Tradition.* Urbana: University of Illinois Press, 2008.

Waldau, Paul, and Kimberly Patton, eds. *A Communion of Subjects: Animals in Religion, Science and Ethics.* New York: Columbia University Press, 2006.

Laura Hobgood-Oster

RESTAURANTS

A growing number of people are choosing to eat vegetarian when dining out at restaurants. Restaurants are recognizing that people are opting to eat vegetarian meals, regardless of whether they follow a strict vegetarian diet, due to an interest in personal health, the environment, animals, or religion. Therefore, restaurants are adding many more vegetarian options to their menus, and every day new vegetarian restaurants are opening up in cities across the world.

Vegetarian restaurants first appeared in the United States at the end of the 19th century. The first documented vegetarian restaurant, opened in 1885, was called Vegetarian Restaurant No. 1 and was located in the Hotel Byron on West 23rd Street in New York City. It was sponsored by the New York Vegetarian Society, which advocated a lifestyle free of meat eating and alcohol consumption. Vegetarian restaurants opened in Boston and Los Angeles shortly thereafter. Generally, these restaurants served nut- and grain-based food products.

The development of vegetarian restaurants in England was similar to that in the United States. In Manchester in the 1850s, there were Barnesley's Vegetarian and Temperance Hotel and Mrs. Hollinworth's vegetarian dining room. By 1886, there were 12 vegetarian restaurants throughout London. The customers were not always vegetarian; they represented the new lower-middle class that included shop assistants and thoughtful members of the artisan class. Vegetarian restaurants in 19th-century London were considered cheap, respectable, and safe places to eat for both men and women. Vegetarian restaurants can be considered a factor in the revival and growth of the vegetarian movement in 19th-century England.

In the 20th century, vegetarian restaurants proliferated as the cost of meat rose. People flocked to vegetarian restaurants and hotels, while nonvegetarian restaurants added meatless dishes such as spaghetti and omelets to their menus. During World War I, vegetarian cafes flourished and chains began to form, due to a growing awareness of vegetarianism as an economical and nourishing way of eating. Vegetarian restaurants did so well during the rationing years because they showed their customers how vegetables could make a satisfying meal. The Physical Culture Restaurant in New York City offered a bowl of vegetarian soup and whole wheat bread for one cent and a more varied menu for five cents. By 1911, there were 20 branches of Physical Culture in the United States, including locations in Boston, Philadelphia, Pittsburgh, Buffalo, and Chicago. The chain, however, declined when the management changed.

By the 1930s, there were 15 Schildkraut's Vegetarian Restaurants in New York City and two Schildkraut vacation resorts in New York State. Owned and operated by Sadie Schildkraut, these restaurants featured a style of preparing vegetables so that customers would think they were eating meat. In the early 1920s, two raw food vegetarian restaurants opened in Los Angeles, and a chain of vegetarian cafeterias appeared in the southern United States.

An estimate of the number of vegetarian restaurants in North America today is in the thousands. Big cities around the world have at least a few vegetarian restaurants. New York City, Toronto, London, Berlin, Paris, Prague, Bangkok, Mumbai, Thailand, Melbourne, Auckland, Cairo, Cape Town, Buenos Aires, and Mexico City all host vegetarian restaurants that repeatedly appear on "best vegetarian restaurants" lists. These lists are easily accessible on the Internet and in travel guides. "Happy Cow" (http://www.happycow.net) is the leading Internet resource that lists and rates vegetarian restaurants from all over the world. In addition, many vegetarian-advocacy organizations produce directories that include a list of vegetarian restaurants and maps that are often specific to a given city.

Vegetarian restaurants in the United States, available in both general and ethnic formats, include typical sit-down restaurants; take-out, fast food, and salad restaurants; buffets and pay-by-weight options at natural food stores; and even all-you-can-eat restaurants. Nonvegetarian restaurants will often make dishes to order and omit animal ingredients for vegetarians, or dairy and eggs for vegans. The server in the restaurant will usually know whether a specific dish can be modified to suit the customer's needs.

Many ethnic restaurants serve traditional dishes that are also vegetarian. For example, Mediterranean restaurants serve falafel, hummus, eggplant moussaka, tabouli, and stuffed grape leaves. Italian restaurants offer pasta in olive oil, pesto sauce, marinara sauce, bruschetta, minestrone soup, and vegetable lasagna. Chinese restaurants serve many dishes that are suitable for vegans. They also offer dishes such as tofu and mixed vegetables, hot and sour soup, vegetable and noodle entrees, fried rice, and vegetarian egg and spring rolls. Ethnic African restaurants serve various types of bean and vegetable rotis with rice, while Mexican restaurants offer such items as burritos, tacos, enchiladas, and tortillas with refried beans, guacamole, and rice. Vegetarian pizza is almost always available at restaurants serving pizza. Often, pizzas without cheese, or with soy cheese, can be made. Fast food and North American–style restaurants increasingly have vegetarian options such as veggie burgers, roasted-vegetable sandwiches, french fries, onion rings, and salads.

Occasionally, vegetarian restaurants increase their marketability by publishing a cookbook that features the restaurant's specialty items. Examples of this include the *New Moosewood Cookbook* (2000) from the Moosewood Restaurant in Ithaca, New York; the *Candle Cafe Cookbook* (2003) from the Candle Cafe in New York City; *Rebar* (2001) from Rebar Modern Food in Victoria, British Columbia; and *Juice for Life* (2003) from Fresh in Toronto, Ontario.

See also Consumer Products; Cookbooks; Domestic Science and Scientific Eating; Ethnic and Racial Groups, U.S.; Health Food Stores and Food Cooperatives; Internet, The; Katzen, Mollie; Macfadden, Bernarr; Social Acceptance; World Wars in England.

Further Reading

The American Dietetic Association. *Being Vegetarian.* Chicago: Chronimed, 1996.
Gregory, James. *Of Victorians and Vegetarians: The Vegetarian Movement in Nineteenth-Century Britain.* New York: Tauris, 2007.
Iacobbo, Karen, and Michael Iacobbo. *Vegetarian America: A History.* Westport, CT: Praeger, 2004.
Kimball, Chad T., ed. *Vegetarian Sourcebook.* Holmes, PA: Omnigraphics, 2002.
Spencer, Colin. *The Heretic's Feast.* London: Fourth Estate, 1995.
Whitaker, Jan. "Restaurant-ing through History." http://victualling.wordpress.com/2008/08/08/early-vegetarian-restaurants/.

Vanessa M. Holm

S

SALT, HENRY S. (1851~1939)

Henry Stephens Salt was a British social reformer, literary critic, and outspoken advocate of vegetarianism and animal rights. Salt attended Eton as a King's Scholar before continuing his education at Cambridge University; upon graduation he was invited back to Eton to serve as a housemaster. Salt married Kate Joynes in 1879 and appeared ready to settle into a respectable middle-class life as a teacher and scholar.

Salt chafed under a school culture that emphasized tradition over new ideas, however, and soon became involved in a network of social and political reformers who challenged many of the accepted conventions of Victorian society. Salt read extensively—especially Shelley and Thoreau—and stopped eating meat around 1883 after reading Howard Williams's *The Ethics of Diet*. Increasingly committed to the ideals of socialism and vegetarianism and disillusioned with his career at Eton, Salt resigned in 1884. Seeking a simpler and more authentic existence, he moved with Kate into a small cottage near Tilford, Surrey, which quickly became a convivial meeting place for an eclectic group of like-minded individuals, including Fabian leaders Beatrice and Sidney Webb, anarchist Prince Kropotkin, poet Edward Carpenter, and playwright George Bernard Shaw. Salt frequently published short pieces on literature, politics, and social change and also embarked on an ambitious program of research and writing that produced biographies of Shelley, Thoreau, and the poet James Thomson by 1890.

Meanwhile, his commitment to vegetarianism intensified. In 1885 Salt was named a vice president of the Vegetarian Society (known today as the Vegetarian Society of the United Kingdome), and the following year he published *A Plea for Vegetarianism and Other Essays,* an anthology of essays highlighting some of his signature approaches to vegetarian advocacy. Especially evident were his favoring of rational arguments over polemical or emotional appeals, and his insistence that a vegetarian diet was more than a mere dietary preference. Salt contended instead that vegetarianism was in fact a crucial element of a broader agenda of interconnected social reform impulses that would ultimately lead to a more humane, just, and civil society, something he began calling "humanitarianism."

In 1891 Salt cofounded the Humanitarian League, an organization designed to put these ideas into practice by uniting vegetarians, antivivisectionists, prison and educational reformers, animal advocates, and opponents of capital and corporal punishment. The following year *Animals' Rights, in Relation to Social Progress* was published, a cogent and logically consistent case for extending rights to animals that would become one of Salt's better-known works. In 1895 the Humanitarian League began publication of the monthly journal *Humanity* with Salt as editor and frequent contributor, and in 1899 he published his second major vegetarian treatise, *The Logic of Vegetarianism,* which refined and expanded on many of his earlier arguments.

Although the Humanitarian League continued to operate through the 1910s, Salt dissolved it permanently in 1919, distraught by the brutality of World War I, the recent death of Kate, and his fear that civilization was regressing into barbarity rather than moving toward an enlightened, humanitarian future. He continued to write, however, penning two autobiographies and two books about wildflowers that evinced a growing environmental awareness. On November 20, 1931, the habitually modest Salt enjoyed one of his proudest moments at a meeting of the London Vegetarian Society, when Indian independence leader Mohandas Gandhi expressed his honor at sharing the dais with Salt and explained how *A Plea for Vegetarianism* had convinced him as a young man to embrace vegetarianism for moral reasons rather than out of cultural obligation.

Salt died in 1939 at the age of 88, retaining a steadfast commitment to his humanitarian principles until the end. In a prepared statement read at his funeral, Salt disavowed established religion but affirmed his faith that eventually humanity would be governed by a "creed of kinship," in which the interrelation of all life was acknowledged and the rights of humans and animals alike were honored. Though for decades both his name and his cause were largely forgotten, Salt's remarkably sophisticated arguments were rediscovered during the emerging vegetarian and animal rights movements of the 1970s. Philosopher Peter Singer—author of the seminal 1975 book *Animal Liberation*—has praised Salt for anticipating most of the contemporary debate regarding vegetarianism and animal rights and noted his 19th-century contributions to the modern movement.

See also Activism and Protests; Animal Rights and Animal Welfare; Antivivisection; Ethical Vegetarianism; Gandhi, Mohandas; Reform; Singer, Peter; Transcendentalism.

Further Reading

Hendrick, George. *Henry Salt: Humanitarian Reformer and Man of Letters.* Urbana: University of Illinois Press, 1977.

Hendrick, George, and Willene Hendrick, eds. *The Savour of Salt: A Henry Salt Anthology.* Fontwell Sussex, UK: Centaur, 1989.

Salt, Henry S. *The Logic of Vegetarianism: Essays and Dialogues.* London: Ideal Publishing, 1899.

Salt, Henry S. *Seventy Years among Savages.* London: George Allen and Unwin, 1921.

Winsten, Stephen. *Salt and His Circle.* London: Hutchinson, 1951.

Gary K. Jarvis

SEVENTH-DAY ADVENTISTS

The Seventh-day Adventist Church, a Protestant denomination with roots in the American Millerite movement of the 1840s, became closely associated with vegetarianism through the writings of Ellen G. White. Now an international organization with more than 15 million members, it promotes the health benefits of vegetarianism through magazines and books and operates food factories in several countries.

Joseph Bates (1792–1872), a former sea captain, developed the new denomination along with James White (1821–1881), previously a Millerite preacher, and his wife, Ellen (1827–1915). While active in the Millerite movement, Bates had adopted vegetarianism, along with other dietary changes, through the influence of health reformer Sylvester Graham. Although his abstemious living became well known within early sabbatarian Adventism, Bates did not promote his dietary philosophy. Several Adventists, however, became interested in health reform during the 1850s and made contact with the physician James Caleb Jackson of Dansville, New York, who operated a water-cure establishment and advocated vegetarianism. In the early 1860s, James White began publishing articles, one of which promoted vegetarianism, by health reformers in the denomination's paper, the *Review and Herald.*

In June 1863, Ellen White, a visionary since December 1844, had a vision in which she learned that care for one's health is a religious duty. She reported this experience in the fourth volume of *Spiritual Gifts* (1864), in which she condemned meat eating along with the use of tobacco, coffee, tea, and medical drugs, later expanding these themes in *Health: How to Live* (1866). James suffered a stroke in 1866, however, and the Whites spent several weeks at Jackson's water cure. This experience led them to start a magazine, the *Health Reformer,* and open the denomination's own Western Health Reform Institute in Battle Creek, Michigan, in 1866. Ellen continued thereafter to promote vegetarianism among church members, arguing that meat consumption contributed to both disease and excitement of the animal passions.

John Harvey Kellogg (1852–1943), an Adventist medical doctor who had studied at the University of Michigan and New York's Bellevue Hospital, took over the *Health Reformer* in 1874, renaming it *Good Health,* and became director of the Health Institute in 1876, after which it became known as the Battle Creek Sanitarium. He soon became the denomination's leading advocate of vegetarianism and other health practices, writing books that were marketed widely, ending the serving of meat at Adventist camp meetings and educational institutions, and developing meat analogues and other health food products. By the early 20th century, vegetarianism was well embedded in Adventism, although it never became a standard of membership.

Drawing on Kellogg's experience, the denominationally owned Loma Linda Food Company began producing meat substitutes for the Adventist market in the 1930s; Worthington Foods, a privately owned company, was established in 1939 to manufacture similar products. Worthington is currently owned by the Kellogg Company, which markets its Morningstar brand to the general public.

See also Alternative and Holistic Medicine; Battle Creek Sanitarium; Consumer Products; Graham, Sylvester; Kellogg, John Harvey; Periodicals; Physiological Benefits; Reform; Religious Beliefs and Practices; Youth.

Further Reading

Numbers, Ronald L. *Prophetess of Health: A Study of Ellen G. White.* 3rd ed. Grand Rapids, MI: William B. Eerdmans, 2008.

Schwarz, Richard W. *John Harvey Kellogg: Pioneering Health Reformer.* Reprint. Hagerstown, MD: Review and Herald, 2006.

Gary Land

SHAKERS, THE

The Shakers, also known as the United Society of Believers in Christ's Second Appearing, are a North American utopian communal society founded by English Quaker Ann Lee in 1747. Shakers believe that celibacy, industriousness, separation from worldly practices, and simple living are the path to Christian sanctification. Throughout the 19th century, Shakers debated the adoption of a meatless diet—a process that caused significant tensions as individual beliefs challenged the communal principle on which Shakerism was founded.

Prior to these 19th-century debates, a typical Shaker meal consisted primarily of seasonal foods, both of animal and plant origin. Beef, pork, mutton, fish, clams, chicken, eggs, potatoes, applesauce, peppers, and pickled cucumbers were common favorites and varied according to the geographic location of each Shaker community. Although Shaker theology indicated that the sexes were spiritually equal, sisters and brethren strictly adhered to traditional gender roles in their communal lives. The majority of women's work occurred within the household. Many female cooks became vocal opponents of vegetarianism, arguing that they were inconvenienced by having to cook separate meals for each individual's dietary preferences, that is, a contradiction of the *communal* principle, and that their authority and role within the family were challenged by the brethren, who were primarily responsible for promoting a meat-free diet. These "kitchen sisters" also thought that the quality and flavor of their traditional Shaker dishes would suffer without the addition of animal fat—an issue that was later resolved by allowing

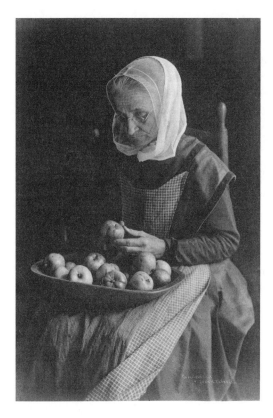

An elderly Shaker woman peels apples for applesauce, ca. 1907. (Courtesy of the Library of Congress)

animal fats to be used for cooking and housekeeping, despite a more general restriction on the consumption of animal flesh.

Two historical events mark the vegetarian debates within Shakerism. The Lead Ministry of the New Lebanon Family, seen at the time as the highest authority for Shakers, first recommended abstention from meat in 1820. This recommendation emphasized the connection of body and soul, the purifying nature of vegetarianism, and the damaging effects of meat (particularly pork) on temperament, health, self-control, and spiritual development. Food regulations were already in place— such as abstaining from raw or unripe fruit and nuts, unseasoned cucumbers, and freshly baked bread—and were designed to increase one's control over one's natural impulses. The Millennial Laws of 1821 formalized the official move toward vegetarianism but allowed each family to progress at its own pace. In November 1841, during a revivalist period in Shakerism, one "gift," or spiritual manifestation, was recorded by the New Lebanon family. According to interpreters of this gift, the Lord required believers to eradicate the use of pork and pork products over a 10-year period. Believers received further gifts in this period, often vague and exclusive, which contributed to overall confusion and frustration concerning how, when, and why believers should abstain from flesh and flesh-derived products. The Millennial Laws of 1845, moral and organizational in nature, attempted to implement strict "corporate asceticism" by banning meat and fish on the Sabbath, nearly prohibiting contact between the sexes, and restricting relationships with nonhuman pets. Shaker debates over a meatless diet coincided with the career of Presbyterian food reformer Sylvester Graham. It has been posited that Graham's program of abstinence as a means of controlling unhealthy and immoral impulses complemented the preexisting Shaker quest for "physical and moral perfection through diet and health" (Puskar-Pasewicz). Graham's teachings on temperance, vegetarianism, and sexual chastity were particularly appealing to young Shakers. Shaker encounters with vegetarian ideology and practice were infused with an ongoing tension between the larger order and individuals, yet by the 1870s vegetarianism was commonplace among Shaker communities, due in large part to the newfound support of Shaker sisters. Their authority over and influence on Shaker foodways and their commitment to food reform were vital for a meatless diet to succeed in these communal, utopian families.

See also Alternative and Holistic Medicine; Bible and Biblical Arguments; Colonies, Communal Societies, and Utopias; Domestic Science and Scientific Eating; Family Dynamics; Graham, Sylvester; Meatless Diets before Vegetarianism; Religious Beliefs and Practices.

Further Reading

Brewer, Priscilla J. *Shaker Communities, Shaker Lives.* 2nd ed. Hanover, NH: University of New England Press, 1986.

Puskar-Pasewicz, Margaret. "Kitchen Sisters and Disagreeable Boys: Debates over Meatless Diets in Nineteenth-Century Shaker Communities." In *Eating in Eden: Food and American Utopias*, edited by Etta M. Madden and Martha L. Finch, 109–24. Lincoln: University of Nebraska Press, 2006.

Stein, Stephen J. *The Shaker Experience in America: A History of the United Society of Believers.* New Haven, CT: Yale University Press, 1992.

Hayley Rose Glaholt

SHELLEY, PERCY BYSSHE (1792–1822)

The English Romantic poet Percy Bysshe Shelley championed many radical causes in the early 19th century. One of these causes was vegetarianism, which was fueled by a growth in humanitarian sentiment around the abolition of slavery, which had led to a reconsideration of the relationship between humans and animals. This cause was also fueled in part by an increasing British interest in the philosophies and lifestyles of its new imperial possessions in India. Shelley's *A Vindication of Natural Diet* (1813, first written as an appendix to the poem "Queen Mab") and *On the Vegetable System of Diet* (probably written in 1815 but not published until 1920) marked perhaps the first time a public figure had written systematically, albeit briefly, on vegetarianism as a philosophy and a practice.

Shelley's poems do have scattered vegetarian references such as this from "Queen Mab":

No longer now
He slays the lamb that looks him in the face,
And horribly devours his mangled flesh;
Which, still avenging nature's broken law,
Kindled all putrid humours in his frame,
All evil passions, and all vain belief,
Hatred, despair, and loathing in his mind,
The germs of misery, death, disease, and crime.
No longer now the winged habitants,
That in the woods their sweet lives sing away,
Flee from the form of man; but gather round,
And prune their sunny feathers on the hands
Which little children stretch in friendly sport
Towards these dreadless partners of their play.

Or this from the "Revolt of Islam":

Never again may blood of bird or beast
Stain with its venomous stream a human feast,
To the pure skies in accusation steaming.

This last passage is especially important as playwright George Bernard Shaw, perhaps the most celebrated of English vegetarian authors, claimed that these lines had opened his eyes to the iniquities of meat eating and the need to become a vegetarian. Shelley's wife, Mary Shelley, made the monster in *Frankenstein* a vegetarian, as one way to portray him as transcending the fallen state of humanity.

Further Reading

Kenyon-Jones, Christine. *Kindred Brutes: Animals in Romantic-Period Writing.* London: Ashgate, 2001.
Perkins, David. *Romanticism and Animal Rights.* New York: Cambridge University Press, 2003.

John Simons

SINGER, PETER (1946~)

Peter Singer is one of the most well-known, respected, and controversial philosophers of the 20th and 21st centuries. Born on July 6, 1946, in Melbourne, Australia, where his parents, Viennese Jews, settled in 1938 after escaping Germany, Singer earned a bachelor's of arts (honors) and a master's of arts from the University of Melbourne and a bachelor's of philosophy from the University of Oxford. He has held academic positions at several universities, including University College, Oxford; New York University; and Monash University. Singer currently has two academic appointments as the Ira W. DeCamp Professor of Bioethics, University Center for Human Values, Princeton University and as laureate professor, University of Melbourne, Centre for Applied Philosophy and Public Ethics.

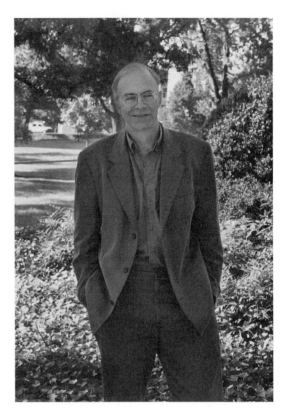

Princeton University professor Peter Singer near his office in Princeton, New Jersey, 2001. (AP Photo/Brian Branch-Price)

Singer is not only a leader of the contemporary animal ethics movement but also a prominent utilitarian and bioethicist known by both philosophers and non-philosophers for his views on the sanctity, or nonsanctity, of human life, and the obligation to help those in poverty. Singer has authored or edited over 40 books, as well as hundreds of articles in professional journals, books, and nonprofessional publications and has been interviewed many times on television and radio. He is a humanist laureate in the International Academy of Humanism and was included in "The Time 100," *Time* magazine's list of the world's most influential people in 2005, in addition to numerous other awards and honors.

Animal Liberation, originally published in 1975, is Singer's seminal work in animal ethics that solidified him as one of the founders of the animal liberation movement. According to Singer, speciesism, an attitude of prejudice or bias in favor of the members of one's own species and against the members of other species, is just as morally wrong as racism and sexism. Singer argues that this is because sentience, the capacity to feel pain and suffer, is the morally relevant quality, not species, race, sex, or even reason. Accordingly, the principle of equality requires that the suffering of a being, regardless of its species, be counted equally with the like suffering of any other being.

Singer combines the notion of sentience with his theory of preference utilitarianism, a version of utilitarianism according to which an agent ought to act so as to maximize preferences or interests, which leads to the conclusion that in most cases, the use of animals for food, especially those that are raised in confined

Factory Farming of Chickens

While the following description of modern chicken farming is probably not entirely new to 21st-century readers, this information was relatively shocking in 1975 when Peter Singer's *Animal Liberation* was first published. Since then, not much has changed, except that Americans' consumption of chicken has increased.

Today in the United States, 102 million broilers—as table chickens are called—are slaughtered each week after being reared in highly automated factory-like plants that belong to the large corporations that control production. Eight of these corporations account for over 50 percent of the 5.3 billion birds killed annually in the U.S.

The essential step in turning chickens from farmyard birds into manufactured items was confining them indoors. A producer of broilers gets a load of 10,000, 50,000, or more day-old chicks from the hatcheries, and puts them into a long windowless shed—usually on the floor, although some producers use tiers of cages in order to get more birds into the same size shed. . . . [E]very aspect of the birds' environment is controlled to make them grow faster on less food. . . . Broiler chickens are killed when they are seven weeks old (the natural lifespan of a chicken is about seven years.). . . . [T]he birds weigh between four and five pounds; yet they still may have as little as half a square foot of space per chicken—or less than the area of a sheet of standard typing paper.

. . . Feather-pecking and cannibalism are, in the broiler producer's language, "vices." They are not natural vices, however; they are the result of the stress and crowding. . . . Chickens are highly social animals, and in the farmyard they develop a hierarchy, sometimes called a 'pecking order'. . . . a flock of ninety chickens can maintain a stable social order. . . . but 80,000 birds crowded together in . . . a single shed is obviously a different matter. . . . [T]o control them the poultry farmer must make their conditions still more unnatural. Very dim lighting is one way of doing this. A more drastic step, though one now very widely used in the industry, is "debeaking."

. . . Debeaking used to be performed with a blowtorch. . . . [T]oday specially designed guillotinelike devices with hot blades are the preferred instrument. The infant chick's beak is inserted into the instrument, and the hot blade cuts of the end of it. The procedure is carried out quickly, about fifteen birds a minute. Such haste means that the temperature and sharpness of the blade can vary, resulting in sloppy cutting and serious injury to the bird.

. . . [M]oreover the damage done to the bird by debeaking is long term: chickens mutilated in this way eat less and lose weight for several weeks. The . . . injured beak continues to cause pain. . . . The birds never see daylight, until the day they are taken out to be killed; nor do they breathe air which is not heavy with the ammonia from their own droppings. The ventilation is adequate to keep the birds alive in normal circumstances, but if there should be a mechanical failure they soon suffocate. . . . Even if the birds escape these hazards, they may succumb to any of a number of diseases that are often prevalent in the broiler houses. . . . When the birds must stand and sit on rotting, dirty, ammonia-charged litter, they also suffer from ulcerated feet, breast blisters, and hock burns.

Source: Peter Singer. *Animal Liberation.* Rev. ed. New York: Ecco, 2002, pp. 98–105.

animal feeding operations, and for research, is morally wrong. This is because the interests that factory farm and research animals have in avoiding the pain and suffering they are subjected to are greater than the interests that humans have in using animals for food and research. In addition, it is prima facie wrong to kill sentient beings, even painlessly, because they have an interest in living or because they experience pleasure and pleasure is valued. Therefore, killing food and research animals, even painlessly, is morally acceptable only in cases in which the interests or pleasures of those who benefit from the deaths of the animals outweigh the interests or pleasures of the animals.

Critics of Singer's view include utilitarians who argue that the pleasure humans get from using animals for food or research outweighs the pain and suffering of animals. Others reject his argument that speciesism is akin to racism and sexism or that the morally relevant quality is sentience. Some commentators claim that Singer's theory does not go far enough to prohibit the use of animals for food and research because it is not an abolitionist view. Additionally, there are those who find his position on the painless killing of animals problematic because it only prima facie prohibits the killing of sentient beings. For example, the killing of sentient beings is acceptable if the preferences of other sentient beings outweigh the preferences of the being to be killed or in some cases if the sentient being can be replaced by another sentient being whose life will be equally pleasant.

See also Activism and Protests; Animal Rights and Animal Welfare; Ethical Vegetarianism; Francione, Gary L.; Newkirk, Ingrid; Reform.

Further Reading

Jamieson, Dale, ed. *Singer and His Critics.* Oxford: Blackwell, 1999.
Schaler, Jeffrey A., ed. *Peter Singer under Fire: The Moral Iconoclast Faces His Critics.* Chicago and LaSalle, IL: Open Court Press, 2009.

Singer, Peter. *Animal Liberation: The Definitive Classic of the Animal Movement.* Harper Perennial ed. New York: HarperCollins, 2009.

Singer, Peter. *Practical Ethics.* Cambridge: Cambridge University Press, 1993.

Monica L. Gerrek

SKINNY BITCH

Former model agent Rory Freedman and former model Kim Barnouin first met at a talent agency in 1996. Their mutual passion for animal rights and healthy living provided the basis for cowriting *Skinny Bitch: A No-Nonsense, Tough-Love Guide for Savvy Girls Who Want to Stop Eating Crap and Start Looking Fabulous.* The book, a manifesto promoting a holistic approach to a healthy lifestyle and well-being, carries a clear vegan message. Using animal rights rhetoric, the authors promote a diet that avoids the consumption of animal products, such as dairy, eggs, and meat, thus contributing to a healthier lifestyle, as well as aiding the environment and animal welfare. The book was an international best seller translated into 20 languages and a #1 *New York Times* best seller with over two million copies in print.

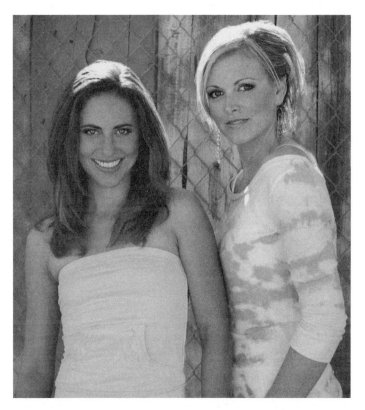

Skinny Bitch authors Rory Freedman and Kim Barnouin. (AP Photo/HO/Running Press)

When it was first published in 2005, only 10,000 copies were originally printed. The profanity-laced healthy eating guide gradually climbed the U.K. bestseller charts during 2007, after celebrity Victoria Beckham was photographed picking up a copy of the book at a trendy Los Angeles boutique. The diet book proved successful, having a drastic impact on book sales on either side of the Atlantic nearly two years after first being published. A catchy title, sassy writing style, and the seductive cover of a slender, tight-hipped figure were all strategies used to market the book to an image-conscious female audience in search of a an alternative diet book.

The book communicates the message of veganism using tough-love tactics, a cheeky tone, and the frequent use of four-letter words, with book chapters titled "Rotting, Decomposing Flesh Diet" and "Dairy Disaster," while coffee is referred to as "crack cocaine" and fizzy drinks are "liquid Satan."

Aimed at young women and teenagers, the book provoked controversy, with critics claiming inaccurate scientific data, the promotion of an ideal female body, irresponsible diet guidelines, and a hypocritical stance regarding processed food, while simultaneously advocating processed meat-substitute products. It has also been criticized by some not so much as a diet book but as propaganda for veganism, promoted with all the zeal of a convert. The book title has also been criticized as misleading, yet the underlying message of the vegan diet guide is that a healthy body weight is achievable as the result of a deeper understanding of the food industry and nutritional science.

Following the success of *Skinny Bitch,* several more books in the series were published: *Skinny Bitch in the Kitch,* a collection of vegan recipes; *Skinny Bitch Bun in the Oven,* advice for a healthy pregnancy; *Skinny Bitchin,* a life motivation guide, and *Skinny Bastard,* targeted at male readers.

Barnouin gave up her career as a model in 1999 in pursuit of a master's of science degree in holistic nutrition from Clayton College of Natural Health; she is currently working on her PhD. Freedman became an animal rights advocate and kindergarten enrichment-program teacher in Wyckoff, New Jersey, in 2002.

See also Agribusiness; Animal Rights and Animal Welfare; Childbearing and Infant Feeding; Consumer Products; Ethical Vegetarianism; Organic Foods and Technology; Physical Fitness and Athleticism; Physiological Benefits; Reform; Social Acceptance; Veganism; Vegetarians and Vegans, Celebrity.

Further Reading

Dugan, Emily. "Tough-Love Diet Book in the Spotlight after Plug from Victoria Beckham." *The Independent,* May 26, 2007. http://www.independent.co.uk/arts-entertainment/books/news/toughlove-diet-book-in-the-spotlight-after-plug-from-victoria-beckham-450425.html.

Freedman, Rory, and Kim Barnouin. *Skinny Bitch.* Philadelphia: Running Press, 2005.

Hirschkorn, Ursula. "Do I Want to Be a Skinny B***h? Fat Chance." *The Daily Mail,* May 24, 2007. http://www.dailymail.co.uk/femail/article-457277/Do-I-want-Skinny-B—h-Fat-chance.html#ixzz0a7njQ2sj.

Rich, Motoko. "A Diet Book Serves Up a Side Order of Attitude." *New York Times,* August 1, 2007. http://www.nytimes.com/2007/08/01/books/01skin.html?pagewanted=1&_r=1&ref=books.

Rich, Motoko. "'Skinny' Authors Have New Goal: Making Men Buff." *New York Times,* April 22, 2009. http://www.nytimes.com/2009/04/23/books/23skinny.html.

Nomi Abeliovich

SOCIAL ACCEPTANCE

Vegetarianism is considered an alternative lifestyle choice by most people living in Western nations. Veganism is even less known and has been criticized as a U.S.-centric movement. Vegetarianism is a dietary choice as much as an ethical one, making it more palatable among nonvegetarians. When people become and remain vegan or vegetarian for dietary reasons, it is met with less resistance. Because of the many health benefits of a vegetarian diet, it has long been prescribed to lower cholesterol, reduce the risk of heart disease and hypertension, and help manage conditions like diabetes.

In some countries or regions of the world, however, veganism and vegetarianism are common. Veganism is popular in Finland, where many people are lactose intolerant. Because of the widespread acceptance of Buddhist, Hindu, and Jain beliefs in India, the country has one of the largest proportions of vegetarians in the world. The United Kingdom has also reported that more than 10 percent of the country's population is vegetarian. Other significant concentrations of vegans are found in Sweden, Germany, and the Netherlands. To address growing numbers of vegetarians and vegans worldwide, several countries' medical associations have created alternate food pyramids with serving suggestions for meat-free and plant-based diets.

For some major religions like Buddhism and Hinduism, vegetarianism is part of an individual spiritual path and legitimized through their teachings. The Buddha was believed to be a vegetarian, and many well-known spiritual leaders are also vegetarians. Jainism requires that all followers be vegetarian. The Seventh-day Adventist Church, a Christian denomination dating back to 1863, recommends vegetarianism for health reasons. Other religions that advocate nonviolence also respect vegetarian principles. In the 1960s, Eastern Hindu-influenced groups in the United States, like Hare Krishnas, made vegetarianism better known, although they were often confused with hippie culture, which was also strongly supportive of vegetarian principles. Rastafarians often adhere to a vegetarian or vegan diet, and some Jews do so as well, as vegetarianism closely adheres to kosher principles.

Despite their growing numbers, vegetarians and vegans are not always widely accepted in mainstream society. A relatively small percentage of celebrities and public figures are openly vegetarian or vegan. Professional athletes are rarely vegetarian, and those who choose to eliminate meat and/or dairy from their diets are often scrutinized because of the widely held belief that people who eat vegetarian food will be protein-deficient.

Vegetarians can also face rejection in their private lives when family members and friends do not understand their choices. This is further complicated when critics of animal rights movements equate vegetarianism and veganism with violent animal rights protest tactics or dogmatic rhetoric. Individuals involved in animal advocacy often eschew popular pastimes that include animal tourism, such as circuses and zoos, which is sometimes viewed as intolerant. While some vegetarians and vegans are involved in various forms of animal rights advocacy and resistance, animal rights welfare organizations and activism are not inherently violent. In fact, as most people who abstain from consuming animal products consider themselves to be compassionate and nonviolent, it is an unusual contradiction and false assumption. Vegetarian and vegan parents who raise their children with the same diet can also face scrutiny. Some critics believe that fetuses and growing children will not get proper nutrition during critical stages of development.

Though slow to gain acceptance, as more people learn about vegetarianism, vegetarian and vegan food is made more widely accessible, both in stores and restaurants. Some U.S. cities have vegetarian or vegan restaurants, and many restaurants now feature several vegetarian-specific menu items. In Europe, vegetarianism is often confused with pesco-vegetarianism, and foods labeled "vegetarian" may still contain fish-based ingredients. Several U.S. cities also have vegetarian or vegan associations that organize events to celebrate their diets and lifestyles, which in turn work to support local vegetarian establishments.

Vegetarian and vegan cookbooks have become popular sellers in the United States, and as the world becomes more aware of the effects of global warming, plant-based diets are seen as a way to combat greenhouse gases. Cruelty-free clothing is also gaining popularity, made from natural, organic, and nonanimal materials. As public awareness grows about colony collapse disorder in beehives, abstaining from honey—a common vegan practice—is more widely received. In 2009, First Lady Michelle Obama planted an organic vegetable garden at the White House, drawing attention to the importance of pesticide-free vegetables as part of a balanced diet. For some, her actions also signaled resistance against factory farming and big agriculture.

Since 2001, veggie pride parades have become popular in large urban areas all over the globe as a way for vegetarians and vegans to bring attention to and gain acceptance for their lifestyle choices. Some critics believe the reappropriation of the gay pride theme is a slight against the LGBTQ community, for whom sexuality and lifestyle are not a choice. The term "veggie" also conflates all types of vegetarians and vegans and sometimes includes pescatarians, who eat fish, and this can be a point of contention among strict vegans. New media tools like blogging and social software have made it increasingly easy for vegetarians and vegans to connect and also seek increased exposure in an effort to gain greater social acceptance. Vegetarians and vegans regularly form virtual groups on social networking Web sites like Facebook, and the Internet also facilitates everything from recipe sharing to e-mail campaigns to local, state, and federal representatives regarding animal welfare legislation.

See also Agribusiness; Animal Rights and Animal Welfare; Backlash; Childbearing and Infant Feeding; Childrearing; Consumer Products; Cookbooks; Eastern Religions, Influences of; Ethical Vegetarianism; Europe; Family Dynamics; Germany; Global Warming; Health Food Stores and Food Cooperatives; India; Internet, The; Jainism; Netherlands, The; Organic Foods and Technology; Physical Fitness and Athleticism; Physiological Benefits; Policy; Reform; Religious Beliefs and Practices; Restaurants; Seventh-day Adventists; United Kingdom; Veganism; Vegetarianism, Types of; Vegetarians and Vegans, Celebrity.

Further Reading

Fraser, Gary. *Diet, Life Expectancy, and Chronic Disease: Studies of Seventh-day Adventists and Other Vegetarians.* New York: Oxford University Press, 2003.

Gregory, James. *Of Victorians and Vegetarians: The Vegetarian Movement in Nineteenth-Century Britain.* New York: Tauris, 2007.

Iacobbo, Karen, and Michael Iacobbo. *Vegetarians and Vegans in America Today.* Westport, CT: Praeger, 2006.

Stuart, Tristram. *The Bloodless Revolution. A Cultural History of Vegetarianism from 1600 to Modern Times.* New York: W.W. Norton, 2007.

Tilston, John. *How To Explain Why You're a Vegetarian to Your Dinner Guests.* Victoria, BC: Trafford, 2006.

Torres, Bob, and Jenna Torres. *Vegan Freak: Being Vegan in a Non-Vegan World.* Colton, NY: Tofu Hound Press, 2005.

Brittany Shoot

T

TELEVISION AND FILMS

Vegetarian and vegan characters in television and film have become increasingly common in the past several decades. They appear in both network and cable television shows, in both comedies and dramas. Often, vegetarian or vegan actors are cast in the roles. Some have a hand in creating vegetarian characters or guiding their scripts and character development.

Throughout various incarnations of the *Star Trek* television series, Vulcan characters are often portrayed as vegetarian because of their logical reasoning to eat healthy foods. Dr. Spock was the first regularly appearing vegetarian character in a television series. Part of the original cast of *Star Trek: The Original Series* (1966–1969), Spock is half-human and half-Vulcan. On *Star Trek: Voyager*, the character of Chakotay was a vegetarian. In *Star Trek: The Next Generation* and *Enterprise*, there are again vegetarian Vulcan characters.

Darlene Connor, a character in the television series *Roseanne*, converts to vegetarianism in a 1994 episode of the show, "Lanford Daze." Connor's character was played by Sara Gilbert, who is a vegan. Lisa Kudrow's character Phoebe Buffay on the television series *Friends* was a vegetarian for the entirety of the show's run. Over the course of several seasons, various characters try to persuade Buffay to eat meat. She gives in to her own meat cravings during her pregnancy in season four and then resumes her vegetarian diet. In the series *V.I.P.*, Pamela Anderson plays the show's vegetarian lead character, named Vallery Irons. Anderson is also a vegetarian in real life. Vegetarian actress Jorja Fox has played multiple vegetarian characters in prime-time television dramas. Formerly part of the cast of *ER*, Fox's character Dr. Maggie Doyle was a vegetarian. Her character on *C.S.I.*, Sara Sidle, is also a vegetarian. Emily Deschanel, a real-life vegan, plays a vegetarian character, Dr. Temperance Brennan, on the television series *Bones*.

American and Canadian cartoons have also included several prominent and recurring vegetarian characters. *Count Duckula* was a television cartoon (1988–1993) about a vegetarian vampire duck. The show's theme song played on the fact that he would not sink his teeth into people or animals because he was a vegetarian. In the Canadian (U.S. syndicated) cartoon *Braceface,* the show's main character Sharon Spitz is a vegetarian. Originally, the character was voiced by actress Alicia Silverstone, who is a vegan. Most notably, in the animated television series, *The Simpsons,* daughter Lisa Simpson is a vegetarian. In an episode called "Lisa the Vegetarian" that originally aired October 15, 1995, Lisa becomes a vegetarian after bonding with a sheep on a family trip to a petting zoo. It is also later revealed that another character on the show, Apu Nahasapeemapetilon, is a vegan. Lisa made People for the Ethical Treatment of Animals' 2004 list of "most animal-friendly TV characters of all time." Sir Paul McCartney guest-starred in the episode on the condition that Lisa's character remains a vegetarian for the rest of the series. The episode later won an Environmental Media Award for "Best Television Episodic Comedy."

Often, television characters are vegetarians but without the explicit label or without delving further into the issue. Sometimes a character's vegetarianism is mentioned in only one episode. In the 1966 cartoon *Kimba the White Lion,* Kimba's character is a vegetarian, though it is never explicitly stated. The show ran in the United States and Japan, where it was known as *Jungle Emperor.* Part of the original cast of *Beverly Hills, 90210,* Shannon Doherty's character Brenda Walsh becomes a vegetarian in season four in a 1994 episode entitled "A Pig Is a Boy Is a Dog," but Doherty left the show and the issue was not explored further. The cartoon *The Powerpuff Girls* includes an episode called "Collect Her," in which Bubbles states that she is a vegetarian, but the show does not revisit the issue in later episodes.

Vegetarians in movies are often treated as a comic foil, and their characters are often weak, silly, and engaged in a variety of New Age or "alternative" practices. Sometimes, they are referred to as "hippies." Ian Miller (played by John Corbett) in *My Big Fat Greek Wedding* is a vegetarian, much to the confusion of his fiancée's Greek family. When an aunt asks them over for dinner and it is explained that Ian is a vegetarian, the aunt responds, "What do you mean he don't eat no meat? Oh, that's okay. I make lamb." In the film *High Fidelity,* the two main characters, Rob and Laura, break up. Laura then becomes involved with her neighbor, a New Age hippie vegetarian (played by Tim Robbins) who lights a lot of incense, practices martial arts, and listens to world music. In *The Night We Never Met,* starring Matthew Broderick and Brooke Smith, Smith plays an over-the-top angry, self-righteous militant vegetarian. Among her more extreme pronouncements, she refuses to drink wine because it is made with yeast. In the 1999 *But I'm A Cheerleader,* Natasha Lyonne's character Megan is a 17-year-old lesbian whose sexuality is apparent to her family because of her interest in, among other things, vegetarianism. In *But I'm A Cheerleader,* which is a dark satirical comedy, all nonnormative behavior is treated as deviant by the adults in charge.

Occasionally, vegetarians are treated with more respect in films. In the 2005 British stop-motion animation film, *Wallace and Gromit: The Curse of the Were-Rabbit,* inventor Wallace and his dog Gromit run a humane pest-control business, Anti-Pesto, and must find a way to protect vegetables from hungry rabbits.

Wallace invents a machine to brainwash the rabbits, but instead they end up creating a were-rabbit who roams the town eating any vegetable it can find. The film's directors, Steve Box and Nick Park, have referred to their creation as the "first vegetarian horror film." In the 2007 dark comedy *Shooting Vegetarians,* main character Neil is a vegetarian forced to go into the family butcher business. Instead of giving in to his family's pressure, he takes the job but uses subversive tactics to spread the word about vegetarianism to the shop's customers.

See also Activism and Protests; Animal Rights and Animal Welfare; Backlash; Family Dynamics; Reform; Social Acceptance; Vegetarians and Vegans, Celebrity.

Further Reading

Marranca, Richard. "Vegging Out with Kung Fu and Star Trek." *Vegetarian Journal* 26, no. 4 (October 2007): 22–23.

Brittany Shoot

TRANSCENDENTALISM

Transcendentalism, a philosophical, religious, and literary movement of mid-19th-century America, began with the ideas of Ralph Waldo Emerson, George Ripley, George Putnam, and Frederick Henry Hedge, who began meeting regularly in Cambridge, Massachusetts, in 1836. Not long after, others such as Margaret Fuller, Bronson Alcott, and Henry David Thoreau became affiliated with the movement. The transcendentalists upheld the overarching goal of improving society through an emphasis on individual spiritual improvement and self-discipline, thus transcending the mundane mess of the material world. Although primarily opposed to reform societies and utopian communities, some transcendentalists advocated that social reform was possible, in part, through individuals partaking of a vegetable diet. Among the transcendentalists, Alcott and Thoreau contributed the most substantial commentary on vegetarianism, both as an ideal and as a practice.

Alcott (1799–1888) was the cofounder of the transcendentalist utopian community Fruitlands in 1843 with Englishman Charles Lane. In 1835, Alcott had stopped eating meat, and in 1842, upon his return from England with Lane, just prior to launching the communitarian effort, he insisted that his family and community members begin what was called a "Pythagorean diet." The diet excluded not only meat but also eggs, milk, butter, cheese, and honey. Beverages other than water were excluded because they were not the results of local production. Likewise, rice and molasses, which depended on slave labor, were excluded. One goal of the diet was to be self-sufficient in a way that would harm no animals, including humans, thus reflecting a spiritual transcendence of individuals over the material realm. Alcott's basis for vegetarianism has been compared with that of his cousin, William A. Alcott, the first president of the American Vegetarian Society.

William, who became a man of medicine, was a follower of Sylvester Graham and the evangelical minister William Metcalfe, with more traditional Christian values driving him, but Bronson remained drawn to classical humanitarianism, continually emphasizing individualized reform and a spiritual vision that incorporated the humane treatment of animals and the abolition of slavery as essential to purifying humanity.

Henry David Thoreau

Although Henry David Thoreau was not a committed vegetarian, during his two-year sojourn in the woods near Walden Pond from March 1845 to September 1847, he voiced the following concerns about the ethical, economic, and even aesthetic reasons to abstain from meat and fish:

> I have found repeatedly, of late years, that I cannot fish without falling a little in self-respect. I have tried it again and again. I have skill at it, and, like many of my fellows, a certain instinct for it, which revives from time to time, but always when I have done I feel that it would have been better if I had not fished. . . . There is unquestionably this instinct in me which belongs to the lower orders of creation; yet with every year I am less a fisherman, though without more humanity or even wisdom; at present I am no fisherman at all. . . . Beside, there is something essentially unclean about this diet and all flesh, and I began to see where housework commences, and whence the endeavor, which costs so much, ... to keep the house sweet and free from all ill odors and sights. Having been my own butcher and scullion and cook, as well as the gentleman for whom the dishes were served up, I can speak from an unusually complete experience. The practical objection to animal food in my case was its uncleanness; and, besides, when I had caught and cleaned and cooked and eaten my fish, they seemed not to have fed me essentially. It was insignificant and unnecessary, and cost more than it came to. A little bread or a few potatoes would have done as well, with less trouble and filth. . . . The repugnance to animal food is not the effect of experience, but it is an instinct. It appeared more beautiful to live low [a 19th-century term for diets that reduced or abstained from meat consumption and other foods thought to be overstimulating] and fare hard in many respects. . . . I believe that every man who has ever been earnest to preserve his higher or poetic faculties in the best condition has been particularly inclined to abstain from animal food, and from much food of any kind.

Source: Henry David Thoreau. *Walden; or, Life in the Woods.* Reprint. Mineola, NY: Dover, 1995, pp. 138–39.

Undoubtedly influenced by the Alcotts, Thoreau (1817–1862) included his views on vegetarianism in his letters and notebooks, refined and published in his well-known book *Walden* (1854). As the exposition of Thoreau's experiment living in the woods near Concord, Massachusetts, from 1842 to 1844, *Walden* reveals in the chapter "Higher Laws" his attitude toward animal food. Overall, he decries the "slimy, beastly life" of "eating and drinking," actions that reflect the "reptile" nature that is awake in humans while their "higher nature slumbers." He derides the messiness of killing, cleaning, and cooking animals, which leads to a loss of appetite; such "repugnance" to animal food should be instinctual. He also abstains from stimulating and intoxicating beverages. Finally, he predicts that America and England will crumble as did Greece and Rome, if their citizens do not reform their dietary indulgences.

See also Alcott, William A.; American Vegetarian Society; Colonies, Communal Societies, and Utopias; Ethical Vegetarianism; Graham, Sylvester; Metcalfe, Rev. William; Physiological Benefits; Pythagoras; Reform; Religious Beliefs and Practices.

Further Reading

Alcott, Louisa May. *Transcendental Wild Oats and Excerpts from the Fruitlands Diary.* Boston: Harvard Common Press, 1981.

Gura, Philip F. *American Transcendentalism: A History.* New York: Hill and Wang, 2007.

Jones, Buford. "'The Hall of Fantasy' and the Early Hawthorne-Thoreau Relationship." *PMLA* 83, no. 5 (October 1968): 1429–38.

Salomon, Louis B. "The Least-Remembered Alcott." *New England Quarterly* 34, no. 1 (March 1961): 87–93.

Thoreau, Henry David. *Walden; or, Life in the Woods.* Boston: Ticknor and Fields, 1854.

Etta M. Madden

UNITED KINGDOM

Background of Vegetarianism   The first vegetarians in the British Isles were members of the Roman ruling elite in the first century AD, who subscribed to the Greco-Roman philosophy of Stoicism, most famously represented by Seneca, who said that "to abstain from the flesh of animals is to foster and to encourage innocence." Seneca practiced vegetarianism for at least parts of his life. The followers of Pythagoras also practiced vegetarianism (including abstention from beans, which they believed could, in certain circumstances, become the repositories of human souls). Pythagoreans were likely among the Roman inhabitants of the British Islands.

Only a few vegetarians might have remained among the Romano-British population after the Romans withdrew from Britain in the wake of invading and migrating tribes from what are now Germany and Denmark. Perhaps the odd warrior had sworn an oath to abstain from eating meat until he had accomplished some feat. The next vegetarians were the monks and nuns of the Christian churches, which were established from 597 on. These monastics practiced vegetarianism as part of the religious discipline of prayer and fasting. Before 1057, when the Great Schism took the British Church out of the orbit of Byzantium and into that of Rome, the laity also might have practiced vegetarian fasting disciplines on a weekly basis and also during the fasts that precede Christmas and Easter.

In the modern era, vegetarianism became the province of scattered enlightened individuals. During the Renaissance, vegetarianism would have been relatively rare, although the revival of Neoplatonic philosophy would have led to renewed interest in the work of the Hellenistic writers Plotinus and Porphyry, both of whom discussed the benefits of a vegetarian regime. By the 18th century, however, there was much more interest in Thomas Tryon (1634–1703), a Pythagorean philosopher who had also studied Indian culture, forming a group of "Hindu Vegetarians." Sir Isaac Newton himself probably practiced at least a meat-reducing diet while the austere neoclassical poet Alexander Pope drew attention to the inhumanity of meat eating. This stress on inhumanity would unleash a much more systematic expression of vegetarian philosophy in the 18th and 19th centuries and lay the ground for the establishment of formal mechanisms by which vegetarians could come together and by which vegetarianism could be promoted and its ideas and practices disseminated in the 20th and 21st centuries.

One concern of the 18th-century vegetarian thinkers was humans' duty not only to the animal kingdom but also to fellow people, and thus vegetarianism became an aspect of new evangelical forms of Christianity. This included the Methodism of John Wesley, who was a vegetarian although he did not expect this of his followers, and the increasing distaste for slavery, which, at that time, was being used as a mechanism to develop trade and industry in the British colonies in the Caribbean and North and South America and elsewhere. For example, the Reverend Humphrey Primatt published in 1776 *The Duty of Mercy and Sin of Cruelty to Brute Beasts,* which drew attention to the fact that animals suffer just as humans do, and so, as it is sinful to cause pain to humans, it is likewise sinful to cause pain to animals. Primatt did not necessarily promote vegetarianism, but his systematic analysis of the relationships between sins against humans and sins against creation made vegetarianism an inevitability. It also made it inevitable to desist from the enslavement and cruel treatment of men and women based solely on the color of their skin. This line had already been followed by Tryon in his *Friendly Advice to the Gentleman Planters of the East and West Indies* (1684), where, again, a connection was made between human rights, Christian duty, and the right response to the animal creation. John Newton, the author of the hymn "Amazing Grace," was a reformed slave trader who also saw vegetarianism as an important component of his Christianity.

Primatt's work can also be contextualized by other 18th-century treatises such as John Hildrop's *Thoughts upon the Brute Creation* (1742), Robert Morris's *A Reasonable Plea for the Animal Creation* (1746), Richard Dean's *An Essay upon the Future Life of Brutes* (1767), James Granger's *An Apology for the Brute Creation* (1772), John Lawrence's *A Philosophical Treatise on Horses and the Moral Duties of Man towards the Brute Creation* (1796–1798), George Nicholson's *On the Conduct of Man to Inferior Animals* (1797), John Oswald's *The Cry of Nature* (1791), and Thomas Young's *An Essay on Humanity to Animals* (1798). Although these books are largely about the development of a more humane attitude toward animals, they often also promote vegetarianism. Especially interesting in this regard is the work of John Oswald. Oswald served as a soldier for many years in colonial India and had become enthralled by Indian culture to such an extent that he had adopted the Hindu practice of vegetarianism. Oswald was also, most unusually for his time, able to look at the comparative merits of Eastern and Western societies with an open mind and was prepared to admit the superiority of Indian culture in some aspects, not least the immensely more humane attitude toward animals it expressed through its vegetarianism. This steady stream of publications throughout the 18th century was obviously of sufficient strength to alarm some of the more conservative elements in British society. It stimulated a satirical response in the form of Thomas Taylor's skit *A Vindication of the Rights of Brutes* (1792).

In the 19th century the first major contributor to the debate was Isaac Gompertz, who wrote two books, *Moral Inquiries on the Situation of Man and Brutes* (1824) and *Fragments in Defence of Animals* (1852). Like Primatt, Gompertz did not distinguish between humans and nonhumans, on the grounds of their equal capacity to suffer. Gompertz also recommended a vegetarian diet and went so far as to provide some rather unappetizing-looking recipes—vegetables, for example, should be boiled so as to "prevent any crispness." He also recommended other measures to ensure a lifestyle that minimized the exploitation of animals; this included not riding horses and eschewing horse-drawn transportation. For Gompertz, a gentleman, this was an astonishingly radical step. Gompertz's first book also coincided more or less with the first law against the cruel treatment of animals. This law was specifically aimed to protect cattle whose sufferings on their way to market and in the slaughterhouse had become, increasingly, a matter of public scandal. The Act to Prevent the Cruel and Improper Treatment of Cattle was passed in 1822 and was promoted by the humanitarian member of Parliament Robert Martin. The climate created by Martin's Act also enabled Gompertz to develop the journal of the newly formed Society for the Prevention of Cruelty to Animals, of which he was secretary. This publication was called *The Animals' Friend or the Progress of Humanity,* and it is significant that although the SPCA (later the RSPCA) never promoted vegetarianism, it chose a vegetarian to fill its key senior post. It is also of interest that Gompertz was Jewish and thus extended the debate about animal welfare and vegetarianism away from the Christian-Hindu connection within which it had been articulated. Other strong advocates of vegetarianism in the early 19th century were John Frank Newton in *The Return to Nature* (1811) and his friend the poet Percy Bysshe Shelley in *A Vindication of Natural Diet* (1812). William Drummond's *The Rights of Animals and Man's Obligations to Treat Them with Humanity* (1838) and Edward Nicholson's *The Rights of an Animal* (1879) were also valuable contributions to the debate.

In the beginning of the 19th century, the first significant vegetarian organization appeared. This was the Reverend William Cowherd's Bible Christian Church, which was founded in Salford, Lancashire, in 1809 This church was the impetus for the American Bible Christian Church, which was inaugurated in 1817 by the Reverends William Metcalfe and James Clark. The church advocated but did not require strict vegetarianism. The first vegetarian cookbook also came out of this movement; it was written by Martha Brotherton, the wife of Joseph Brotherton, a member of Parliament. One of Cowherd's most influential followers was James Simpson, a vegetarian mill owner from Accrington who spent many hundreds of pounds promoting the Christian vegetarian cause.

The British and Foreign Society for the Promotion of Humanity and Abstinence from Animal Food was founded in 1843. The Vegetarian Society, the main organization for vegetarians in the United Kingdom today, was founded in 1847 at a meeting at the vegetarian hospital that had been established at Ramsgate, Kent, the year before, and this society gradually grew away from its strong connections with Bible Christian Church. By 1848 there were 478 members, and in 1849 a meeting was held to establish a group in London. In 1849 the cheap magazine the *Vegetarian Messenger* was circulating in an edition of 5,000 copies and in 1851 was using the slogan "Live and Let Live."

In 1875 another society, the Dietetic Reform Society, was formed, and this linked vegetarianism to other kinds of consumption as its members also abstained from alcohol and tobacco. And in 1877 the London Food Reform Society was created and merged with the Vegetarian Society in 1885. *The Vegetarian* newspaper commenced publication in 1888. Many other regional societies were either independent or local groups affiliated with the Vegetarian Society. These included the Manchester and Salford Vegetarian Advocates Society (1849), the Liverpool Vegetarian Association (1852)—Liverpool was also the first city to have a dedicated animal welfare group—the Birmingham Vegetarian Association (1853), the Paisley Vegetarian Association (1857), the Brighton Vegetarian Association (1858), and the Sheffield Vegetarian Association (1861); between 1853 and 1855 vegetarian associations were formed in other cities as well. By the end of the 19th century, vegetarianism had become a truly national movement.

Many of the original societies expanded, merged, or changed their names. There was also a growth in societies devoted to specific social groups or to activities. For example, the Vegetarian Amateur Athletic Club was founded in London in 1890 and the Manchester and District Vegetarian Cycling Club in 1899. The Women's Vegetarian Union started in 1895, and the Children's Vegetarian Society for Manchester in 1899 was followed in the next year by the Junior Scottish Vegetarian Society. In 1902 the Quaker movement spawned the Friends Vegetarian Society.

Perhaps the most important literary expression of the vegetarian movement in Britain in the 19th century is found in the work of Henry Salt, most notably in "A Plea for Vegetarianism" (1888), which helped convert Mohandas Gandhi to vegetarianism, *The Humanities of Diet* (1897), *The Logic of Vegetarianism* (1899), and, especially *Animals' Rights* (1892). Salt also edited two periodicals: *Humanity* (later the *Humanitarian*) and the *Humane Review*. These magazines were mouthpieces of the Humanitarian League, an organization that brought together a complex of radical ideas including socialism, pacifism, feminism, vegetarianism, and animal rights. This complex of causes, espoused by high-profile figures such as the feminist writer Frances Power Cobbe and playwright George Bernard Shaw, was to remain a feature of vegetarian organization and discourse throughout most of the 20th century, having its roots in both traditional British radical concerns and the new pressures imposed by a mass-industrialized and increasingly urbanized society.

Salt was involved in all manner of radical causes relating to animal welfare, as manifested through the practice of humanitarian vegetarianism, and other political concerns. For example, he campaigned against the export of live animals to the slaughterhouses of continental Europe, hunting, the use of fur and feathers in the fashion industry, and vivisection. All of these causes are still part of the landscape of the vegetarian movement in the United Kingdom today, and although progress has been made on some, there is still work to do on others.

Salt continued to work well into the 20th century, and during this period the intense and varied activity of vegetarians in the Victorian era was replaced by a gradual consolidation and establishment of the various vegetarian associations into the Vegetarian Society and a continued, though much less frenetic, growth of more local groups. The most interesting of these are the Vegan Society (1944), the Jewish Vegetarian Society (1965), the Young Indian Vegetarians (1984), the Lesbian Vegan Group (2002), and the Christian Vegetarian Association (2004). These show the ways in which vegetarianism has continued to grow within British society; as attitudes toward cultural and sexual diversity have changed, minorities have been able to develop organizations that enable them to articulate vegetarianism and veganism with the other concerns for their group. Since the 1980s the Vegetarian International Voice for Animals (VIVA!) has added a vibrant and colorful voice through its various campaigns. The vegetarian movement also has its own charities: The Vegetarian Housing Association (formerly Homes for Elderly Vegetarians) and the Vegetarian Charity (to support young vegetarians) formed in 1986 from a merger of the Vegetarian Children's Charity and Jersey Vegetarian Home for Children. The Vegetarian Society also runs an internationally renowned academy, the Cordon Vert Cookery School, which offers training and qualifications in the highest levels of vegetarian cooking and nutrition.

Vegetarianism continues to flourish in the United Kingdom with extensive and well-founded organizations. And although the actual number of vegetarians appears to be declining, vegetarianism still has a high profile and remains a familiar concept to and a familiar practice of millions of people.

Beliefs and Conditions   Given that the British—and especially the English—are so closely associated with roast beef—the French call them *Les Rosbifs,* and their ceremonial guards are called Beefeaters—it is surprising that the proportion of vegetarians in the British population is higher (or has until quite recently been higher) than the proportion of vegetarians in any other part of the developed world. The only other country that comes anywhere near having the same proportion of vegetarians is Germany, which is another country with a culture in which meat, especially pork, is highly privileged.

There are a number of reasons for this surprising phenomenon. First, British culture has a very long tradition of nonconformism and radical thought—what in modern times might be called alternative lifestyles—which, from time to time, have been associated with or have associated themselves with vegetarianism. Second, the broadly Protestant character of British society from the 16th to the 20th century allowed a theology to flourish that was more tolerant of speculation regarding the position of animals in creation and the possibility that they had souls and that humans had a duty of care toward them than would have been possible in a society that was predominantly Roman Catholic.

Third, during the 1990s especially, a number of serious contaminations of the British food chain took place. These ranged from the presence of the poisonous bacteria salmonella in eggs to *E. coli,* a potentially fatal bacterial agent, in meat to, most serious of all, the suspicion that the mad cow disease, which had entrenched itself in the British cattle herd, could jump species and emerge as the fatal variant Creutzfeldt-Jakob's disease in humans who ate meat from animals that had been infected with bovine spongiform encephalopathy (BSE). In addition, the major outbreak of foot and mouth disease at the beginning of the 21st century exposed British people to the sight of massive bonfires composed of the bodies of infected or potentially infected cows and sheep, and many in the United Kingdom were sickened at the obvious excesses of the meat-farming industry. Thus, a strain of vegetarianism associated mainly with disease avoidance came into being. Indeed, so strong was the temporary effect of the foot and mouth disease epidemic that in 2001 29 percent of people surveyed said that they were considering not eating meat and 35 percent that they intended to stop eating red meat. These figures did not translate into practice in any statistically meaningful way. In practice, few of the people who said this appear to have actually given up eating meat.

Fourth, there is also in British culture a long tradition of public affiliation with animal welfare. The United Kingdom was the first country to develop a public body devoted solely to the protection of animals and the promotion of their welfare (the RSPCA), and the fact that this was established prior to the related body devoted to the protection of children (the NSPCC) says a great deal about British attitude toward animals. To some extent, the history of the foundation of the RSPCA bears out the statement that only in a country where cruelty to animals was endemic would a society for their protection be necessary. In addition, the British Parliament passed, very early on, laws to protect animals and to criminalize cruelty toward them. Thus, a strain of what might properly be called "humanitarian vegetarianism" came into being.

Fifth, the advanced consumer culture that developed in the United Kingdom since the 1970s and came into full power in the 1980s and 1990s also promoted self-definition by lifestyle choice, and thus vegetarianism as a fashion accessory was born. At the same time extreme body shapes and, especially, the desire to be abnormally thin promoted vegetarianism as a way of avoiding high-calorie food. At the same time, the cult of health and natural living caused many to associate meat—rightly or wrongly—with various undesirable conditions such as cancer and heart disease, and this also created a group of health-driven vegetarians.

Sixth, immigration, especially from the Indian subcontinent in the years following World War II, introduced new populations, some of whom had long-standing cultural and religious motivations for being vegetarian. Finally, the rise of environmentalism as a mainstream political concern has caused many people to question the wastefulness of a farming industry based on meat rather than on vegetables and cereals, and this has led, if not to an increase in vegetarianism, then certainly to a reduction in the animal-based components of many people's diets.

Vegetarian Practices Although vegetarianism grew during the 1980s and 1990s, there is evidence that vegetarianism as a mass phenomenon has peaked and is now in decline. Between 1984 and 1999 the numbers of vegetarians as a proportion of the British population increased from 2.1 percent to 5 percent with some increase each year. Since 1999, however, the number of vegetarians has declined. In 2006, for example, only 2 percent of the population were identified as vegetarians, although a survey in 2007 resulted in a figure of 3 percent (with 2 percent declaring themselves vegan). This still, however, represents a relatively large number of people, say 2.5 million, which compares dramatically with the number of people who declared themselves vegetarian for rationing purposes during World War II. (In 1945 they numbered 100,000.) Even taking into account the relative decline in numbers in recent years, vegetarianism—whether as a lifestyle choice, an artifact of identity politics, a commitment to health or welfare, or simply a humane desire not to live by exploiting animals—has developed a high profile in British life, and vegetarianism in Britain is mainstream.

Vegetarianism is not a phenomenon that is uniformly distributed across British society or even evenly distributed across the British Isles, and there is no such thing as a typical vegetarian. For example, women are twice as likely to be vegetarians as are men. There are more vegetarians in the south and north than in the midlands of England. While there are roughly the same proportion of vegetarians in English, Welsh, and Scottish populations—about 2 percent in 2007—there are very few in Northern Ireland. People under 35 years old are more than twice as likely to be vegetarians than are older age groups. Women between 16 and 29 years old currently constitute the highest proportion of vegetarians and have been since the early 1990s. Better-off professionals are more likely to be vegetarian than are less wealthy people with blue-collar jobs.

However, these figures begin to look less reliable when considering how people choose to define themselves, for example, as lacto-ovo vegetarians, pesco-vegetarians, and vegans. In 2007, for example, 8 percent of those surveyed said that they ate fish. Some 7 percent described themselves as "partly vegetarian," which is meaningless. Another 5 percent said that they ate vegetarian food; presumably they meant that sometimes they ate dishes that were not meat-based. So while vegetarianism is actually in decline in modern Britain, paradoxically, there may actually be more self-declared vegetarians than ever.

Thus the position of vegetarianism is contemporary Britain is curious in that it would seem that the idea of calling oneself a vegetarian is attractive and confers some form of imagined status or interest to one's personal identity. In fact, there is a weak relationship between the act of calling oneself a vegetarian and the more difficult task of actually living a vegetarian life. But the British are eating less meat and extending their dietary options to include many more meals that do not require meat as a main course.

In the 20th century at least, the traditional British diet was relatively limited, and the standard form of most meals consisted of a piece of meat or fish with potatoes and a vegetable. There can be no doubt that vegetarianism, or at least the thought that it is possible to eat well without eating meat every day, has had a profound effect on the British diet. This diet has been changing since the 1960s for other reasons, too. The growth of cheap holiday travel to continental Europe in the 1970s opened the British up to a wider range of foods, and items such as pizza and pasta became commonplace staples. The entry of American or American-style fast food outlets like McDonald's and Burger King changed the face of the British town, and, for the first time, a wide variety of fast food became available beyond the traditional fish and chips. Finally, the growth of the Chinese and Indian communities led to a corresponding growth in restaurants serving ethnic food, supplemented by an increasing number of Thai restaurants; these have changed the British palate by serving carefully modified and unchallenging versions of various national cuisines designed to appeal to the British taste. Indeed, in 2001, chicken tikka masala—a kind of curry said to have been invented in an Indian restaurant in Glasgow, Scotland, probably in the 1960s—had become Britain's most popular dish. Indian food, with its important vegetarian strand, had been known to the British for many years due to their rule over India during the Imperial era (roughly 1757–1946). Indeed, curry first appeared on a menu in London as early as 1773, and the first Indian restaurant, the Hindostanee Coffee House (it was not a coffeehouse but rather a restaurant that served Indian food and offered the opportunity to smoke Indian tobacco from hookahs), opened in 1809, well before the first fish and chip shop opened in London in 1860.

It could be argued, therefore, that the position of vegetarianism in Britain since the 1980s has been as much the result of a more widespread change in the British diet and in British attitudes toward food as the result of a sudden conversion to animal welfare or concerns about personal health and hygiene. Although pure vegetarianism appears to be on the wane, prepared vegetarian foodstuffs that are designated as vegetarian continue to be one of the fastest-growing sectors of the food market. Every British supermarket now stocks a significant range of vegetarian foods, and these include prepared products such as burgers and sausages composed of meat substitutes such as soy, wheat protein, Quorn, or tofu; prepared meals such as curries and pasta dishes; cheese made with vegetarian rennet; and also a smaller range of vegan products such as soy- and tofu-based milk, cream, ice cream, and mayonnaise. Many large companies have made their products suitable for vegetarians. For example, the brewery Guinness used to use isinglass, a substance derived from the swim bladders of sturgeon, as an ingredient in its beer. Now it no longer does, presumably because it knows that its market is significantly expanded if its products are acceptable to both vegetarians and nonvegetarians. In 2008 the Mars confectionary company faced a consumer outcry when it stated that it could no longer guarantee that its chocolate was made with nonrennet-based dairy products and quickly backtracked on its decision. The green plant sign showing that the product is suitable for vegetarians is now commonplace on all manner of prepared foods.

The food industry has responded vigorously to this social trend, and between 1999 and 2001 the annual growth rate in the sector producing vegetarian foods increased from 12.2 percent to 16.6 percent. Although this has now fallen to around 5 percent, this still represents a very important area of profit for the industry and one that it envisages will continue to grow in value (in 2006 this sector was worth £670 million, or about US$987 million), if not in absolute terms, for the foreseeable future. Industry analysts believe that this growth is partly the result of successful government public-health campaigns to encourage people to eat more fruit and vegetables and partly due to the residual effects of the bovine spongiform encephalopathy scare and the foot and mouth disease epidemic. The industry concludes that a new pattern of eating, designated "meat reducing," has emerged in the United Kingdom and is compensating for the decline in the number of actual vegetarians. Nevertheless, it is probable that many of these meat reducers actually describe themselves as vegetarian when surveyed. In fact, the 2004 survey determined that of those who had described themselves as vegetarian, only 42 percent actually abstained from meat and fish.

The many self-defined vegetarians who live either on foods of non-British origins or on the prepared foods designated by the food industry for meat reducers now clearly outnumber the two original vegetarian communities—those who were vegetarian for religious or political purposes and, even more numerous, especially in the 1960s and 1970s, the "whole fooders" who introduced brown rice and lentils to the British vegetarian diet and whose descendants are now at the forefront of the organic farming movement and the consumer reaction against genetically modified produce. The clearest signifier of the decline of the whole-food school of vegetarianism was the closure of the flagship whole-food vegetarian restaurant Cranks, which had been the London shopwindow for this group since 1961 before the more diversified style of vegetarian foodways killed it off in 2001. There is still a small Cranks restaurant in the art colony of Dartington, Devon, but its main business now consists in the marketing of branded prepared food, as a whole-food approach to vegetarianism is no longer viable in London. In this respect, the fate of Cranks might stand as a symbol of the development of vegetarian foodways in Britain since the late 1990s.

See also Agribusiness; Animal Rights and Animal Welfare; Bible Christians, English; Eastern Religions, Influences of; India; Reform; Religious Beliefs and Practices; Salt, Henry S.; Shelley, Percy Bysshe; Vegetarian Society of the United Kingdom; World Wars in England.

Further Reading

Spencer, Colin. *The Heretic's Feast: A History of Vegetarianism.* London: Fourth Estate, 1994.

Stuart, Tristram. *The Bloodless Revolution: A Cultural History of Vegetarianism from 1600 to Modern Times.* New York: W.W. Norton, 2007.

Walters, Kerry, and Lisa L. Portmess, eds. *Ethical Vegetarianism: From Pythagoras to Peter Singer.* Albany: State University of New York Press, 1999.

Williams, Howard. *The Ethics of Diet: A Catena of Authorities Deprecatory of the Practice of Flesh-Eating.* Urbana: University of Illinois Press, 2003.

Wynne-Tyson, Jon. *The Extended Circle: An Anthology of Humane Thought.* London: Cardinal, 1990.

John Simons

VEGANISM

Veganism is a practical philosophy oriented toward living without directly or indirectly harming or exploiting animals and actively seeking to end that harm and exploitation where it exists. Veganism is most commonly associated with eschewing foods of animal origin. These include animals' flesh and other body parts, as well as the products of animals' biological processes, such as milk, eggs, or honey. Instead, vegan diets tend to include a variety of plant foods, such as fruits, vegetables, legumes, nuts, seeds, and whole grains. Veganism, however, extends beyond diet to encompass concern to avoid complicity in, and to actively oppose, the exploitation of animals for clothing, cosmetics, toiletries, sport, entertainment, vivisection, or any other purpose. Veganism, therefore, is a voluntary, purposeful way of life that is distinct from involuntary subsistence on a plant-based diet for reasons of poverty or lack of availability of animal-based foods.

The word "vegan" was coined by Donald Watson, the cofounder, with Elsie Shrigley, of the world's first Vegan Society in the United Kingdom in 1944. Watson derived the term "vegan" from the first and last syllables of "vegetarian," arguing that veganism began with vegetarianism but took it to its logical conclusion. Watson and Shrigley formed the Vegan Society in the immediate context of the Vegetarian Society's refusal to devote space in its publications to dairy-free living. There had already been debates within the U.K. vegetarian movement in the preceding decades of the 20th century about the cruelty involved in dairy and egg production. Also, the first vegan cookbook, which included essays on the health, ethical, aesthetic, and economic advantages of a plant-based diet, was published in Britain in 1910: *No Animal Food* by Rupert H. Wheldon. Since 1944, many societies inspired by veganism have appeared throughout the world, including in India, Indonesia, the United States, and Australia as well as in much of Europe, and the vegan movement has become a global phenomenon annually celebrated on November 1, World Vegan Day, and in the nomadic International Vegan Festival, first held in Denmark in 1981.

Reasons for Veganism   The first manifesto of the U.K. Vegan Society argued that veganism was intended to lead to "a more reasonable and humane" society and not only guide individual ethical choices. This rested on a contention that dependence on animal exploitation led to the moral impoverishment of human society, just as had dependence on human slavery. The combination of care of the self and care for the wider environment, including the human and other animals who share it, is a leitmotif of veganism. This is reflected in the supporting reasons for veganism, which draw on animal ethics, environmentalism, concerns with global food security, human health, spirituality, and aesthetic preference for plant-based foods. One or more of these reasons usually provides a prominent motivation for individual vegans.

The global consumption of animal products has tended to rise as average incomes increase throughout the world, suggesting that veganism is a choice that goes against the grain of mainstream dietary preferences. However, the interpretation that this indicates an innate preference for animal-based foods needs to treated with caution, as the desirability of animal-based foods may, at least partly, be shaped by cultural forces. Scholars such as Carol J. Adams have argued that the consumption of animal-based foods is linked to hierarchical relations of gender, ethnicity, and class. Adams, for example, argues that meat eating symbolizes male dominance and that there is a resonance in contemporary Western cultures between the ways that nonhuman animals, women, and people of color are objectified. Therefore, veganism represents a form of compassionate opposition to a way of viewing the world that perpetuates forms of human domination, as much as it does the domination of other animals.

Veganism also draws on several strands of Western secular animal ethics, which, in spite of differences of philosophy and tactics, tend to advocate veganism as one of their practical conclusions. These include the utilitarian approach developed by Peter Singer; the rights-based approach developed by Tom Regan; feminist care ethics, advocated by Adams, Josephine Donovan, and others; the abolitionist approach developed by Gary L. Francione; and arguments for animal liberation, associated with the work of Steve Best.

Spiritual and religious traditions have also been influential on veganism. The American Vegan Society, founded in 1960 by H. Jay Dinshah, draws on the principles of *ahimsa,* a Sanskrit term that may be interpreted as "dynamic harmlessness" and that is associated with the nonviolent practice of Mahatma Gandhi. Hinduism, Buddhism, Sikhism, and Jainism all share an affiliation with veganism through traditions of ethical concern about the proper relationship between humans and other animals. The affinity between Abrahamic traditions (Judaism, Christianity, and Islam) and veganism is less well known, but veganism is compatible with, and has adherents from, all major world faiths, as demonstrated, for instance, in Andrew Linzey's work on the connections between Christian theology and animal ethics.

A concern for the environmental and social justice consequences of an animal-based diet can be traced at least as far back as Plato, but concerns have grown in prominence in recent years in the context of environmental degradation and food security. Through reducing global dependence on animal farming, veganism is argued to be able to contribute to slowing the rate of greenhouse gas emissions, making more efficient use of land and water resources, reducing pollution, ameliorating deforestation and soil erosion, and reducing the rate of decline in biodiversity. Many of these environmental benefits are also argued to have positive consequences for human food security, through making more efficient use of land, water, and plant-food resources. As well as shifting consumption toward plant foods, stock-free, or vegan-organic, farming methods provide a model for sustainable plant-food production through minimizing carbon footprints, maintaining soil fertility through use of crop rotation and green manures, and avoiding reliance on animal-based or synthetic chemical inputs.

The association of high levels of animal-product consumption with some chronic degenerative diseases, especially in developed Western nations, suggests the human health benefits of veganism as well. While the available evidence suggests that a balanced vegan diet is at least as healthy as any other, there is thus far insufficient research to warrant a conclusion that vegan diets are healthier than any others. Nevertheless, many vegans testify to perceived improvements in their physical and psychological health.

See also Ahimsa; Dinshah, H. Jay; Eastern Religions, Influences of; Ethical Vegetarianism; Francione, Gary L.; Physical Fitness and Athleticism; Physiological Benefits; Reform; Religious Beliefs and Practices; Singer, Peter; Vegetarianism, Types of; Vegetarian Society of the United Kingdom; Watson, Donald.

Further Reading

Adams, Carol J. *The Sexual Politics of Meat: A Feminist-Vegetarian Critical Theory.* 10th anniversary ed. New York: Continuum, 2000.

Amato, Paul R., and Sonia A. Partridge. *The New Vegetarians: Promoting Health and Protecting Life.* New York: Plenum, 1989.

Best, Steve, and Anthony J. Nocella, eds. *Terrorists or Freedom Fighters? Reflections on the Liberation of Animals.* New York: Lantern Books, 2004.

Donovan, Josephine, and Carol J. Adams, eds. *The Feminist Care Tradition in Animal Ethics.* New York: Columbia University Press, 2007.

Francione, Gary L. *Rain without Thunder: The Ideology of the Animal Rights Movement.* Philadelphia: Temple University Press, 1996.

Leneman, Leah. "No Animal Food: The Road to Veganism in Britain, 1909–1944." *Society and Animals* 7 (1999): 1–5.

Marcus, Erik. *Vegan: The New Ethics of Eating.* Ithaca, NY: McBooks, 2001.

Regan, Tom. *The Case for Animal Rights.* London: Routledge and Kegan Paul, 1983.

Singer, Peter. *Animal Liberation: A New Ethics for Our Treatment of Animals.* New York: Avon Books, 1975.

Stepaniak, Joanne. *Being Vegan: Living with Conscience, Conviction, and Compassion.* Los Angeles: Lowell House, 2000.

Vegan Society. http://www.vegansociety.com/home.php.

Matthew Cole

VEGETARIANISM, TYPES OF

Although vegetarianism is often viewed as a fad, the practice of abstaining from animal flesh can be traced back to ancient Greece and India. As vegetarianism has become more mainstream in recent decades, new or revived varieties have emerged. These new or revived types of vegetarianism are motivated to protest animal cruelty but are also a political statement about the environmental damage perpetuated by the factory farm system, the health benefits of vegetarianism, religious ideals, and gender equality.

The traditional definition of vegetarianism is the practice of eating no fish or animal flesh. Two subgroups have been recently recognized, perhaps to make the definition of veganism clearer. A lacto-ovo vegetarian is perhaps the most common type of vegetarian; this person does not eat meat or fish but does eat dairy products and eggs. Pesco-vegetarians eat fish in addition to a traditional vegetarian diet.

Veganism, a more restrictive diet, excludes all animal products including milk, eggs, and honey. Vegans are divided into two subcategories: lifestyle vegans and dietary vegans. Lifestyle vegans eschew all animal products in their diet and life, such as not wearing leather or fur or using consumer products made with ingredients derived from animals. Dietary vegans exclude animal products only from their diet.

The raw food movement is another offshoot. Most raw foodists (or living foodists) eat vegan diets and do not heat foods above 116 degrees Fahrenheit. They argue that eating raw food is good for one's health because cooking destroys certain beneficial enzymes.

The most permissive new type of vegetarianism is called "flexitarianism," or semivegetarianism. The term "flexitarian" was coined in 1992 and is a combination of the words "flexible" and "vegetarian." In 2003, "flexitarian" was named a word of the year by the American Dialect Society. Flexitarians are not vegetarians

---

Types of Vegetarianism

Lacto-ovo vegetarians avoid meat, poultry, and fish but eat plant foods, dairy products, and eggs.

Lacto-vegetarians avoid meat, poultry, and fish as well as eggs but eat plant foods and dairy products.

Ovo-vegetarians avoid meat, poultry, and fish as well as dairy but eat plant foods and eggs.

Vegans or total vegetarians avoid all animal foods including meat, dairy, honey, and eggs and eat plant foods only.

Pesco/pollo-vegetarians eat seafood and chicken but avoid other meats.

Flexitarians or semivegetarians occasionally eat meat, fish, and/or poultry.

but might prefer to identify that way because they have a mostly vegetarian diet but eat some animal products. Flexitarians are not a well-defined group of people, because they may not identify as vegetarian at all, simply preferring a diet low in animal foods. Their motivations and practices also vary. They may eschew red meat while continuing to consume poultry or fish or may consume small amounts of meat-based foods, such as chicken broth. They may also eat meat only in restaurants and refuse to prepare it at home. Some flexitarians will consume only meat that is produced humanely. Flexitarians are often acting out of a concern for health but may also want to take advantage of the lower expense of eating a mostly vegetarian diet.

Two other less popular variations on vegetarian diets are macrobiotic diets and fruitarianism. *Macrobiotic* means "large life," and those who eat macrobiotic diets eat whole foods in limited quantities. They eat grains, vegetables, beans, and fruit. Fruitarianism has a variable definition, but generally fruitarians eat only grains and fruits. Therefore, fruitarianism is a subcategory of veganism. Some practitioners will not eat food that has been harvested from live plants because it kills the organism, so they consume what is naturally shed.

Strict vegetarians and vegans may not identify with or validate people who identify as flexitarians or pesco-vegetarians. While flexitarians and pesco-vegetarians might view themselves as committed to preventing animal cruelty or environmental degradation, their practices are seen by stricter vegetarians and vegans as not entirely consistent and therefore have the possibility of undermining the movement.

See also Agribusiness; Animal Rights and Animal Welfare; Ecofeminism; Ethical Vegetarianism; Global Warming; Meatless diets before Vegetarianism; Physiological Benefits; Religious Beliefs and Practices; Social Acceptance; Veganism.

Further Reading

Harris, John. "The New Vegetarianism: Meat Is More Murderous Than Ever." *The Guardian,* June 19, 2008, p. 34.

Spencer, Colin. *The Heretic's Feast: A History of Vegetarianism.* London: University Press of New England, 1995.

The Vegetarian Society of the United Kingdom. http://www.vegsoc.org.

Yabroff, Jennie. "No More Sacred Cows: Vegetarians Who Eat Meat." *Newsweek,* December 31, 2009.

Ansley Watson

VEGETARIANS AND VEGANS, CELEBRITY

Since the 1950s, celebrities have used their star power and the media to appeal to the public about animal rights and vegetarianism. Celebrity vegetarians and vegans have included musicians, actors, athletes, writers, spiritual leaders, and scholars.

Sir James Paul McCartney, the English singer-songwriter and former member of the Beatles, has been a practicing vegetarian since meeting his late wife, Linda (Eastman) McCartney, in 1975. Linda McCartney authored several vegetarian cookbooks and was an outspoken animal rights activist who claimed that if "slaughterhouses had glass walls, the whole world would be vegetarian." In the 1990s, she released a line of frozen vegetarian meals licensed under her name and lent her voice to television segments for People for the Ethical Treatment of Animals (PETA). After she died from breast cancer in 1995, Paul McCartney asked that fans support her memory by donating to breast cancer research that did not entail animal testing, or by becoming vegetarian. The late George Harrison, the former lead guitarist for the Beatles, was also a vegetarian.

Canadian model and actress Pamela Anderson is a controversial opponent of animal cruelty who has repeatedly protested against fur, seal hunting, and American fast food giant Kentucky Fried Chicken. Her tactics often include nude modeling—"I'd rather go naked than wear fur"—or wearing a lettuce bikini on a Times Square billboard in 2006. Her activism has drawn criticism for its blatant use of female sexuality to convince others about the merits of vegetarianism. She has been a vegetarian since her mid-teens and has worked as a longtime PETA spokeswoman. Miss Black USA 2003 Elizabeth Muto also participated in PETA's lettuce-bikini campaign.

Actress Alicia Silverstone has been a vegan since 1998 and often works on animal rights campaigns. In 2009, she published *The Kind Diet,* a book about nutrition and health that promotes plant-based diets. Actor Toby McGuire, best known for his role as Spider-man in the 2002 film named for the superhero, has been a vegetarian since age 14 and often avoids dairy and eggs as well. He has admitted to eating honey and milk chocolate and therefore refuses to call himself a vegan. Actor Joaquin Phoenix has been a vegan since childhood. In 2003, he narrated the documentary *Earthlings for Nation Earth,* a film about human dependence on animals for food, clothing, experiments, and entertainment. The film was scored by Moby. Actress Natalie Portman is also an animal rights activist and vegetarian. Actress Anne Hathaway is a vegetarian. Actress and model Liv Tyler is a vegan. Actress and activist Daryl Hannah has been a vegetarian since childhood. Comedienne Ellen DeGeneres and her partner, actress Portia de Rossi, are both vegan. Comedian and social justice activist Dick Gregory has been a vegetarian since the 1970s. Television actresses Emily Deschanel (*Bones*) and Gillian Anderson (*The X Files*) are vegans, as are the actors Casey Affleck, Jason Schwartzman, Woody Harrelson, and Kevin Nealon. Actor Alec Baldwin and actress Mary Tyler Moore are committed animal rights activists. Director and producer Peter Bogdanovich (*The Last Picture Show, The Godfather Part II*) is a vegetarian, and director Richard Linklater (*Dazed and Confused, Waking Life, A Scanner Darkly*) is also a vegetarian. Actress Susan Sarandon was a vegetarian for many years but now eats meat.

Professional athletes are less likely to be vegetarian because many believe it will be difficult to get the necessary protein intake without eating meat. Wladek "Killer" Kowalski was a Canadian professional wrestler who in the 1960s went vegetarian and claimed to be the only vegetarian in professional wrestling. In addition to avoiding meat, he abstained from dairy products and alcohol. Dave Scott is a triathlete best known for his record-breaking six repeated Ironman competition wins throughout the 1980s. During that time, he was a strict vegetarian. More recently, professional athletes have been adopting and sustaining vegetarian diets after reading popular literature on the subject. Tony Gonzalez, a football player who has played for the Kansas City Chiefs and Atlanta Falcons, adopted a vegan diet after suffering from Bell's palsy in 2007. An acquaintance recommended that he read *The China Study: The Most Comprehensive Study of Nutrition Ever Conducted* by T. Colin Campbell, and it convinced him to switch to a plant-based diet for health reasons. Major League baseball player Prince Fielder has been an outspoken vegetarian since 2008 and has been the target of antivegetarian backlash within the professional sports community. Fielder went vegetarian after reading the book *Skinny Bitch,* believing that being vegetarian was an ethical choice. Seba Johnson, the first black female Alpine ski racer, was raised since birth as a vegan and was once disqualified from a World Cup ski race because she refused to wear a racing suit that included leather patches.

Writers have long influenced others' thinking about vegetarianism. Many famous writers are vegetarians, even if they do not explicitly write about their diet or food. Alice Walker, a renowned African American writer best known for *The Color Purple,* is a vegetarian. Other famous female vegetarian writers include Charlotte Bronte, Mary Wollstonecraft Shelley, and Joanne Shaw. Leo Tolstoy wrote several influential essays on vegetarianism. German poet Rainer Maria Rilke, Czech author Franz Kafka, Irish playwright George Bernard Shaw, and American philosopher Henry David Thoreau were all vegetarian. It is said that the French philosopher Voltaire, the Greek philosopher Plato, the Chinese Taoist philosopher Lao Tse, the Chinese philosopher Confucius, and the Buddha were all vegetarian. Writer and literary critic J.M. Coetzee is a vegetarian. Contemporary American novelist Jonathan Safran Foer has been a vegetarian since he was nine years old and has started writing nonfiction about animal consumption. Safran Foer recorded the narration for the 2006 documentary *If This Is Kosher . . . ,* an exposé about the kosher certification process and vegetarianism. Vegan chef and cookbook author Isa Chandra Moskowitz began as a vegetarian and is a longtime vegan.

While some musical acts like Minor Threat, Dead Prez, and Propagandhi include references to animal-free diets in their lyrics, many artists are known for being both performers and vegetarians or vegans. Moby, née Richard Melville Hall, is a musician and DJ also known for his animal rights advocacy and status as a longtime vegan. Musician Prince is a practicing vegan and has been voted the "world's sexist vegetarian" in a PETA online poll. Ziggy Marley, a practicing vegetarian, is a reggae musician and the son of Bob Marley, the famous Jamaican reggae singer-songwriter. Masta Killa and RZA are American rappers best known for their work as part of the Wu Tang Clan and are both vegetarian. Masta Killa has been a vegetarian for most of his adult life and has starred in advertisements for PETA2, the youth outreach branch of PETA. The singer Pink has engaged in various campaigns against animal cruelty and has spoken out against wearing fur and the practice of mulesing. Rapper and producer Dr. Dre, singer Chris Martin of Coldplay, The Pretenders frontwoman Chrissie Hynde, singer-songwriter k.d. lang, musician Morrissey, British musician Stuart Murdoch (Belle and Sebastian), Pearl Jam frontman Eddie Vedder, and rapper Andre 3000 from OutKast are all vegetarians. Singer-songwriter Joss Stone was raised from birth as a vegetarian. Female singer-songwriters Erykah Badu, Sinead O'Connor, Fiona Apple, Joan Jett, and Alanis Morissette are vegan. Singer Grace Slick (Jefferson Airplane, Starship) practices relaxed veganism, occasionally indulging in foods that contain animal products. Radiohead frontman Thom Yorke is a vegan.

Political figures can often use their power to influence others about their own beliefs regarding vegetarianism. Newark, New Jersey, mayor Cory Booker is a vegetarian and does not drink alcohol or smoke. Former Cleveland mayor and U.S. Congressman Dennis Kucinich (D-Ohio) is a longtime vegan, as is his wife Elizabeth. Kucinich often works for legislation to promote better treatment of animals. Chelsea Clinton, the daughter of former president Bill Clinton and Secretary of State Hillary Rodham Clinton, is a vegetarian. Antiwar activist and former U.S. congressional candidate Cindy Sheehan is a vegan. Janez Drnovsek (1950–2008), former president of Slovenia, became a vegan after contracting cancer. He also vigorously advocated for environmentalism and animal rights to the extent that one commentator called him "Slovenia's Gandhi."

In the business world, Serbian inventor and engineer Nikola Tesla was a vegetarian, and businessman and Apple Computer cofounder Steve Jobs is also a vegetarian. American physician and corn flakes cereal coinventor John Harvey Kellogg was a vegetarian. Technology entrepreneur and venture capitalist Joi Ito is a vegan.

A number of models have spoken out about animal rights and vegetarianism. Former French model Brigitte Bardot has been a vegetarian since 1986. She condemns seal hunting and the consumption of horsemeat. Former model Heather Mills (the former Heather Mills McCartney) has a lengthy history of working for animal rights. She is a critic of fur, seal hunting, dairy consumption, and carbon emissions from animal agriculture. Model Petra Nemcovais also a vegan.

Perhaps most obvious are vegetarians who work directly with and on behalf of animals. Vegetarian chef Marie Oser and vegan chef and restaurateur Alissa Cohen are two well-known cooks who avoid meat and animal ingredients while advocating for animal-free diets. Primatologist Jane Goodall is an animal welfare activist and former president of the Scottish organization Advocates for Animals. She is the recipient of many prizes and numerous honorary university degrees for her work for animals and on behalf of the environment.

See also Activism and Protests; Agribusiness; Alternative and Holistic Medicine; Animal Rights and Animal Welfare; Antivivisection; Consumer Products; Cookbooks; Ethical Vegetarianism; Global Warming; People for the Ethical Treatment of Animals; Physical Fitness and Athleticism; Physiological Benefits; Policy; Reform; Religious Beliefs and Practices; *Skinny Bitch*; Social Acceptance; Television and Films; Veganism.

Further Reading

Coetzee, J. M. *The Lives of Animals*. Princeton, NJ: Princeton University Press, 2001.

Johnson, Seba. "Lessons My Mother Taught Me." *Satya Magazine*, October 2002.

McCartney, Linda. *Linda's Kitchen: Simple and Inspiring Recipes for Meatless Meals*. New York: Bulfinch, 1995.

Walters, Kerry, and Lisa Portmess, eds. *Religious Vegetarianism: From Hesiod to the Dalai Lama*. Albany: State University of New York Press, 2001.

Brittany Shoot

VEGETARIANS AND VEGANS, NOTED

Plant-based diets have existed in many cultures throughout recorded history. Themes such as the moral consideration of other species, nonviolence, and human health have been found in writings over the millennia. Religious leaders and writers have had the greatest influence in maintaining and expanding the practice of vegan and vegetarian diets, evidenced by the edicts in Buddhism, Hinduism, Judeo-Christianity, and other religions and major belief systems. Activists, artists, authors, philosophers, and politicians have also promoted plant-based diets for their moral and social advantages, while physicians, health reformers, and scientists have written about the physical benefits of eating only plants.

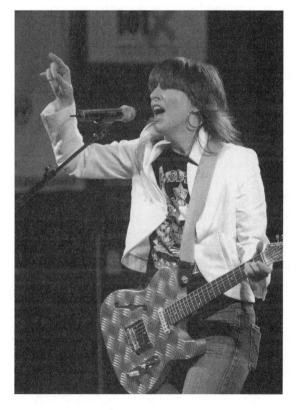

Chrissie Hynde performs in 2006. Hynde has a vegan restaurant in her hometown of Akron, Ohio. (AP Photo/Jack Plunkett)

A number of people who have identified their diet as vegan, vegetarian, ascetic, or another form of abstention from eating animal flesh and who have either committed their lives to advocating for a plant-based diet or made other profound contributions to society that make their diet historically significant are mentioned here.

Leo Tolstoy (1828–1910), the famous Russian author of literary classics such as *War and Peace* and *Anna Karenina,* was also an important proponent of vegetarianism. He is also said to have influenced Mahatma Gandhi's ideas about vegetarianism. In his 1892 essay titled "The First Step," Tolstoy wrote,

> Once, when walking from Moscow, I was offered a lift by some carters who were going to Serpukhov. . . . On entering a village we saw a well-fed, naked, pink pig being dragged out of the first yard to be slaughtered. It squealed in a dreadful voice, resembling the shriek of a man. Just as we were passing they began to kill it. A man gashed its throat with a knife. The pig squealed still more loudly and piercingly, broke away from the men, and ran off covered with blood.
>
> Being near-sighted I did not see all the details. I saw only the human-looking pink body of the pig and heard its desperate squeal, but the carter saw all the details and watched closely. They caught the pig, knocked it down, and finished cutting its throat. When its squeals ceased the carter sighed heavily. "Do men really not have to answer for such things?" he said.
>
> So strong is humanity's aversion to all killing. But by example, by encouraging greediness, by the assertion that God has allowed it, and above all by habit, people entirely lose this natural feeling.
>
> I only wish to say that for a good life a certain order of good actions is indispensable. . . . And if he be really and seriously seeking to live a good life, the first thing from which he will abstain will always be the use of animal food, because, to say nothing of the excitation of the passions caused by such food, its use is simply immoral, as it involves the performance of an act which is contrary to moral feeling—killing; and is called forth only by greediness and the desire for tasty food. . . .
>
> And the progress of vegetarianism is of this kind. That progress is expressed in the actual life of mankind, which from many causes is involuntarily passing more and more from carnivorous habits to vegetable food, and is also deliberately following the same path in a movement which shows evident strength, and which is growing larger and larger— viz. vegetarianism. That movement has during the last ten years advanced more and more rapidly.

. . . This movement should cause special joy to those whose life lies in the effort to bring about the kingdom of God on earth. . . . because it is a sign that the aspiration of mankind towards moral perfection is serious and sincere, for it has taken the one unalterable order of succession natural to it, beginning with the first step.

One cannot fail to rejoice at this, as people could not fail to rejoice who, after striving to reach the upper story of a house by trying vainly and at random to climb the walls from different points, should at last assemble at the first step of the staircase and crowd towards it, convinced that there can be no way up except by mounting this first step of stairs.

Source: International Vegetarian Union. http://www.ivu.org/history/tolstoy/step.html.

Religious Leaders and Scholars   Buddha (ca. 563–483 BC), whose name was Siddhartha Gautama, taught that *ahimsa* (nonviolence) and mercy are necessary for enlightenment. As humans seek to escape suffering, Siddhartha reasoned that humans should not cause others to suffer. The *Lankavatara,* an authoritative record of Mahayana Buddhism's teachings, quotes him as saying, "Meat eating in any form, in any manner, and in any place is unconditionally and once for all prohibited. . . . Meat eating I have not permitted to anyone, I do not permit, I will not permit."

Mani (ca. AD 210–276) founded Manichaeism, which thrived in Persia and extended as far as Rome and China between the third and seventh centuries. Mani taught compassion and asceticism, the latter meaning the pursuit of spiritual purity through abstention from alcohol, sex, and eating animals.

Elijah Muhammad (1897–1975) developed and led the Nation of Islam for four decades. He believed that before Noah's Flood, people were vegetarian and lived for hundreds of years. So Muhammad taught that in conformity with Allah's will, eating only fruits and vegetables was the best diet and that, at a minimum, all members of the Nation of Islam should be vegetarian during the month of Ramadan.

Hsing Yun (1927–) is an internationally renowned and politically active Buddhist monk. As a central figure in the reformation of Buddhism, he developed humanistic Buddhism, which directs Buddhists to make positive contributions to society through improving themselves and their community. Humanistic Buddhism promotes veganism through its tenets of altruism and universality.

Richard Schwartz (1934–) is the president of Jewish Vegetarians of North America (JVNA) and the Society of Ethical and Religious Vegetarians. He has authored over 100 articles on vegetarian-related topics and frequently gives talks and interviews. He is the associate producer of a JVNA-sponsored documentary film, *A Sacred Duty: Applying Jewish Values to Help Heal the World,* which discusses veganism from a Jewish perspective.

Andrew Linzey (1952–) is the director of the Oxford Centre for Animal Ethics and the preeminent theologian on the status of nonhuman animals. He contradicts Thomas Aquinas's premise that nonhumans are irrational objects for human convenience. His major works, including *Animal Rights: A Christian Assessment* (1976), *Christianity and the Rights of Animals* (1987), *Animal Theology* (1994), and *Why Animal Suffering Matters* (2009), argue that vegetarianism is obligatory for Christians.

Philosophers, Educators, and Authors Pythagoras (ca. 580–500 BC) was a Greek mathematician whose philosophy would be considered today as a blend of spirituality and science. His philosophy recognized moral value in nonhuman animals and therefore prohibited any adverse treatment, including their killing for food or religious rituals. He is regarded as Europe's first prominent vegetarian.

Confucius (551–479 BC) was an extremely influential philosopher in the East, comparable to Socrates' influence in the West. Compassion was central to his philosophy. Confucius taught that the path to love was parallel to vegetarianism and that the consumption of animals reinforced ideas of violence and warfare.

Socrates (ca. 470–399 BC) is the father of Western philosophy. He opposed consuming animals because the cruelty involved would tend to make humans violent and because war was the natural result of nations competing for the greater resources that are required in an animal-based diet.

Apollonius of Tyana (ca. 3 BC–AD 97) was a charismatic neo-Pythagorean sage who traveled extensively. He was said to be a magician, healer, and prophet who became famous for good deeds. He was vegan because of Pythagorean principles: He walked barefoot or wore bark for sandals, refused to have a horse killed to honor him, and refused a goat statue as a tribute because it was made of beeswax.

Porphyry (234–305) was the second-most famous ancient Greek vegetarian. He wrote *De Abstinentia* (On abstinence) and *De Non Necandis ad Epulandum Animantibus* (On the impropriety of killing living beings for food), among several other books on language, music, philosophy, religion, and science.

Percy Bysshe Shelley (1792–1822) was an English romantic poet who was criticized as an idealist but admired by later poets and political activists such as George Bernard Shaw, Karl Marx, Mohandas Gandhi, and Henry David Thoreau. Shelley was well known for his vegetarian advocacy. He wrote defenses of vegetarianism and attacks on meat eating.

Bronson Alcott (1799–1888) was an educator and philosopher in New England. Many of his ideas that were considered extreme in his time are popular today, such as egalitarianism, sustainable living, and veganism. He founded Fruitlands in 1843 as a utopian vegan community and the Concord School of Philosophy in 1879, which frequently hosted discussions of vegetarianism.

Leo Tolstoy (1828–1910) is the most famous Russian novelist and was a social reformer, pacifist, and famous for his vegetarianism. He believed that the only way to abolish oppression and violence was to absolutely refuse to commit either. He wrote *The First Step* (1909), which described how refusing to harm animals was the first step toward recognizing that humans and nonhumans share the same soul and that eating flesh prevented spiritual perfection.

Mark Twain (1835–1910), a novelist, social critic, and humorist, was a vegetarian and opposed vivisection, stating that no sentient being should be made to suffer for another.

George Bernard Shaw (1856–1950) started his career as a novelist but earned international fame as a playwright for his political satire, verbal wit, and attacks on social hypocrisy. He told an antivivisection activist that not opposing barnyard vivisection as well as laboratory vivisection was absurd.

Mohandas Gandhi (1869–1948) was a lawyer and revolutionary who was instrumental in ending the British occupation of India. His parents' Hindu and Jain beliefs in nonviolence were foundational in Gandhi's vegetarianism, but after reading Henry Salt's "A Plea for Vegetarianism," Gandhi made it one of his missions. He believed that nonhumans were as precious as humans. For humans to embrace peace, he reasoned that they should not harm human or nonhuman animals.

Franz Kafka (1883–1924) is one of the most influential Western writers, though much of his work is incomplete and was published posthumously against his dying request. He adopted veganism for ethical reasons and health, becoming a raw foodist after contracting tuberculosis.

Isaac Bashevis Singer (1902–1991) was best known as a short-story writer. Vegetarianism was extremely important to Singer, and he incorporated it into many of his writings. He believed that eating animals was a denial of all ideals and all religions. He compared the Nazi genocide of Jews with humans committing genocide on nonhumans.

Brigid Brophy (1929–1995) was an English author who is credited with starting the animal rights movement in England. She argued that society was duplicitous, as it encouraged altruism and sentimentality unless money could be made by being cruel to nonhuman animals.

Alice Walker (1944–) is a novelist and poet, most famous for *The Color Purple* (1982). In her autobiography, *Anything We Love Can Be Saved* (1997), she writes about why she chose the life of an activist and to be vegan.

John Robbins (1947–) wrote *Diet for a New America* (1987), an indictment of the meat and dairy industries. Since then, he founded EarthSave International, an activist organization advocating veganism for its environmental benefits. He also wrote *Food Revolution* (2001), explaining how human health directly relates to the environment's health. He has lectured internationally and is widely regarded as one of the most eloquent speakers on the benefits of veganism.

Carol J. Adams (1951–) is an author of many books and articles that explain and help define the links between feminism, veganism, and nonviolence. Her landmark book, *The Sexual Politics of Meat: A Feminist-Vegetarian Critical Theory* (1990), discusses meat eating's association with men, war, and the subjugation of women and nonhuman animals. Her work advocates neither the traditional rights approach of Tom Regan, nor the utilitarian approach of Peter Singer, but instead a feminist care approach that recognizes how oppression is interconnected.

Joan Dunayer (1951–) authored *Animal Equality: Language and Liberation* (2001) and *Speciesism* (2004). The first book on language and speciesism, *Animal Equality* shows that biased, misleading words perpetuate injustice toward nonhuman animals. *Speciesism* critiques "old speciesism" (which accords rights only to humans) and "new speciesism" (which accords rights to humans and a favored class of nonhumans), offering guidelines for nonspeciesist philosophy, law, and activism.

Physicians, Health Reformers, and Scientists   Leonardo da Vinci (1452–1519) is widely regarded as a universal genius, excelling in several disciplines of art and science. He refused to consume animals and recognized the suffering that humans caused them. He was known to buy birds from markets and set them free.

Albert Schweitzer (1875–1965) was a physician and philosopher well known for his reverence for all life. He believed that nature was ethically neutral, and it was the duty of humans to be better than nature. He said that humans are truly ethical only when they help others and refuse to harm others.

Albert Einstein (1879–1955), a world-famous physicist, was vegetarian only late in his life. He agreed with vegan principles for its moral standing and believed that the physical effect of vegetarianism would be beneficial on everyone's temperament.

Herbert Shelton (1895–1985), a naturopathic doctor, fought against the meat bias of the food and medical industries by promoting Natural Hygiene, using natural foods for superior nutrition. He believed that raw vegan food and therapeutic fasts were the best combination for human health, and he wrote several books on both topics. Among his many criticisms of a meat-based diet, he said that nuts are a natural and superior source of protein for humans whereas meat was unnatural and inferior. In 1956, Shelton was the American Vegetarian Party's candidate for U.S. president.

Alvenia Fulton (1907–1999), a naturopathic doctor, was known as the "queen of nutrition" and a pioneer of health reform through diet. In the 1950s, she opened the first African American natural food store and vegetarian restaurant, located in Chicago. She wrote *The Fasting Primer* (1978), and she collaborated with Dick Gregory on the book *Vegetarianism: Fact or Myth?* (1974).

Carl Sagan (1934–1996), an astronomer and writer, was known for his empathy for all life. He said that humans who exploit or kill nonhumans have a tendency to pretend that their victims do not suffer. Regarding Sagan's novel, *Contact* (1985), philosopher Steve Best argues that Sagan's alien characters from Vega, Vegans, are allegorical to vegans in their mutual philosophy of nonviolence and their mutual feelings of alienation from the necrovorous majority.

T. Colin Campbell (1934–) is a professor emeritus of nutritional biochemistry at Cornell University and a vegan. He coauthored with his physician son, Thomas M. Campbell II, *The China Study*, which chronicles his half-century of research and which is based, in part, on a 20-year study of the diet, lifestyle, and disease characteristics of 880 million Chinese. This research concluded that humans who consume protein in excess of the minimum amount needed, especially animal protein, are the most likely to get heart disease, cancer, and other diseases.

Michael Klaper, a physician, has become an authority on nutrition after his chronically ill patients dramatically improved on a regimen of a vegan diet, exercise, and stress reduction. As the director of the Institute of Nutrition Education and Research located in California, Klaper is conducting the Vegan Health Study to research the long-term effects of a vegan diet. Klaper has authored several books and lectured on nutrition, contributed to Public Broadcasting Service productions on diet, and hosts a radio program on health.

John McDougall (1947–), a physician, has developed a 10-day retreat where his patients who are suffering from heart disease, cancer, and other severe illnesses learn about and practice the benefits of a vegan diet. McDougall has authored several books, videos, and other publications on nutrition and is often sought as an expert.

Alan Long (1925–), a biochemist and nutritionist, wrote the *Green Plan* (1976) and has published studies on vegetarian-related subjects. He also served as an advisor to Vegetarian and Green Agriculture (VEGA), the International Vegetarian Union, and farming practices in the United Kingdom. He testified against McDonald's in the infamous "McLibel" trial (1997), a lawsuit intended to ruin vegan activists that instead resulted in a condemnation and judgment against McDonald's.

Dean Ornish (1953–), a physician, is the founder and president of the Preventive Medicine Research Institute. Since the 1970s, Ornish has been reversing all stages of coronary disease in his patients without drugs or surgery, using lifestyle changes such as a vegan diet, exercise, and clean water. His program has recently expanded to include some forms of cancer. He has written several books on nutrition, has been published in medical journals, and has a monthly column in *Newsweek* magazine. He was a consultant to U.S. President Bill Clinton.

Queen Afua founded the nationally recognized Heal Thyself Natural Healing Center, which teaches holistic healing and natural living. She specializes in women's health and practices from an Afrocentric perspective. She has authored several books, such as *Heal Thyself: For Health and Longevity* (2002), and has lectured at universities and government institutions.

Noted Nonvegetarians

Women's rights activist Susan B. Anthony (1820–1906) supported the vegetarian movement, attending lectures by Sylvester Graham and hosting vegetarian dinners at her house. She wrote in her diary, however, about her continuing to eat turkeys, cows, and other animals.

Nazi leader Adolf Hitler's (1889–1945) vegetarianism was a myth. News of Hitler's plant-based diet was propaganda to portray him as an ascetic, sacrificing luxuries of meat, alcohol, and tobacco for the people, yet some biographers and journalists described his fondness for flesh, including that of pigs and turtles.

Sources: Berry, Ryan. "At Home With The Fuhrer." In *Hitler: Neither Vegetarian Nor Animal Lover*. New York: Pythagorean Publishers, 2004; Eberle, Henrik and Uhl, Matthias. *The Hitler Book: The Secret Dossier Prepared for Stalin from the Interrogations of Otto Guensche and Heinze Linge, Hitler's Closest Personal Aides*. Bergisch Gladbach, Germany: Verlagsgruppe Lüebbe, 2005; Huth, Mary M. "Food For Thought." *Miss Anthony's Kitchen*, a monthly newsletter of the Susan B. Anthony House, December, 2007.

Activists, Advocates, and Others   Joe Rollino (1905–2010) was a strongman who, weighing 150 pounds at his peak, moved 3,200 pounds with his back. He reportedly moved 635 pounds with one finger and 450 pounds with his teeth. Receiving awards for valor and bravery in World War II, he would take repeated runs onto the battlefield, returning with two injured soldiers under each arm on each trip.

Rosa Parks (1913–2005), whose civil disobedience catapulted the civil rights movement in the United States, maintained a vegetarian diet. She embraced a philosophy of egalitarianism and what she called quiet strength.

Cesar Chávez (1927–1993) was a civil rights activist who cofounded the United Farm Workers. Through his decades of activism, he organized for labor, immigration, education, and voting rights. He ardently supported animal rights and was a committed vegan.

Karen Davis (1944–) founded United Poultry Concerns in 1990, an organization dedicated to the respectful treatment and protection of chickens and other birds traditionally used for food. United Poultry Concerns led the successful campaign to stop the force-molting of laying hens by starvation, a procedure used to manipulate egg production. She is the author of several books including *Prisoned Chickens, Poisoned Eggs: An Inside Look at the Modern Poultry Industry* (1996). Davis maintains a sanctuary for chickens, turkeys, and ducks in Virginia.

Alex Hershaft (1950–) is best known for founding the Farm Animal Reform Movement (FARM) in 1976, a vegan advocacy organization. FARM established several vegan holidays, such as World Vegetarian Day, World Farm Animals Day, the Great American Meatout, and Gentle Thanksgiving. Through FARM, Hershaft organizes national animal rights conferences. In 1981, Hershaft organized the Action for Life Conference that formally launched the U.S. animal rights movement.

Bob Linden (1951–) created the "Go Vegan with Bob Linden" radio show, the first mainstream media program covering veganism, animal rights, and the environment, which is broadcast throughout the United States and is available internationally on his Web site. Linden began his career in news and entertainment broadcasting but changed to advocacy in 2001. He has also organized vegan festivals and had Vegan Earth Day recognized by the U.S. Congress.

Bruce Friedrich (1969–) is the vice president of policy and government affairs for People for the Ethical Treatment of Animals (PETA) and has masterminded many of its most successful vegan advocacy campaigns, including producing PETA's very popular *Meet Your Meat* video. He coauthored *The Animal Activist's Handbook* (2009) and has contributed to other animal rights books. Friedrich is a popular speaker on veganism and animal rights topics.

Kim Stallwood (1955–) is a veteran animal activist who has promoted veganism since 1976. He is an author, scholar, and advisor on animal rights issues. He is European director of the Animals and Society Institute, which advances the status of nonhuman animals in public policy. He has held leadership positions with some of the world's foremost organizations in the United Kingdom and United States, including Compassion in World Farming, the British Union for the Abolition of Vivisection, and PETA. He edited the *Animals' Agenda* and produced two anthologies of articles from the magazine, *Speaking Out for Animals* (2001) and *A Primer on Animal Rights* (2002).

Carolena Nericcio (1960–) created American Tribal Style Belly Dance, recognized worldwide and attracting people of diverse cultures. Nericcio uses her celebrity status to promote veganism and compassion for all human and nonhuman animals. She was vegetarian for most of her life but became vegan when she recognized the cruelty of the milk and egg industries. lauren Ornelas [*sic*] (1970–) is the founder and director of the Food Empowerment Project. She is also the former executive director of Viva!USA, a national nonprofit vegan advocacy organization. Collaborating with activists across the United States, she achieved systemic change within Whole Foods Market, Trader Joe's, and Pier 1 Imports, after campaigning to end their use of duck meat and feathers.

Paul Shapiro (1979–) founded the vegan advocacy organization Compassion Over Killing and served as its campaign director for 10 years. He conducted undercover investigations of factory farms, livestock auctions, and slaughterhouses, which he used to create several documentaries. He also helped lead the organization's national advertising campaign of pro-vegan commercials on youth-oriented stations. Shapiro later became a campaign director with the Humane Society of the United States to advocate veganism.

See also Activism and Protests; Agribusiness; Ahimsa; Alternative and Holistic Medicine; Animal Rights and Animal Welfare; Antivivisection; Ethical Vegetarianism; Global Warming; Meatless Diets before Vegetarianism; People for the Ethical Treatment of Animals; Physiological Benefits; Policy; Reform; Religious Beliefs and Practices; Veganism.

Further Reading

International Vegetarian Union. http://www.ivu.org/people.

Phelps, Norm. *The Longest Struggle: Animal Advocacy from Pythagoras to PETA*. New York: Lantern Books, 2007.

Jerold D. Friedman

VEGETARIAN SOCIETY OF AMERICA (1886–CA. 1920)

The Vegetarian Society of America (VSA) was an organization based in the United States that from 1886 until the early 1920s attempted to unite American vegetarians under a common heading. The VSA promoted a vegetarian lifestyle in an age of what was perceived as increasing industrialization that led to unsanitary lifestyles and moral decay.

The lineage of the VSA can be traced back as far as 1817 with the founding of the Bible Christian Church in Philadelphia. The Bible Christians drew their belief in vegetarianism from God's granting to humanity the fruits of the earth (particularly in Genesis 1:29) and in turn made this a cornerstone of their church. In 1850, the church contributed to the founding of the American Vegetarian Society, a forerunner of the VSA. The American Vegetarian Society enjoyed the support of some of the era's most notable reformers but was in existence for only

15 years. However, one reformer, Henry S. Clubb, understood that the demise of the American Vegetarian Society left a substantial void in American culture and politics, and he worked to inaugurate a new era of vegetarianism in the United States.

Clubb, who had been a founding member of the Vegetarian Society of the United Kingdom, immigrated to the United States in 1850 to aid in vegetarianism's spread. Interested in holistic social reform, Clubb was a charismatic activist and—like many reformers of his day—wrote extensively in support of not only vegetarianism but also abolition, temperance, the benefits of octagon-shaped housing, sanitation, phrenology, hydropathy, and the precursor to the sustainable communities described in the writings of Charles Fourier. These reform efforts resulted from popular misgivings about the rapid industrialization of the United States following Reconstruction, which Clubb and others saw as a significant contributor to spreading ill health in the nation. In the summer of 1886, Clubb gathered a group of nearly 200 vegetarians for a picnic in Alnwick Grove Park, near Philadelphia, celebrating the vegetarian lifestyle as an alternative to the social and moral decay of the times. Those assembled, moved by the large number of supporters, established a steering committee of 14 prominent reformers, which in turn selected Clubb as their president. After a few organizational meetings over the following months, the committee officially founded the VSA in their meeting on November 30, 1886.

Using the Bible Christian Church at 936 Franklin Street in Philadelphia as its headquarters, the VSA managed an impressive agenda of activities. First and foremost, it was publisher and clearinghouse for Clubb's extensive dispatches about social reform through vegetarianism. A robust print culture in the United States, still largely undeveloped during the time of the American Vegetarian Society, provided a loosely affiliated network of outlets; favorable notices regarding the VSA's existence soon began to appear in ladies' homemaking magazines, agricultural digests, and other reformers' publications. The VSA also began publication of its own magazine, *Food, Home and Garden,* which provided a template for vegetarian publishing that remains today, printing testimonies of vegetarian converts, profiles of famous vegetarians, dispatches on the latest health and science, recipes, reports from vegetarian gatherings, and news of upcoming events. After establishing itself in the media, the society began holding annual meetings, attracting celebrities as keynote speakers such as John Harvey Kellogg, famed dietary reformer and inventor of the now-ubiquitous grain cereal as an alternative to the meat-heavy Victorian breakfast. Emboldened by the success of these domestic meetings, Clubb was instrumental in working with his connections in England at the Vegetarian Federal Union to organize the International Vegetarian Congresses in the 1890s to put American vegetarianism on the world stage. He was also instrumental in bringing the 3rd International Congress to the 1893 World's Columbian Exhibition in Chicago. This event went a long way toward exposing vegetarianism to a large and diverse audience, given that that the Columbian Exposition was the largest public event in U.S. history, drawing over 27 million visitors during its run.

The infusion of contemporary scientific discourse into the VSA's meetings and publications successfully professionalized vegetarianism in the United States, which had been in many ways a radical or fringe movement. In this way, the society gave American vegetarians affiliated with the association a coherent structure and a recognizable front, a diverse pool of learned people from whom to draw advice, a base made up of concerned nonspecialists, and the moral support that membership afforded. At the same time, however, these benefits were always somewhat diffuse. The center of the VSA remained the energetic Clubb, and as such, the organization retained his weaknesses, albeit minor, as well. While an excitable orator and tireless writer, Clubb was less attentive to the day-to-day business of running the organization, his enthusiasm at times outstripping his managerial skills, especially given the relatively small resources the society had at its disposal. Furthermore, Clubb, though tolerant and interested in scientific research inasmuch as it confirmed his faith's dictates, remained devoted to biblical exegesis and the Christian doctrines that founded his vegetarianism, an attitude at odds with the rationalism pervasive in late 19th-century America. The seemingly objective claims of scientists—including some, like Kellogg, still friendly with the society—grated against Clubb's ideological underpinnings drawn from Christianity about the need to reject animal products. Despite the Bible Christians' effort, however, as time passed, the secular, scientific rationale came to overshadow biblical imperatives.

Most difficult for the VSA to overcome, however, was Clubb's seemingly inexhaustible will to grow the movement, which had difficulty sustaining itself with its still rather meager pockets of supporters. While the British Vegetarian Society from which Clubb had come had flourished as a result of its diverse network of local chapters, an embedded organizational bureaucracy, and a relatively small geographic region, the VSA lacked any such cohesion, unable to overcome the obstacles of a decentered population and great distance between chapters in an age of little communication technology. Clubb nevertheless reached out into the loose network of emerging local societies. In an attempt to foster connections, Clubb negotiated with the Chicago chapter, based in a city on the rise in the national consciousness, to merge the publication of its *Vegetarian Magazine* with *Food, Home and Garden,* maintaining the title of the former. This move, however, only solidified the waning of Philadelphia as a center of American culture and population as well as vegetarian reform. Indeed, Philadelphia itself had begun to present direct logistical challenges to the VSA. After a sausage factory opened next door to the church in 1890, disgusted members sought to move; however, the only willing buyer was, in a fit of unfortunate irony, a pork-processing facility. Through an agent the Bible Christians sold their building and moved to a small, custom-built chapel in North Philadelphia.

Enthusiasm for the tenets of the religious movement that had fostered early American vegetarianism sharply declined among members of the VSA. At the turn of the 20th century, moral and religious tracts continued to be published, but vegetarian meetings were dominated by scientific discourse espousing the nutritional values of abstaining from meat. Moreover, in 1906, the publication of Upton Sinclair's novel *The Jungle* electrified the nation against the dominant modes of food production, especially in slaughterhouses, which imperiled workers' health and the safety of food products. By 1909, Clubb—aged 82—was the last pastor of a Bible Christian Church in the United States. Though he still made it a point to publish pamphlets and tracts bearing the name Vegetarian Society of America from his pastoral seat, after this time dispatches and meetings ceased. Clubb died in 1921 at the age of 94, and with him the VSA died as well.

See also Alternative and Holistic Medicine; American Vegetarian Society; Bible and Biblical Arguments; Bible Christians, Philadelphia; Clubb, Henry S.; Colonies, Communal Societies, and Utopias; Periodicals; Reform; Religious Practices and Beliefs; Vegetarian Society of the United Kingdom.

Further Reading

Clubb, Henry S., ed. *Food, Home and Garden* magazine. Philadelphia: Vegetarian Society of America, 1897.

History of Vegetarian Societies in North America. International Vegetarian Union Web Site. http://www.ivu.org/history/societies/usa.html.

Iacobbo, Karen, and Michael Iacobbo. *Vegetarian America: A History.* Westport, CT: Praeger, 2004.

Unti, Bernard. "Vegetarian Roots." *Vegetarian Times* 152 (1990): 52–58, 82.

Tom Hertweck

VEGETARIAN SOCIETY OF THE UNITED KINGDOM

The Vegetarian Society of the United Kingdom was founded on September 30, 1847, and is the oldest continuing national vegetarian society in the world. Its goals were "to induce habits of abstinence from the flesh of animals as food, by the dissemination of information upon the subject, by means of tracts, essays, and lectures, proving the many advantages of a physical, intellectual, and moral character, resulting from vegetarian habits of diet; and thus to secure, through the association, example, and effort of its members, the adoption of a principle which will tend to true civilization, to universal brotherhood, and to the increase of human happiness generally." Joiners were required to have abstained from meat for one month and to cooperate in "promulgating the knowledge of the advantages of a vegetarian diet."

About 150 people attended this inaugural meeting chaired by Joseph Brotherton, the Liberal member of Parliament for Salford, near Manchester. Local associations, each with their own secretary and meetings, were established in various parts of the country, and the *Vegetarian Messenger* became the society's official journal. Many original members were either Bible Christians, Concordists, or connected with Northwood Villa, the hydropathic institute near Ramsgate, Kent, where the inaugural meeting convened. The Bible Christian Church had been established in Salford in 1809 by the Reverend William Cowherd, a scholar and former Anglican who ran a dissenting academy. The Concordium was a vegetarian community formed in the late 1830s at Alcott House, Ham Hill, near Richmond, where a previous conference had prepared the formation of the society following an earlier unsuccessful attempt in 1843. Henry S. Clubb, both a Bible Christian and a Concordist, was founding secretary of the Manchester and Salford association and later immigrated to New York. He became a radical abolitionist journalist, before being elected founding president of the Vegetarian Society of America in 1886.

Many of the society's early members in Manchester and Salford were working class, and many were teetotalers. The mid-Victorian values of rational free choice and moral improvement by self-help provided good ground for the seeding of vegetarianism, as did the sense of personal bodily discipline inculcated by factory work. During the 1870s and 1880s, however, vegetarianism took deeper root among white-collar professionals, especially clerical and retail workers. The society gained many new and younger members, including playwright George Bernard Shaw, but fewer from the industrial working class. Cosmopolitan London became the center of vegetarianism, with over 30 new vegetarian restaurants. Vegetarians frequently opposed vivisection and vaccination and advocated other social and political reforms such as women's suffrage. Many continued to campaign for an end to capital punishment and supported the peace movement.

These cultural shifts intensified existing rivalries between the Manchester and Salford association and the London association, especially over the definition of vegetarianism. Working-class Manchester and Salford had been the center of vegetarianism in the 1850s, but in London a range of food and dietary reform groups were developing. Under Professor Francis Newman, brother of Cardinal John Henry Newman and president of the society from 1873 to 1883, associate membership was granted to people who were not completely vegetarian. Moreover, an independent vegetarian group, the London Dietetic Reform Society, was constituted in 1875 with more relaxed membership rules. Newman was succeeded as president by J.E.B. Mayor, professor of Latin at Cambridge University. During Mayor's presidency, the London group affirmed that it was an association of the national society, but in 1888, it declared a separate London Vegetarian Society with a new journal, the *Vegetarian*. Arnold Hills, a raw foodist and wealthy shipbuilder, became president, and committee members included Thomas Allinson, promoter of whole-grain bread, and Mohandas Gandhi, then a young London law student. The following year they established the Vegetarian Federal Union, intended to bring together all societies and associations in the United Kingdom and overseas. This was superseded in 1908 when the International Vegetarian Union was launched.

During World War I, vegetarianism was seen as promoting household economy. Throughout the interwar period, it formed part of various progressive education schemes and consolidated its middle-class profile. In World War II, householders were systematically encouraged to grow vegetables in their gardens and allotments. The government recognized vegetarianism by allowing registered vegetarians special rations, including extra cheese, fat, and nuts. But in 1944, the breakaway Vegan Society UK was established following disagreements about the ethics and dietary necessity of dairy products.

During the 1950s, calls grew for the Vegetarian Society, headquartered in Manchester, and the London Vegetarian Society to work more closely together. In 1958, their two journals merged, and in 1969 the societies formally amalgamated as the Vegetarian Society of the United Kingdom. In this period, vegetarianism was frequently regarded as part of a wider counterculture encompassing feminism, alternative medicine, and New Age religion. Some older connections, such as with temperance and theosophy, virtually disappeared. Vegetarian restaurants had a reputation for simplicity, cheapness, and good staff relations, and the animal rights movement provided vegetarianism with a major new impulse.

The society currently has affiliated groups across the country and premises at Parkdale, in Altrincham near Manchester. It defines a vegetarian as someone who does *not* eat any meat, poultry, game, fish, shellfish or crustaceans, or slaughter by-products. Ongoing activities include National Vegetarian Week, a food-labeling scheme, an awards scheme, nutritional research, and campaigns. The society's Cordon Vert School for cookery was founded in 1982 by Sarah Brown, who also presented *Vegetarian Kitchen,* a popular television series. Vegetarian options are now the norm in restaurants. With a growing awareness that current levels of meat consumption are ecologically unsustainable, there is new interest in vegetarianism.

See also Alternative and Holistic Medicine; Antivivisection; Bible Christians, English; Bible Christians, Philadelphia; Clubb, Henry S.; Dinshah, H. Jay; Ecofeminism; Ethical Vegetarianism; Gandhi, Mohandas; Global Warming; International Vegetarian Union; Periodicals; Policy; Reform; Religious Beliefs and Practices; Restaurants; Social Acceptance; Transcendentalism; United Kingdom; Vegetarian Society of America; World Wars in England.

Further Reading

Gregory, James R.T.E. *Of Victorians and Vegetarians: The Vegetarian Movement in Nineteenth-Century Britain.* London: Tauris, 2007.

International Vegetarian Union. www.ivu.org.

Twigg, Julia. *The Vegetarian Movement in England, 1847–1981: A Study in the Structure of Its Ideology.* PhD diss., London School of Economics, 1981. www.ivu.org/history/thesis/index.html.

The Vegetarian Society of the United Kingdom. www.vegsoc.org.

David Grumett

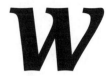

WATSON, DONALD (1910–2005)

Born September 2, 1910, in Mexborough, South Yorkshire, England, Donald Watson coined the term "vegan" to describe individuals who abstain from the consumption and use of animal products and founded the Vegan Society to promote this idea. Watson spent much of his life as a woodworker or teaching woodwork. His father was a headmaster of a nearby school. His uncle and grandmother ran the family farm, and, at an early age, Watson, who had thought of the farm as an idyllic place, witnessed the slaughter of a pig. This began his reassessment of the human-nonhuman relationship, which continued through Watson's adolescence.

In 1924, at age 14, Watson became a vegetarian. Twenty years later, in 1944, he founded the Vegan Society, although he had already been practicing a vegan diet and lifestyle for a few years prior. "Vegan" comes from the beginning and ending letters of the word "vegetarian." Watson thought that veganism was the logical conclusion of rejecting animal products for reasons of morality and health. He maintained that dairy products, such as milk, eggs, and cheese, were every bit as cruel and exploitive of sentient animal life as was slaughtering animals for their flesh: "The unquestionable cruelty associated with the production of dairy produce has made it clear that lacto-vegetarianism is but a half-way house between flesh-eating and a truly humane, civilised diet, and we think, therefore, that during our life on earth we should try to evolve sufficiently to make the 'full journey.'" He also avoided wearing leather, wool, or silk and used a fork, rather than a spade, in his gardening to avoid killing worms.

Watson was opposed to hunting, fishing, blood sports, and the use of animals in experiments or for testing purposes. Although he claimed to have respect for those who liberated animals from laboratories or engaged in other forms of direct action, he expressed concern that such activities were counterproductive. He was an advocate of organic farming and was critical of genetic modification of plants and animals.

Watson touted and exemplified the health benefits of a vegan diet, but he clearly saw veganism primarily as a moral principle. He regarded the vegan movement as "the greatest movement that ever was" because it provided a solution to the crisis of greed and violence that affected and afflicted humankind and that threatened ecological disaster. Although he was not religious in a traditional sense, he had deeply held spiritual beliefs that included the idea that being a carnivore violated natural law and that violence against nonhuman animals was a violation of spiritual laws that brought psychological unhappiness and ill health. Watson maintained that compassion was the only useful part of religion and that veganism involved practicing compassion.

Watson was committed to nonviolence in general. He had objector status during World War II. He lived an active and healthy life until his death in 2005 at age 95. Watson predicted, as did playwright George Bernard Shaw about his own funeral, that it would be attended by "all the spirits of all the animals" that Watson had never eaten.

See also Activism and Protests; Animal Rights and Animal Welfare; Ethical Vegetarianism; Organic Farming and Technology; Physiological Benefits; Reform; Veganism.

Further Reading

"Interview with Donald Watson on Sunday 15 December 2002." http://www.abolitionistapproach.com/media/links/p2528/unabridged-transcript.pdf.
The Vegan News, November 1944.
The Vegan Society. http://www.vegansociety.com/home.php.

Gary L. Francione

WORLD HUNGER

A shortage of food is a looming crisis in view of exponential population growth. At present, an estimated 850 million people are undernourished. With the growth of the human population, this number is likely to grow in view of the limited availability of fertile land and freshwater resources. Food security will become even a bigger issue in the future. Vegetarianism can be seen as one quick solution to the problem.

When Julius Caesar (ca. 50 BC) ruled Rome, the world population was about 250 million people. It grew to about 500 million by the time Christopher Columbus arrived in the Americas in 1492. The world population was about 750 million when Thomas Jefferson signed the Declaration of Independence in 1776. It was two billion at the time of the World War II. Presently, the world population is approximately six billion and is growing exponentially at the rate of about 1.5 percent a year, with a doubling period of 47 years, adding about 80–90 million people (roughly the population of Germany today) to the earth annually. According to most estimates, however, the growth rate is expected to decrease, and the population will be about nine billion by 2050. This increase of population by 50 percent, from six billion to nine billion, will require a corresponding increase of food production to feed people.

Because the earth is a closed system, sustainable food practices are needed. There is a need to find effective methods to deal with the population growth. It is recognized that new technologies need to be developed for food production, and some would argue for new family planning practices and a change from the meat-based Western diets. It has been suggested that more than half of commercially grown corn can be used to feed humans directly instead of feeding the animals humans raise to eat. Similarly, about 56 percent of all freshwater is used for irrigation and raising livestock. Farm animals consume about one trillion gallons of water per year; much of it can be saved, however, by adopting a meatless diet.

In the developing countries, daily meat consumption per person is about 1.68 ounces (47 grams), and about 7.9 ounces (224 grams) in the developed countries. The world consumption of meat was about 71 million tons in 1961 and increased to 284 million tons in 2007. This four-fold increase in consumption means that about 70 percent of all agricultural land on the planet, or about 30 percent of the earth's ice-free land, is used to support livestock industries. Furthermore, one pound of beef in a U.S. feedlot creates about 14.8 pounds of carbon dioxide (CO_2). This is equivalent to the amount of CO_2 produced while driving 20.6 miles in a typical car. The release of CO_2 is known to cause global warming.

Past methods of increasing food production have had limited success. Fertile cropland is being destroyed at a high rate, by about one-third in the last 50 years. In addition, the problems of erosion are difficult to resolve; it can take several centuries to convert eroded land into fertile soil suitable for agriculture production.

See also Agribusiness; Ethical Vegetarianism; Global Warming; Policy.

Further Reading

Shah, Mahendra, and Maurice F. Strong. *Food in the 21st Century: From Science to Sustainable Agriculture.* Washington, DC: World Bank, 2000.
Steinfeld, Henning, et al. *Livestock's Long Shadow: Environmental Issues and Options.* Rome: Food and Agriculture Organization of the United Nations, 2006.

Alok Kumar

WORLD WARS IN ENGLAND

Wartime vegetarianism is mainly documented by the Vegetarian Society of the United Kingdom, including accounts given by vegetarians serving in the armed forces and recorded in the movement's archives. Most reports from World War I show that no special provision was made for vegetarians serving in the forces, so their diet seldom was adequate. Increasing shortages during the war put special stress on most vegetarians, who owed their survival to food parcels sent from home.

On the home front, a food economy legacy dominated in all warring countries, with the result that in 1917, two to three meatless days per week were adopted almost everywhere, which found natural favor among vegetarians. In the United States, Wisconsin was the first state to organize such a scheme to support the federal government's "Food Will Win the War" campaign. A State Council of Defense as well as a County Council of Defense were set up to help educate citizens on the war and the sacrifices that were demanded of them. In Britain, the government used prominent vegetarians Leonora Cohen and Dugald Semple, among others, to spread propaganda for such food innovations as barley rissoles (a kind of croquette) and nut foods. In 1918, meat rationing was introduced in Britain at the level of three-quarter pound per person per week. Vegetarians were allowed extra fat and butter instead of extra cheese, but from August 1918 they faced a fruit shortage due to the British government's decision to give priority to jam making.

Vegetarian activities declined considerably in the immediate postwar period. Beginning in the late 1920s, however, mostly middle-class and lower-middle-class people contributed to the increase of membership in the Vegetarian Society. From 1937 to 1942, British vegetarian societies continually negotiated with the government that dietary concessions be made for the 50,000 soldiers registered as vegetarians in World War II. An additional supply of cheese and fats and a special allowance of nuts were then gained. The government's policy was seemingly centered on increasing home production of the four major staples, namely, milk, potatoes, oatmeal, and vegetables; controlling prices and supplies; and rationing foods like meat, fats, and sugar. While key staple foods like potatoes and bread were not rationed, many vegetarians duly regarded the wartime diet as embodying many of their own ideals. They also regarded it as an important stage in the official recognition and wider acceptance of their diet. The prewar, newer knowledge of nutrition, highly advocated by such prominent figures as J.C. Drummond and Sir John Orr, shaped the thinking about what an adequate diet was, and it clearly included a vegetarian component. There was an emphasis on ensuring the fullest possible production of milk, potatoes, and vegetables by offering to farmers guaranteed markets and attractive prices for these products, not only during World War II but also for at least a three-year period after the war. The government's intention was to secure an adequate diet for all even after the war ended. The success of this financial policy undoubtedly contributed to the social and cultural acceptability of vegetarianism.

See also Agribusiness; Domestic Science and Scientific Eating; Policy; United Kingdom.

Further Reading

Burnett, John. *Plenty and Want: A Social History of Food in England from 1815 to the Present Day.* London: Routledge, 1989.

Whittier, Peggy. "Wheatless Mondays and Meatless Tuesdays." *New York History Review. An Anthology of New York State History.* October 1917, 5 and 9.

P. Arouna Ouédraogo

YOUTH

Since the late 18th century and increasingly in the last few decades, youth in North America have expressed an interest in adopting a vegetarian diet. Some reasons for this include their increasing concern for the environment, animal welfare and rights, personal health, and religious affiliations. Changing social attitudes and a growing acceptance of different dietary choices have made it easier for youth to move toward vegetarianism.

Historically, most of the world's population has eaten a vegetarian diet. Only in Western countries, where meat and animal products are affordable to most people, has a diet based on meat been typical. However, pauper children working for mill owners in the 19th century were often vegetarian in the sense that meat was considered too expensive to feed to child workers, especially girls. Vegetarianism became the diet of the lower classes during this time because of its low cost. Exceptions, however, certainly existed, and some early vegetarians who joined burgeoning vegetarian groups throughout the 19th century were decidedly middle class. As vegetarianism moved into the 20th century, it became increasingly a diet of the upper and middle classes, as it was a style of eating that was known and accepted for its economy as well as its nutritional value.

A 2007 survey issued to approximately 9,000 adults by the Centers for Disease Control and Prevention found that 367,000 Americans under the age of 18 are vegetarian. This translates to about 1 in every 200 children. This is the first study done by the U.S. government that estimates how many young people avoid meat. Other surveys suggest the number could be four to six times higher among older youth, who have more control over what they eat. According to this study, vegetarian youth today are most often female, from higher-income families, and living on the East or West coasts.

Some youth follow a vegetarian diet for religious reasons. Vegetarianism and spirituality are connected in a number of religions that originated in ancient India, for example, Hinduism, Jainism, and Buddhism. Some Seventh-day Adventists and Hare Krishnas as well as Christian and Jewish sects also promote vegetarian diets.

Overall, youth are adopting a vegetarian diet mainly because of their growing awareness of environmental and animal rights issues. The environment is a prominent topic in the news and pop culture media, and young people can access information from advocacy groups via the Internet. Many young people are becoming involved in school-based vegetarian clubs, and colleges and universities are opting to include vegetarian and vegan food in cafeterias. This is partly because of school-based vegetarian groups and youth-targeted information about vegetarianism. In 1995, the University of California at Berkeley became the first college to offer vegan options at every meal. This action was the result of joint efforts between campus organizations and individuals wishing to take part in the campaign.

In recent decades, activist information directed toward children has proliferated. In the 1990s, much of the literature and other material coming out of environmental and animal rights organizations was written for and geared toward an adult audience. Today, a number of these same organizations feature Web sites, magazines, stickers, and literature created just for youth. This is not a completely new development in the history of vegetarian activism; earlier groups like the Vegetarian Society of America in the late 19th and early 20th centuries also printed testimonies by vegetarian children and promoted the formation of children's clubs. In this way, youth have often been prepared to be activists who have the ability to influence their society.

There are conflicting opinions regarding the extent to which youth should be involved in vegetarian activism. Some newspapers denounce animal rights groups for directing their messages toward children. Other media outlets assess the extent to which children are taking positive action in society as a result of the information provided by these same organizations. Since Web information is often the easiest for children to immediately access, it is important to consider the effects that Internet information has on youths' actions. One of the most popular vegetarian Web sites directed toward children is from People for the Ethical Treatment of Animals (PETA), www.petakids.com. PETA is the most internationally known animal rights organization, and most media attention focused on vegetarian youth activists is based on this organization's information.

Vegetarian eating can be healthy, nutritious, and delicious for children and young adults. Children raised on a vegetarian diet can have an easier time maintaining a healthy weight and have fewer problems with acne, allergies, and gastrointestinal problems than their meat-eating peers. The heights and weights of vegetarian youths are comparable to those of meat-eating children. Furthermore, a balanced vegetarian or vegan diet can often prevent or help manage health problems such as heart disease and obesity, which can start in childhood.

See also Advertising; Animal Rights and Welfare; Childbearing and Infant Feeding; Childrearing; Eastern Religions, Influences of; Family Dynamics; Global Warming; Inter-

Vegetarian/Vegan Sources for Youth

The increasing interest in vegetarianism and veganism among children and teens has resulted in an explosion of books aimed specifically at them and at parents. Here are some published since 1990:

Askew, Claire. *Generation V: The Complete Guide to Going, Being, and Staying Vegan as a Teenager.* Colton, NY: Tofu Hound Press, 2008.

Bass, Jules, and Debbie Harter. *Cooking with Herb, the Vegetarian Dragon: A Cookbook for Kids.* New York: Barefoot Books, 1999.

Bates, Dorothy R., et al. *Munchie Madness: Vegetarian Meals for Teens.* Summertown, TN: Book Publishing Company, 2001.

Bojang, Ali Brownlie. *Why Are People Vegetarian?* Austin, TX: Raintree Steck-Vaughn, 2002.

Bradley, Anne, and Elise Huffman. *Cows Are Vegetarians!* Aptos, CA: Healthways, 1992.

Calvert, Samantha, and Carron Brown. *We're Talking about Vegetarianism.* Hove, UK: Wayland, 1997.

Johnson, Kristi. *Grilled Pizza Sandwich and Other Vegetarian Recipes.* Mankato, MN: Capstone, 2009.

Katzen, Mollie. *Salad People and More Real Recipes: A New Cookbook for Preschoolers and Up.* Berkeley, CA: Tricycle Press, 2005.

Klaven, Ellen, and Adrienne Hartman. *The Vegetarian Factfinder.* New York: Little Bookroom, 1996.

Krizmanic, Judy, and Matthew Wawiorka. *A Teen's Guide to Going Vegetarian.* New York: Viking, 1994.

Newkirk, Ingrid. *Making Kind Choices: Everyday Ways to Enhance Your Life through Earth- and Animal-Friendly Living.* New York: St. Martin's Griffin, 2005.

Parr, Jan, and Sarah Durham. *The Young Vegetarian's Companion.* New York: Franklin Watts, 1996.

Pavlina, Erin. *Vegan Family Favorites: Tasty and Satisfying Recipes Even Your Kids Will Love.* Las Vegas: VegFamily, 2005.

Roth, Ruby. *That's Why We Don't Eat Animals: A Book about Vegans, Vegetarians, and All Living Things.* Berkeley, CA: North Atlantic Books, 2009.

Schwartz, Ellen. *I'm a Vegetarian: Amazing Facts and Ideas for Healthy Vegetarians.* Plattsburgh, NY: Tundra Books of Northern New York, 2002.

Sokoloff, Myka-Lynne, and Lisa Chauncy Guida. *Beans or Burgers? To Be or Not to Be a Vegetarian.* Bothell, WA: Wright Group/McGraw-Hill, 2001.

Winkler, Kathleen. *Vegetarianism and Teens: A Hot Issue.* Springfield, NJ: Enslow, 2001.

net, The; Jainism; People for the Ethical Treatment of Animals; Periodicals; Physiological Benefits; Reform; Religious Beliefs and Practices; Seventh-day Adventists; Social Acceptance.

Further Reading

Kimball, Chad T., ed. *Vegetarian Sourcebook.* Detroit, MI: Omnigraphics, 2002.
Spencer, Colin. *The Heretic's Feast.* London: Fourth Estate, 1995.

Vanessa M. Holm

Selected Bibliography

Adams, Carol J. *Help! My Child Stopped Eating Meat!* New York: Continuum, 2004.

Adams, Carol J. *The Sexual Politics of Meat: A Feminist-Vegetarian Critical Theory.* New York: Continuum, 1990.

Alcott, Louisa May. *Transcendental Wild Oats and Excerpts from the Fruitlands Diary.* Boston: Harvard Common Press, 1981.

Alcott, William A. *Vegetable Diet Defended.* London: J. Chapman, 1844.

Amato, Paul R., and Sonia A. Partridge. *The New Vegetarians: Promoting Health and Protecting Life.* New York: Plenum, 1989.

American Dietetic Association. "Position of the American Dietetic Association: Vegetarian Diets." *Journal of the American Dietetic Association* 93, no. 11 (November 1993): 1317–19.

Anderson, Michael W. "Field of Forgotten Dreams: The Ill-Fated Vegetarian Colony in Kansas." *Kansas Heritage* 7, no. 3 (Autumn 1999), 13–16.

Attwood, Charles R. *Dr. Attwood's Low-Fat Prescription for Kids.* New York: Viking, 1995.

Ball, Matt, and Bruce Friedrich. *The Animal Activist's Handbook.* New York: Lantern Books, 2009.

Baur, Gene. *Farm Sanctuary: Changing Hearts and Minds about Animals and Food.* New York: Simon and Schuster, 2008.

Beers, Diane L. *For the Prevention of Cruelty: The History and Legacy of Animal Rights Activism in the United States.* Athens, OH: Swallow Press, 2006.

Belasco, Warren, and Roger Horowitz, eds. *Appetite for Change: How the Counterculture Took On the Food Industry.* Updated ed. Ithaca, NY: Cornell University Press, 1993.

Belasco, Warren, and Roger Horowitz, eds. *Food Chains: From Farmyard to Shopping.* Philadelphia: University of Pennsylvania Press, 2008.

Best, Steven, and Anthony J. Nocella II. *Terrorists or Freedom Fighters? Reflections on the Liberation of Animals.* New York: Lantern Books, 2004.

Carson, Gerald. *Cornflake Crusade.* Toronto: Rinehart, 1957.

Cavalieri, Paola. *The Animal Question: Why Nonhuman Animals Deserve Human Rights.* New York: Oxford University Press, 2004.

Chapple, Christopher K. *Nonviolence to Animals, Earth, and Self in Asian Traditions.* Albany: State University of New York Press, 1993.

Crossley, Ceri. *Consumable Metaphors: Attitudes towards Animals and Vegetarianism in Nineteenth-Century France.* Oxford: Peter Lang, 2005.

Dombrowski, Daniel A. *The Philosophy of Vegetarianism.* Amherst: University of Massachusetts Press, 1984.

Dwyer, Johanna T. "Health Aspects of Vegetarian Diets." *American Journal of Clinical Nutrition* 48, no. 3 (1988): 712–38.

Elias, Megan J. *Stir It Up: Home Economics in American Culture.* Philadelphia: University of Pennsylvania Press, 2008.

Ernst, Robert. *Weakness Is a Crime: The Life of Bernarr Macfadden.* Syracuse, NY: Syracuse University Press, 1991.

Fee, Elizabeth, and Theodore M. Brown. "John Harvey Kellogg, MD: Health Reformer and Antismoking Crusader." *American Journal of Public Health* 92 (2002): 935.

Fogarty, Robert S. *All Things New: American Communes and Utopian Movements, 1860–1914.* Chicago: University of Chicago Press, 1990.

Forward, Charles W. *Fifty Years of Food Reform: A History of the Vegetarian Movement in England.* London: Ideal Publishing Union, 1898.

Fox, Michael Allen. *Deep Vegetarianism.* Philadelphia: Temple University Press, 1999.

Francione, Gary L. *Animals as Persons: Essays on the Abolition of Animal Exploitation.* New York: Columbia University Press, 2008.

Francione, Gary L. *Animals, Property, and the Law.* Philadelphia: Temple University Press, 1995.

Francione, Gary L. *Introduction to Animal Rights: Your Child or the Dog?* Philadelphia: Temple University Press, 2000.

Francione, Gary L. *Rain without Thunder: The Ideology of the Animal Rights Movement.* Philadelphia: Temple University Press, 1996.

Freedman, Rory, and Kim Barnouin. *Skinny Bitch.* Philadelphia: Running Press, 2005.

Gaard, Greta, ed. *Ecofeminism: Women, Animals, Nature.* Philadelphia: Temple University Press, 1993.

Gandhi, Mohandas Karamchand. *The Moral Basis of Vegetarianism.* Compiled by R. K. Prabhu. Navajivan, India: Ahmedabad, 1959.

Graham, Sylvester. *Lectures on the Science of Human Life.* Boston: Marsh, Capen, Lyon, & Webb, 1839.

Gregerson, Jon. *Vegetarianism—A History.* Fremont, CA: Jain, 1994.

Gregory, Dick. *Dick Gregory's Natural Diet for Folks Who Eat.* New York: Harper & Row, 1973.

Gregory, James. *Of Victorians and Vegetarians: The Vegetarian Movement in Nineteenth-Century Britain.* London: Tauris, 2007.

Griffin, Susan. *Woman and Nature: The Roaring Inside Her.* San Francisco: Harper & Row, 1978.

Grumett, David, and Rachel Muers. *Theology on the Menu: Asceticism, Meat and Christian Diet.* New York: Routledge, 2010.

Guillermo, Cathy Snow. *Monkey Business: The Disturbing Case That Launched the Animal Rights Movement.* Washington, DC: National Press Books, 1993.

Haenfler, Ross. *Straight Edge: Clean-Living Youth, Hardcore Punk, and Social Change.* New Brunswick, NJ: Rutgers University Press, 2004.

Hamilton, Malcolm. "Eating Ethically: 'Spiritual' and 'Quasi-religious' Aspects of Vegetarianism." *Journal of Contemporary Religion* 15, no. 1 (2000): 65–83.

Harris, John. "The New Vegetarianism: Meat Is More Murderous than Ever." *The Guardian,* June 19, 2008.

Henderson, Elizabeth, and Robyn Van En. *Sharing the Harvest: A Citizen's Guide to Community Supported Agriculture.* White River Junction, VT: Chelsea Green, 2007.

Hendrick, George. *Henry Salt: Humanitarian Reformer and Man of Letters.* Urbana: University of Illinois Press, 1977.

Hobgood-Oster, Laura. *Holy Dogs and Asses: Animals in the Christian Tradition.* Urbana: University of Illinois Press, 2008.

Iacobbo, Karen, and Michael Iacobbo. *Vegetarian America: A History.* Westport, CT: Praeger, 2004.

Iacobbo, Karen, and Michael Iacobbo. *Vegetarians and Vegans in America Today.* Westport, CT: Praeger, 2006.

Jamieson, Dale, ed. *Singer and His Critics.* Oxford: Blackwell, 2000.

Kellogg, Ella Eaton. *Science in the Kitchen.* Chicago: Modern Medicine, 1893.

Lappé, Frances Moore. *Diet for a Small Planet.* New York: Ballantine Books, 1971.

Lappé, Frances Moore, and Anna Blythe Lappé. *Hope's Edge: The Next Diet for a Small Planet.* New York: Tarcher, 2002.

Leneman, Leah. "No Animal Food: The Road to Veganism in Britain, 1909–1944." *Society and Animals* 7 (1999): 1–5.

Levenstein, Harvey. *Revolution at the Table: The Transformation of the American Diet.* Rev. ed. Berkeley: University of California Press, 2003.

Luke, Brian. *Brutal: Manhood and the Exploitation of Animals.* Chicago: University of Illinois Press, 2007.

Lyman, Howard F., and Glen Merzer. *Mad Cowboy: Plain Truth from the Cattle Rancher Who Won't Eat Meat.* New York: Scribner, 1998.

Madden, Etta M., and Martha L. Finch, eds. *Eating in Eden: Food and American Utopias.* Lincoln: University of Nebraska Press, 2006.

Marcus, Erik. *Vegan: The New Ethics of Eating.* Ithaca, NY: Mcbooks, 2000.

Maurer, Donna. *Vegetarianism: Movement or Moment?* Philadelphia: Temple University Press, 2002.

Medearis, Angela Shelf. *The Ethnic Vegetarian—Traditional and Modern Recipes from Africa, America, and the Caribbean.* New York: Rodale, 2004.

Melina, Vesanto, and Brenda Davis. *The New Becoming Vegetarian: The Essential Guide to a Healthy Vegetarian Diet.* 2nd ed. Summertown, TN: Book Publishing, 2003.

Metcalfe, William. *Bible Testimony on Abstinence from the Flesh of Animals as Food.* Philadelphia: J. Metcalfe, 1840.

Metcalfe, William. *Out of the Clouds: Into the Light. With a Memoir by His Son, Reverend Joseph Metcalfe.* Philadelphia: J. B. Lippincott, 1872.

Miller, Timothy. *The Quest for Utopia in Twentieth Century America.* Vol. 1, *1900–1960.* Syracuse, NY: Syracuse University Press, 1998.

Miller, Timothy. *The 60s Communes: Hippies and Beyond.* Syracuse, NY: Syracuse University Press, 1999.

Monamy, Vaughn. *Animal Experimentation: A Guide to the Issues.* 2nd ed. Cambridge: Cambridge University Press, 2009.

Nestle, Marion. *Food Politics: How the Food Industry Influences Nutrition and Health.* Berkeley: University of California Press, 2002.

Newkirk, Ingrid. *Free the Animals: The Amazing True Story of the Animal Liberation Front.* New York: Lantern Books, 2000.

Newkirk, Ingrid, and Jane Ratcliffe, eds. *One Can Make a Difference: How Simple Actions Can Change the World.* Cincinnati, OH: Adams Media, 2008.

Nissenbaum, Stephen. *Sex, Diet and Debility in Jacksonian America: Sylvester Graham and Health Reform.* Westport, CT: Greenwood, 1980.

Numbers, Ronald L. *Prophetess of Health: A Study of Ellen G. White.* 3rd ed. Grand Rapids, MI: William B. Eerdmans, 2008.

O'Connell, Anne. *Early Vegetarian Recipes.* Devon, UK: Prospect Books, 2008.

Perkins, David. *Romanticism and Animal Rights.* New York: Cambridge University Press, 2003.

Phelps, Norm. *The Longest Struggle: Animal Advocacy from Pythagoras to PETA.* New York: Lantern Books, 2007.

The Philadelphia Bible Christian Church. *The History of the Philadelphia Bible Christian Church, for the First Century of Its Existence, 1817 to 1917.* Philadelphia: J. B. Lippincott, 1922. http://www.ivu.org/history/usa19/history_of_bible_christian_church.pdf.

Pitzer, Donald E., ed. *America's Communal Utopias.* Chapel Hill: University of North Carolina Press, 1997.

Preece, Rod. *Sins of the Flesh: A History of Ethical Vegetarian Thought.* Seattle: University of Washington Press, 2008.

Puskar-Pasewicz, Margaret. "'For the Good of the Whole': Vegetarianism in Nineteenth-Century America." PhD diss., Indiana University, Bloomington, 2003.

Puskar-Pasewicz, Margaret. "Kitchen Sisters and Disagreeable Boys: Debates over Meatless Diets in Nineteenth-Century Shaker Communities." In *Eating in Eden: Food and American Utopias*, edited by Etta M. Madden and Martha L. Finch, 109–24. Lincoln: University of Nebraska Press, 2006.

Regan, Tom. *The Case for Animal Rights.* Berkeley: University of California Press, 1983.

Ryder, Richard D. *Animal Revolution: Changing Attitudes towards Speciesism.* Rev. ed. New York: Berg, 2000.

Schwartz, Richard H. *Judaism and Vegetarianism.* New York: Lantern Books, 2001.

Schwarz, Richard W. *John Harvey Kellogg: Pioneering Health Reformer.* Hagerstown, MD: Review and Herald, 2006.

Shah, Mahendra, and Maurice F. Strong. *Food in the 21st Century: From Science to Sustainable Agriculture.* Washington, DC: World Bank, 2000.

Shelton, Herbert. *Superior Nutrition.* San Antonio, TX: Dr. Shelton's Health School, 1976.

Shevelow, Kathryn. *For the Love of Animals: The Rise of the Animal Protection Movement.* New York: Henry Holt, 2008.

Singer, Peter. *Animal Liberation: A New Ethics for Our Treatment of Animals.* New York: Avon Books, 1975.

Spencer, Colin. *Vegetarianism: A History.* Cambridge, MA: Da Capo, 2004.

Stein, Stephen J. *The Shaker Experience in America: A History of the United Society of Believers.* New Haven, CT: Yale University Press, 1992.

Steinfeld, Henning, Pierre Gerber, Tom Wassenaar, Vincent Castel, Mauricio Rosales, and Cees de Haan. *Livestock's Long Shadow: Environmental Issues and Options.* Rome: Food and Agriculture Organization of the United Nations, 2006.

Stepaniak, Joanne. *Being Vegan: Living with Conscience, Conviction, and Compassion.* Los Angeles: Lowell House, 2000.

Stepaniak, Joanne. *The Vegan Sourcebook.* 2nd ed. Los Angeles: Lowell House, 2000.

Stepaniak, Joanne, and Vesanto Malina. *Raising Vegetarian Children: A Guide to Good Health and Family Harmony.* Boston: McGraw-Hill, 2003.

Stuart, Tristram. *The Bloodless Revolution: A Cultural History of Vegetarianism from 1600 to Modern Times.* New York: W. W. Norton, 2007.

Stuart, Tristram. *Waste: Uncovering the Global Food Scandal.* New York: W. W. Norton, 2009.

Stull, Donald, and Michael Broadway. *Slaughterhouse Blues: The Meat and Poultry Industry in North America.* Belmont, CA: Thompson, 2004.

Thoreau, Henry David. *Walden; or, Life in the Woods.* Boston: Ticknor and Fields, 1854.

Torres, Bob, and Jenna Torres. *Vegan Freak: Being Vegan in a Non-Vegan World.* Colton, NY: Tofu Hound Press, 2005.

Turner, James. *Reckoning with the Beast: Animals, Pain, and Humanity in the Victorian Mind.* Baltimore: Johns Hopkins University Press, 1980.

Twigg, Julia. "Food for Thought: Purity and Vegetarianism." *Religion* 9 (1979): 13–35.

Unti, Bernard. "Vegetarian Roots." *Vegetarian Times* 152 (April 1990): 52–58, 82.

Waldau, Paul, and Kimberly Patton, eds. *A Communion of Subjects: Animals in Religion, Science and Ethics.* New York: Columbia University Press, 2006.

Walters, Kerry S., and Lisa Portmess, eds. *Ethical Vegetarianism: From Pythagoras to Peter Singer.* Albany: State University of New York Press, 1999.

Walters, Kerry S., and Lisa Portmess, eds. *Religious Vegetarianism: From Hesiod to the Dalai Lama.* Albany: State University of New York Press, 2001.

Whorton, James C. *Crusaders for Fitness: The History of American Health Reformers.* Princeton, NJ: Princeton University Press, 1982.

Whorton, James C. *Nature Cures: The History of Alternative Medicine in America.* New York: Oxford University Press, 2002.

Whorton, James C. "'Tempest in a Flesh-Pot!' The Formulation of a Physiological Rationale for Vegetarianism." *Journal of the History of Medicine and Allied Sciences* 32 (April 1977): 115–39.

Yabroff, Jennie. "No More Sacred Cows: Vegetarians Who Eat Meat." *Newsweek,* December 31, 2009.

WEB SITES

African Hebrew Israelites. http://africanhebrewisraelitesofjerusalem.com/.
    History, resources, and links for the African Hebrew Israelite Nation of Jerusalem

American Vegan Society. http://www.americanvegan.org/.
    Group's home page includes information about upcoming events, how to become a member, the organization's history, and links to relevant books and videos

Animal Rights: The Abolitionist Approach. http://www.abolitionistapproach.com/.
    Created by prominent animal rights activist and moral philosopher Gary L. Francione, the Web site explains the group's mission; gives information about pamphlets, videos, and books related to veganism; and provides a forum for a blog, regularly updated podcasts, and an ongoing counter that lists the number of animals killed in the world as food for human consumption.

Caring Consumer: A Guide to Kind Living. http://www.caringconsumer.com.
    Sponsored by PETA.org, this site provides a database of cruelty-free products and companies, information about current activities and activism, and links for donating to related causes

Compassion in Action Club. www.theciaclub.com.
    Information about the club's origins, membership, events, and how to start your own
    branch
Compassion Over Killing. www.cok.net.
    Group's history and current activism as well as databases for vegan-related resources
Farm Animal Reform Movement (FARM). www.farmusa.org.
    Gives information about the group's background, campaign updates, and how to join,
    as well as resources for how to become a vegetarian
Farm Sanctuary. http://farmsanctuary.org/.
    Group's history and current activities related to anticruelty activism as well as re-
    sources and a special section for kids
Go Vegan with Bob Linden. www.goveganradio.com.
    Information, archives, and new programs for a radio show dedicated to veganism
Howard Lyman: Mad Cowboy. http://www.madcowboy.com/.
    Home page for prominent activist Howard Lyman, a former rancher
International Vegetarian Union. http://www.ivu.org.
    The best online database for issues related to vegetarianism, including the move-
    ment's history and its proponents around the world, as well as current organizations,
    restaurants, stores, resources, and much more
Jewish Vegetarians of North America (JVNA). http://www.jewishveg.com.
    Information about the group as well as numerous resources including an online
    documentary
Michael Greger, M.D. http://www.drgreger.org/.
    Home page of a well-known physician and proponent of vegetarianism
MollieKatzen.com. http://www.molliekatzen.com/.
    Links to buy Katzen's books as well as online recipes, cooking videos, and resources
People for the Ethical Treatment of Animals (PETA). www.peta.org.
    Information about the organization, its current campaigns, news articles, and how to
    get involved
PETAKids.com. http://www.petakids.com/.
    Web site sponsored by PETA, with resources and activities aimed at children
PETA2.com. http://www.peta2.com/.
    Web site sponsored by PETA, aimed at teens and young adults, including news ar-
    ticles and a blog
Physicians Committee for Responsible Medicine (PCRM). http://www.pcrm.org.
    New and archived articles and other resources on issues related to the prevention of
    sickness and disease, the ethical use of animals in medical practice and research, and
    related advocacy
Small Planet Institute. http://www.smallplanet.org/.
    Started in 2001 by Frances Moore Lappé, long-time activist and best-selling author of
    Diet for a Small Planet, and Anna Lappé, her daughter and coauthor of *Hope's Edge,* the
    institute's Web page was created to promote civic activism related to environmental
    and other global issues
Vegan Outreach. www.veganoutreach.org.
    Outlet to distribute illustrated booklets and other materials to promote cruelty-free
    eating and activism on behalf of animals
Vegan Society. http://www.vegansociety.com/home.php.
    Web site for the United Kingdom's national organization to promote veganism and
    provide relevant resources

Vegetarian Resource Group (VRG). http://www.vrg.org/index.htm.
Compilation of resources, such as news articles, polls, recipes, and research, on vegetarianism and related issues such as nutrition, ethics, and world hunger
Vegetarian Society of the United Kingdom. http://www.vegsoc.org.
Information about the United Kingdom's national vegetarian society, also the longest-operating vegetarian society in the world

About the Editor and Contributors

THE EDITOR

Margaret Puskar-Pasewicz is an independent historian whose research focuses on the social and cultural significance of food. She is writing a book on vegetarianism in the United States from 1817 to 1918.

THE CONTRIBUTORS

Nomi Abeliovich is an architect, photographer, and freelance writer.

Julia A. Abramson is associate professor of French at the University of Oklahoma, Norman, and the author of *Food Culture in France* (Greenwood, 2006).

Jen Westmoreland Bouchard is a faculty member in the World Languages Department of Normandale Community College in Bloomington, Minnesota, and the owner of Lucidité Writing.

Eric Boyle is a Stetten postdoctoral fellow at the Office of History at the National Institutes of Health, where he is examining the historical relationships between alternative and orthodox medicine in America since the 19th century.

Garrett Broad is a doctoral student in the Annenberg School for Communication at the University of Southern California. His work examines the role of communication and media in the promotion of healthy communities, with a particular focus on community food security and sustainable food systems. In 2009, he helped to organize the *VBQ for Life*—a free vegan BBQ and health fair in Inglewood, California—the largest-ever all-vegan event in an American community of color.

Samantha Calvert is a PhD candidate in the School of Philosophy, Theology and Religion at the University of Birmingham, England.

Joshua L. Carreiro is a doctoral candidate in the Department of Sociology at the University of Massachusetts. He has published research on media representation of the labor movement and union organization in the whole-foods economic sector.

Shayna Cohen is a senior consultant with Karp Resources.

Matthew Cole is a U.K.-based sociologist whose research interests include veganism and human-nonhuman animal relations.

David Dillard-Wright is assistant professor of philosophy at the University of South Carolina Aiken, where he teaches philosophy, ethics, and religion. His research focuses on animals in continental philosophy and the ethics of sympathy. He has authored *Ark of the Possible: The Animal World in Merleau-Ponty* (2009).

Michael Allen Fox is professor emeritus of philosophy, Queen's University, Kingston, Ontario, Canada, and adjunct professor, School of Humanities, University of New England, Armidale, New South Wales, Australia. He is the author of *The Remarkable Existentialists, The Accessible Hegel, Deep Vegetarianism,* and other works.

Gary L. Francione is distinguished professor of law and Nicholas deB. Katzenbach Scholar of Law and Philosophy at Rutgers University School of Law, Newark, New Jersey. His primary area of scholarly research is animal ethics, and he has written widely concerning the abolition of animal exploitation, the failure of animal welfare regulations, and the importance of veganism. He maintains a Web site at www.abolitionistapproach.com.

Jerold D. Friedman is an attorney who works for animal rights. His principal interests are working with animal advocates on organizing campaigns, providing activists with legal representation, and promoting secular ethics. He is the president of the Animal C.A.R.E. Foundation in Hawaii.

Monica L. Gerrek is a fellow with the Cleveland Fellowship in Advanced Bioethics. Her primary areas of research include animal ethics, bioethics, and ethical theory.

Hayley Rose Glaholt is a doctoral candidate in the Department of Religious Studies at Northwestern University. Her primary focus is religious perspectives on animal ethics, and her dissertation investigates 19th-century Quaker women's involvement in antivivisection activism.

David Grumett is a research fellow in theology at the University of Exeter, United Kingdom.

Ursula Heinzelmann is a Berlin-based journalist and author specializing in food and wine. She is the author of *Erlebnis Essen* (2006) as well as *Food Culture in Germany* (Greenwood, 2008).

Tom Hertweck is a PhD student in the Program for Literature and Environment at the University of Nevada, Reno.

Laura Hobgood-Oster is professor of religion and environmental studies at Southwestern University.

Vanessa M. Holm is a doctoral candidate in environmental studies at York University, Toronto. Her research interests include food policy and politics, "green" consumerism, vegetarianism, and animal rights.

Lisa Hudgins is an independent researcher for the University of South Carolina.

Gary K. Jarvis is an independent scholar in Ann Arbor, Michigan.

Alok Kumar is chair of the Department of Physics at the State University of New York, Oswego.

Gary Land is professor of history and department chair at Andrews University, Berrien Springs, Michigan. Among other works, he has published *Adventism in America: A History* (1986) and *Historical Dictionary of the Seventh-day Adventists* (2005).

Caroline Lieffers is a master's student in history at the University of Alberta.

Andrew Linzey is director of the Oxford Centre for Animal Ethics and a member of the Faculty of Theology in the University of Oxford. He is also honorary professor at the University of Winchester, special professor at Saint Xavier University, Chicago, and the first professor of animal ethics at the Graduate Theological Foundation, Indiana. Linzey has written or edited 20 books, including *Christianity and the Rights of Animals* (1987), *Animal Theology* (1992), and *Why Animal Suffering Matters* (2009).

Lois N. Magner, professor emerita, Purdue University, taught courses in the history of medicine and life sciences. Her publications include *A History of Infectious Diseases and the Microbial World* (2009), *A History of Medicine* (2005), and *A History of the Life Sciences* (2002).

Reed Mangels is a nutrition advisor for the Vegetarian Resource Group, Baltimore, Maryland.

Etta M. Madden is professor of English and on the gender studies faculty at Missouri State University. She is the coeditor with Martha Finch of *Eating in Eden: Food and American Utopias* (2006).

Angela Shelf Medearis is a culinary historian, food columnist, and the author of several best-selling cookbooks including *The Ethnic Vegetarian* and *The New African-American Kitchen*. She is also the executive producer and host of *The Kitchen Diva!*

Shankar Narayan is the founder and president of the Indian Vegan Society and a councilor and regional coordinator (India and South and West Asia) for the International Vegetarian Union.

Jill Nussinow is a chef-educator and vegetarian cookbook author.

P. Arouna Ouédraogo is a senior researcher in the sociology of food consumption at the Institut National de la Recherche Agronomique, France.

Evert Peeters is a postdoctoral researcher at the Centre for Historial Research Documentation on War and Contemporary Society (Belgium). He publishes on the history of alternative politics, gender and sexuality.

Cedar Phillips is an independent historian based in San Francisco.

Ammini Ramachandran is a freelance writer and author of *Grains, Greens, and Grated Coconuts.*

Gwynne K. Langley Rivers is a PhD candidate in history at the University of Illinois, Chicago. Her dissertation is a study on health practices in American communitarian societies in the mid-19th century.

Colleen Taylor Sen is a food writer and author of *Food Culture in India* (2004) and *Curry: A Global History* (2005).

Brittany Shoot is a writer and independent scholar living in Copenhagen, Denmark.

Adam D. Shprintzen is a doctoral student and adjunct instructor of history at Loyola University Chicago.

John Simons is executive dean of arts at Macquarie University in Sydney, Australia. A major recent publication is *Animal Rights and the Politics of Literary Representation* (2002).

Angus Taylor teaches philosophy at the University of Victoria in British Columbia. He is the author of *Animals and Ethics: An Overview of the Philosophical Debate.*

Melissa Tedrowe works in the Department of English at the University of Wisconsin–Madison.

Sabrina Tonutti is a researcher in cultural anthropology at the University of Udine, Italy.

Mandy Van Deven is a freelance writer, grassroots organizer, and founder of the Feminist Review blog. Her writing focuses on gender, sexuality, popular culture, and religion.

Dirk-Jan Verdonk is a program manager for WSPA Netherlands.

Ansley Watson is a graduate student in food systems at New York University. Her research interests include sustainable agriculture and food policy.

Zipporah Weisberg is a PhD student specializing in critical animal studies in the Division of Humanities at York University, Toronto.

Milton W. Wendland is an attorney and a doctoral candidate in American studies at the University of Kansas.

Matthew Winston is a doctoral candidate in Journalism Studies at Cardiff University.

Jen Wrye is a PhD candidate and instructor in the Department of Sociology and Anthropology at Carleton University in Ottawa, Canada. Her research interests include pet food, the sociology of food and eating, animal-human relations, feminist theory, and environmental sociology.

Benjamin E. Zeller is assistant professor of religious studies at Brevard College and chairs the Religion, Food, and Eating Seminar of the American Academy of Religion. He researches new and alternative religions in the United States. He is the author of *Prophets and Protons: New Religious Movements and Science in Late Twentieth-Century America* (2010).

Index